Sports Medicine and Arthroscopic Surgery of the Foot and Ankle

Amol Saxena

Editor

Sports Medicine and Arthroscopic Surgery of the Foot and Ankle

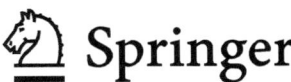 Springer

Editor
Dr. Amol Saxena D.P.M.
Department of Sports Medicine
Palo Alto Foundation Medical
Group-Palo Alto Division
Palo Alto, CA
USA

ISBN 978-1-4471-4105-1   ISBN 978-1-4471-4106-8   (eBook)
DOI 10.1007/978-1-4471-4106-8
Springer Dordrecht Heidelberg New York London

Library of Congress Control Number: 2012943940

Printed on acid-free paper

Springer is part of Springer Science+Business Media (www.springer.com)

Foreword

As a colleague and friend of Amol Saxena, I feel honoured to write the foreword to *Sports Medicine and Arthroscopic Surgery of the Foot and Ankle.*

During my 20 years of experience, I found the specialty of foot and ankle surgery growing unexpectedly. This was due to international collaboration between podiatric, orthopaedic, and trauma surgeons from around the globe.

As a German trauma surgeon I had little to no exposure to reconstructive foot andankle surgery at the time I was trained; the first hallux valgus repair I performed was with Dr. Brian Holcomb, a podiatric surgeon in Georgia. Years later this led to the formation of the German-based foundation, the Association for Foot Surgery. Among others, this foundation created a global platform for all disciplines to train together and shares ideas and experiences concerning foot pathologies. Amol Saxena was one of the invited speakers to the scientific conference in Munich, where he shared all his experience with the surgeons.

As a speaker at many international conferences he took it upon himself to gather international contributing authors for this book. All the authors have extraordinary personal experience with the procedures they describe.

While this book does not exclude scientific background, it emphasizes a practical, hands-on approach. To meet the demand of all foot and ankle surgeons, the book encompasses forefoot and rearfoot deformities as well as trauma and reconstructive surgery of the diabetic foot.

With that in mind I strongly recommend this book for all foot and ankle surgeons of any subspecialty from any nation as this book will shortly be recognized as the state of the art.

Germany   Kai Olms, M.D.

Preface

It is with great pleasure and gratitude that I am able to edit *Sports Medicine and Arthroscopic Surgery of the Foot and Ankle*. The idea for this book came about through my contact and subsequent friendships with two well-known and innovative foot and ankle surgeons – Nicola Maffulli, M.D., Ph.D., and Kai Olms, M.D. – as we discussed the need to share international thought leaders' concepts. As the world progressed into a global economy and the Internet helped connect people of similar interests in the early twenty-first century, I began communicating, writing, and lecturing with these two individuals across the globe. Through these two individuals with their zeal for traveling, teaching, and learning (but not necessarily in that order!), professional friendships and further contacts developed, ideas were shared, and many of the authors of this book became connected.

The globalization of foot and ankle surgery may not be readily apparent; however in this book there are many examples. Recently I personally experienced this as I performed a "Stainsby" procedure on a patient whose second toe was severely dislocated despite metatarsal osteotomy, hammertoe, and soft tissue lengthening. In the past I may have performed an isolated partial metatarsal head resection. However, I was able to relocate the toe, preventing a possible transfer lesion with the Stainsby, which I learned from German authors of chapters in this text, which they in turn "imported" from the British surgeon it is named after. The Italian surgeon Valente Valenti performed a resectional arthroplasty for hallux rigidus in the mid-1970s. His procedure was "imported" to the United States in the mid-1980s and subsequently "exported" back to Germany early in the twenty-first century.

Many older procedures have been re-popularized with regional modifications such as the Hohmann osteotomy first described in Germany in the early 1900s. In the United States, the procedure was performed on the first and fifth metatarsal with no fixation as a minimally invasive technique during the 1970s. Subsequently with the increased utilization of AO fixation from Europe, the desire to have more stability, and predictable healing time, the Hohmann procedure was adapted with inclusion of screw fixation. As the Europeans (particularly the Latin-based speaking countries of Italy, France, and Spain) increased their desire to have smaller incisions, this osteotomy has been increasingly utilized using percutaneous fixation.

Other examples are Ilizarov fixation from Russia, arthroscopy from Japan, and the Weil osteotomy from the United States being adopted by other parts of the world. This often came about by motivated surgeons visiting other surgeons with similar interests and the desire to better serve their patients.

I believe all the authors in this text share this commonality as our patients drive us to learn and excel, and I am grateful for the opportunity to pull this select group together. I am cognizant that many authors created chapters on topics that could be entire texts in their own right. Furthermore, the need to publish in a foreign language provides additional stress, along with combining different writing styles in chapters where similar topics were "blended" together. This adds to this text's uniqueness.

Everyone's life journey, including their career, is a story formed by happenstance and instances of luck, misfortune, and guidance. As a young and often injured runner I found myself in the offices of two early forefathers of sports medicine, Fred Behling, M.D., and Gordon Campbell, M.D., in my hometown of Palo Alto, California. It was through their encouragement and possibly lack of interest in foot surgery, that I pursued podiatry as a profession, as they desired a partner proficient in treating the sports medicine aspects of the foot and ankle. They professed and practiced subspecialization as a way of achieving excellence in patient care. I subsequently joined their practice in 1993 just as they were retiring from the Palo Alto Medical Clinic's Sports Medicine Department, where I currently have three orthopedic sports medicine and one pediatric sports medicine colleagues. All four are among the most productive in their respective fields in the United States, covering professional and high school sports teams, writing chapters, and having high-volume practices. With the support of our department, combined with my other podiatric colleagues within our clinic, I have been able to offer a fellowship for post-residency training in sports medicine and foot and ankle surgery. These fellows have been able to further share in exchanges with some of the international authors of this book and I have hosted colleagues from other countries as well.

As I stated, luck has a part in one's journey and subsequently their training. I am extremely fortunate to have had the training from not only one of the most versatile foot and ankle surgeons but great teacher and human being in John Grady, D.P.M. There are other highly respected authors I've met through contacts that are mentors writing here as well. I was also fortunate to be able to connect and shadow with another legend and thought leader in the foot and ankle world, Sigvard T. Hansen, M.D., early on, whose philosophy on foot and ankle surgeons paralleled mine in life, in that everyone is equal until proved otherwise. It is also exciting to have many of the current and future bright minds of the orthopedic, podiatric, and trauma worlds of foot and ankle surgery all contributing in the name of advancing foot and ankle surgery.

Finally, I am indebted to my family, teachers, and friends for being supportive of not only this project but how my career developed. I am richer for all their positive encouragement, able to be fulfilled professionally, but also personally. I am sure I could not have completed this and other accomplishments without them.

USA   Amol Saxena, D.P.M.

Contents

Contributors

Marque A. Allen, D.P.M. Texas Center for Athletes, San Antonio, TX, USA

Richard T. Bouché, D.P.M. The Sports Medicine Clinic, Northwest Hospital, Seattle, WA, USA

Yelena Boumendjel, D.P.M. Department of Podiatry, Jesse Brown VA Medical Center, Chicago, IL, USA

Timothy P. Charlton, M.D. Department of Orthopaedic Surgery, USC Keck School of Medicine Surgery of the Foot and Ankle, Los Angeles, CA, USA

Peter A.J. de Leeuw, M.Sc. Department of Orthopaedic Surgery, Academic Medical Center, Amsterdam, The Netherlands

Vincenzo Denaro, M.D. Department of Trauma and Orthopaedic Surgery, University Campus Bio-Medico of Rome, Rome, Italy

Nicholas Antonio Ferran, M.B.B.S., M.R.C.S.Ed. Department of Trauma and Orthopaedics, Lincoln County Hospital, Lincoln, Lincolnshire, UK

Brian W. Fullem, D.P.M. Tampa, FL, USA

John F. Grady, D.P.M. Department of Surgery, Foot and Ankle Institute of Illinois, Oak Lawn, IL, USA

Allison N. Granot, P.T., M.P.T., O.C.S., C.S.C.S. Dept of Physical Therapy, Palo Alto Medical Foundation, Palo Alto, CA, USA

George Tye Liu, D.P.M. Department of Orthopaedic Surgery, University of Texas Southwestern Medical Center, Dallas, TX, USA

Umile Giuseppe Longo, M.D. Department of Trauma and Orthopaedic Surgery, University Campus Bio-Medico of Rome, Rome, Italy

Nicola Maffulli, M.D., M.S., Ph.D., F.R.C.S (Orth). Barts and The London School of Medicine and Dentistry, Centre for Sports and Exercise Medicine, Mile End Hospital, Queen Mary University of London, London, UK

Francesco Oliva, M.D., Ph.D. Department of Trauma and Orthopaedic Surgery, University of Rome "Tor Vergata", Rome, Italy

Amol Saxena, D.P.M. Department of Sports Medicine, PAFMG-Palo Alto Division, Palo Alto, CA, USA

Audra M. Smith, D.P.M. Department of Podiatry, Jesse Brown VA Medical Center, Chicago, IL, USA

Daniel R. Stephenson, M.D. Department of Orthopaedic Surgery, University of Southern California, Los Angeles, CA, USA

David B. Thordarson, M.D. Department of Orthopaedic Surgery, University of Southern California, Los Angeles, CA, USA

Christiaan J.A. van Bergen, M.D., M.Sc. Department of Orthopaedic Surgery, Academic Medical Center, Amsterdam, The Netherlands

C. Niek van Dijk, M.D., Ph.D. Department of Orthopaedic Surgery, Academic Medical Center, Amsterdam, The Netherlands

Maayke N. van Sterkenburg, M.D., M.Sc. Department of Orthopaedic Surgery, Academic Medical Center, Amsterdam, The Netherlands

Chapter 1
First Metatarsophalangeal Joint Sesamoidopathy

Richard T. Bouché

1.1 Introduction

Hallucal sesamoids play a critical role in foot function as they protect the flexor hallucis longus tendon, increase the mechanical advantage of the flexor hallucis brevis tendon, facilitate load transmission to the medial forefoot, and minimize joint forces acting on the first metatarsophalangeal joint (MTPJ).[1-4] Disorders of these bones are not uncommon problems that pose a significant challenge to the foot surgeon as there are few good studies available that have studied the effectiveness of conservative and surgical treatments recommended to treat these disorders. These injuries can be disabling particularly for athletic patients and surgical extirpation may be contemplated. Concerning evidence-based medicine for surgical treatment, there are no level 1 or 2 prospective randomized studies to rely on with majority of studies being level 3, 4, or 5. Thus, recommended treatments are either anecdotal or based on limited case studies and few anatomical "bench studies." Because of this lack of knowledge, there have also been many myths that abound pertaining to sesamoid pathology and the treatments rendered thus adding to the confusion. The purpose of this section is to generally review hallucal sesamoidopathy with emphasis on the role of surgery specifically discussing incisional approaches and recommended procedures for specific pathological conditions.

R.T. Bouché, D.P.M.
The Sports Medicine Clinic, Northwest Hospital,
10330 Meridian Ave. N., Suite 300,
Seattle, WA 98133, USA
e-mail: rbouche@nwhsea.org

A. Saxena (ed.), *Sports Medicine and Arthroscopic Surgery of the Foot and Ankle*,
DOI 10.1007/978-1-4471-4106-8_1, © Springer-Verlag London 2013

1.2   Definition

Simply defined, hallucal sesamoidopathy in this section refers to pathology affecting the sesamoids of the first metatarsophalangeal joint (MTPJ) specifically involving the tibial and fibular sesamoids and their articulation with the first meta-tarsal head.

1.3   Anatomy

First MTPJ anatomy should be well known to the foot surgeon and is of paramount importance especially as it applies to surgical procedures performed involving the hallucal sesamoids. It is important to appreciate that these bones are embedded in the tendon slips of flexor hallucis brevis which are bound together by the intersesamoidal ligament and the plantar plate. Like the lesser toe joint plantar plate, the hallucal ses-amoid–plantar plate complex plays a significant role in anchoring the various static and dynamic stabilizers attaching to this region and is an integral part of the longitu-dinal and transverse tie-rod system previously described.[5] Static stabilizers include medial and lateral metatarsophalangeal joint (collateral) ligaments, medial and lateral sesamoidal ligaments (metatarsal [suspensory] and phalangeal components), joint capsule, plantar plate, intersesamoidal ligament, plantar fascial slips, and transverse intermetatarsal ligament.[6] Dynamic stabilizers include flexor hallucis longus (FHL) tendon, flexor hallucis brevis (FHB) tendon slips, abductor hallucis tendon, and oblique and transverse head of adductor hallucis tendon.[6] Having an appreciation of this anchor system allows the surgeon to make rational decisions when deciding on the various types of surgical procedures available related to sesamoidopathy.

Knowledge of the blood supply to the sesamoids is also crucial in making good decisions as it applies to choice of surgical incisions. Sesamoid arteries (one to three branches) arise from the plantar arteries of the hallux (proper plantar artery medi-ally and first metatarsal artery laterally) which arise from either both the medial plantar artery and plantar arch (52% incidence), the plantar arch (24% incidence) or the medial plantar artery (24% incidence).[7]

1.4   Etiology/Pathomechanics

Sesamoidopathy can result from trauma (i.e., fracture, hyperextension or "turf-toe" type injuries, avascular necrosis), overuse (i.e., sesamoiditis), attrition (i.e., age-dependent "wear and tear") and/or iatrogenic (plantar plate disruption from triamci-nolone injections) causes. Predisposing factors can be divided into mechanical (i.e., plantarflexed first metatarsal, shoe irritation from cleats) or systemic (i.e., rheuma-toid disease) categories. The sesamoids are exposed to significant forces during weight bearing (WB) and play a key role in providing static and dynamic stability to the first MTPJ. It has been estimated that 50–75% of WB forces are transmitted through the first MTPJ and these forces can account for up to three times body weight.[8] For these reasons, they are vulnerable to injury that can result in significant compromise in walking and running activities.

1.5 Clinical Evaluation

History, physical examination, differential diagnosis, and diagnostic testing comprise the clinical evaluation, the purpose of which is to establish an accurate diagnosis. A complete and thorough history provides the foundation for the remainder of the clinical examination. Any history relating to hyperextension of the first MTPJ should be scrutinized in detail. Predisposing factors should always be sought. Physical examination should be comprehensive, and if problem is unilateral, the contralateral side can be used for comparison. Exam should always include vascular, neurological, dermatological, and musculoskeletal (general and local) components. Musculoskeletal exam always considers static and dynamic evaluation as well as evaluation of hosiery and shoes. Inspection, joint range-of-motion (static and dynamic), muscle testing, systematic palpation, and provocative testing form the basis for examination. Upon completion of the examination, a broad differential diagnosis should be considered (Table 1.1). Depending on the differential diagnosis, appropriate diagnostic testing can be considered including diagnostic imaging, blood work, electrodiagnostic studies, gait analysis, Harris pressure mat testing, diagnostic injections, etc. Any clinical suspicions should be validated by some form of objective diagnostic testing if possible. From the aforementioned information, a "working diagnosis" can be confidently established and treatment options considered.

1.6 Diagnostic Imaging

Standard weight-bearing X-rays are ordered initially and include axial sesamoid views (Fig. 1.1). Bipartite sesamoids are common and generally have a larger overall configuration than unipartite sesamoids. Proximal migration of sesamoids indicates plantar plate or flexor hallucis brevis tear and is discussed in Chap. 2. Technicium bone scans are sometimes helpful to isolate sesamoid pathology from arthritidies such as gout, rheumatoid arthritis, etc. Increased uptake on the blood flow phase indicates acute fracture while uptake only on the delayed images is associated with sesamoiditis. Computed tomography (CT) scans are helpful to show cystic changes and isolate fractures; however, magnetic resonance imaging (MRI) is becoming more common, as 3 T machines with foot coil can show fractures and avascular necrosis (Fig. 1.2).

Table 1.1 Differential diagnosis

Intra-articular disorders	Chondral/osteochondral lesions
	Subchondral cysts
	Sesamoid displacement
	Plica
Congenital variations	Inherited disorders
	Absence
	Accessory sesamoid
	Symptomatic partism
	Coalition
	Size variations
Overuse	Avascular necrosis (see trauma)
	Sesamoiditis
	Chondromalacia
	FHL/FHB tendinitis
	Bursitis
Sesamoid trauma	Subluxation/dislocation
	Stress fracture
	Acute fracture
	Delayed/nonunion
	Avulsion fracture
	Diastasis
	Ligament/tendon rupture
	AVN dorsal capsular tear/strain (Sand Toe)
	Plantar capsular tear/strain (Turf Toe)
	Metatarsal or phalangeal fracture
	Subluxation/dislocation
Neurologic	Charcot neuroarthropathy
	Neuritis
Arthritis	Fibromyalgia
	Osteoarthritis
	Crystalline deposition disease
	Rheumatoid arthritis
	Seronegative arthritis
Infection	Osteomyelitis
Tumor	Bone
	Soft tissue
	Tumor-like conditions (i.e., Ganglion)
Dermatologic	IPK/callus/porokeratosis
	Epidermal inclusion cyst
	Ulceration
Iatrogenic	Hallux abductus (Valgus)
	Hallux adductus (Varus)
	Sesamoiditis S/P Lapidus procedure
Pain dysfunction syndromes	(i.e., CRPS)
Other	

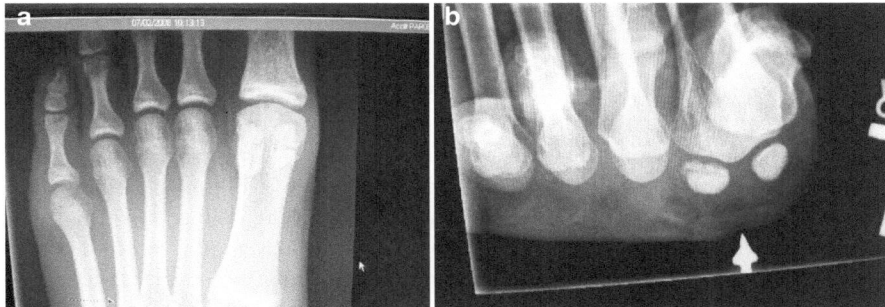

Fig. 1.1 (**a**) Weight-bearing AP X-ray of a patient with a symptomatic bipartite tibial sesamoid. (**b**) Axial sesamoid view depicting a fractured fibular sesamoid (Photo courtesy of Amol Saxena, DPM)

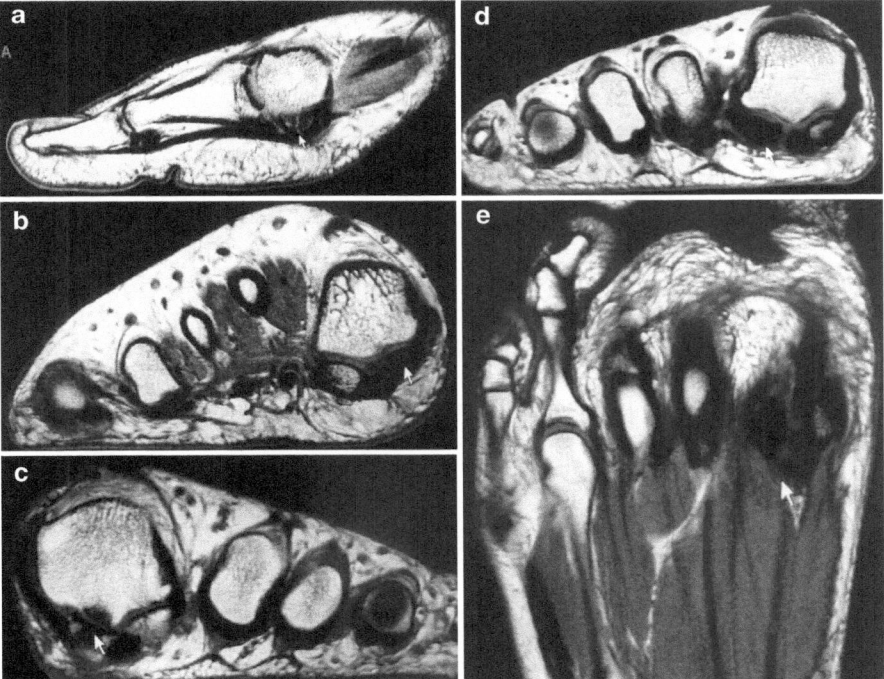

Fig. 1.2 (**a**) Sagittal T1 MRI image of a fractured tibial sesamoid. (**b**) Axial MRI view showing avascular necrosis (*AVN*) of tibial sesamoid. (**c**) Axial MRI of a patient with long-standing tibial sesamoidapathy revealing adjacent metatarsal degenerative disease. (**d**) Axial MRI showing fibular sesamoid fracture. (**e**) MRI showing AVN of fibular sesamoid (Photos courtesy of Amol Saxena, DPM)

1.7   Treatment

Appropriate and specific treatment is predicated on accurate diagnosis. Types of treatment can vary significantly and is pathology and patient-type (sedentary, active, athlete) dependent. As a rule, conservative (nonsurgical) treatment is attempted in most circumstances when there is a reasonable chance it will provide a predictable result. There are exceptions to this rule though, depending on the patient type. For example, high-level amateur or professional athletes may require more definitive and efficient treatment to allow an earlier return to activity. Thus, treatment plans will need to be individualized to each patient depending on their specific expectations and circumstances.

In the case of sesamoidopathy, conservative treatments are anecdotal and have not been studied carefully. For example, in the case of an acute sesamoid fracture, recommended treatments can vary significantly from immediate weight-bearing in an accommodative orthoses or short-leg walking (SLW or below-knee) boot to prolonged non-weight-bearing cast immobilization. Because of the significant difference in treatment approaches, it is not surprising to see a high rate of delayed and nonunions in this type of injury. This disparity in method of conservative treatment can apply to most pathologies that fit under the umbrella of hallucal sesamoidopathy. The author (RTB) has coined the term "sick sesamoid"[9] to apply to hallucal sesamoidopathy that is chronic in nature (>6 months), characterized by intractable pain and dysfunction, unresponsive to comprehensive conservative treatment, and pathology that has been validated by diagnostic testing. In this situation, further conservative treatment is usually futile and the patient can either live with their problem (which many patients do) or they can consider surgery. Many patients live with their problem because they are told by their health professional that sesamoid surgery does not work and the surgery will likely make them worse. This recommendation is commonly made by health professionals in general and is one of the myths that are propagated due to ignorance about this disorder.

1.8   Surgery

Surgery for hallucal sesamoidopathy can be successful and predictable even in athletic patients[10] but it must be approached in a rational manner. Generically, this surgery can be considered emergent (e.g., advanced grade traumatic dorsal first MTPJ dislocation) or elective (e.g., sesamoid planing for intractable plantar skin lesion). Fortunately, most of the cases involving hallucal sesamoids are elective cases. Patients who are considering surgery are not able to live with their problem due to severity, and conservative treatment has not been successful or is not practical based on their individual situation. There are many types of surgery to consider when attempting to address hallucal sesamoidopathy (Table 1.2) and though many

Table 1.2 Surgical options

- Relocation
- Total-excision
- Hemi-excision
- Planing
- Fenestration/osteotomy
- Implant
- MTPJ fusion
- Lengthen PL
- Open reduction, internal fixation (ORIF)
- Percutaneous reduction, internal fixation (PRIF)
- Auto grafting

options are available, few have been universally accepted and recommended. Historically, surgical excision has been the mainstay but has been stigmatized by concern over postoperative complications including persistent pain, weakness, first MTPJ stiffness, and hallux deformity.[11-14] This author (RTB) feels that much of the problem with surgical excision has been related to two factors: poor incision choice and not preserving the flexor hallucis brevis tendon slips.[9,15] The blood supply (see sect. 1.3.2) is vulnerable to injury, and medial and plantar longitudinal central incisions have been recommended[7,9] that are safer. Preservation of the FHB tendon slips is paramount to avoid hallux deformity and weakness of the flexor apparatus.[16,17] Partial sesamoidectomies are preferred over total sesamoidectomies as the potential for postoperative weakness is greatly diminished.[16-18] When considering surgery, there are multiple preoperative concerns to consider including patient type, concurrent foot problems, and determining whether just one or both sesamoids are pathologically involved.

Patients can be classified as sedentary, active, and athletic. Expectations and demands of the athletic patient will be different (and many times more challenging) than the sedentary patient, and these issues need to be thoroughly discussed preoperatively. Concurrent problems need to be recognized and the effect of sesamoid surgery needs to be considered. For example, patients with hallux abducto valgus deformity that require a tibial sesamoidectomy may need to consider a prophylactic bunionectomy procedure to prevent worsening of the deformity. Likewise, patients who have a congenital hallux varus deformity with fibular sesamoid pathology could expect worsening of the deformity with isolated fibular sesamoidectomy alone. Finally, careful clinical evaluation with confirmatory diagnostic testing can determine if one or both sesamoids are pathologic. It has been generally recommended to avoid removing both sesamoids[2,10] though the author feels if both are pathologic, total sesamoidectomy of both sesamoids can be successfully performed if the flexor brevis tendon slips are preserved.[14]

In considering surgical approaches for sesamoidectomy, the ideal surgical approach would be to: provide visualization, protect vital structures, preserve FHB slips, and allow a "clean" excision. Based on these criteria, the author recommends

Fig. 1.3 Medial approach for isolated tibial sesamoidectomy

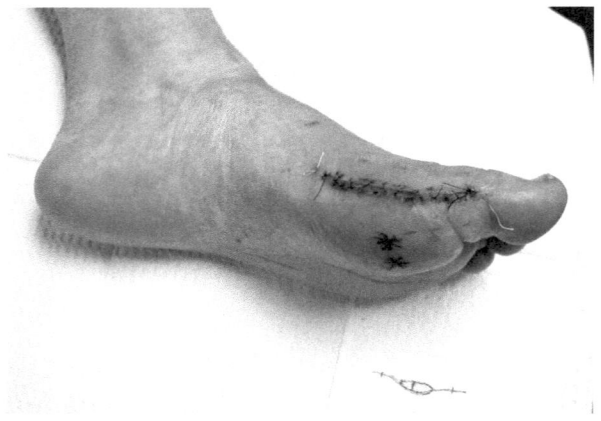

Fig. 1.4 Plantar-central approach for fibular sesamoidectomy and for both sesamoid removal/plantar plate and flexor repair

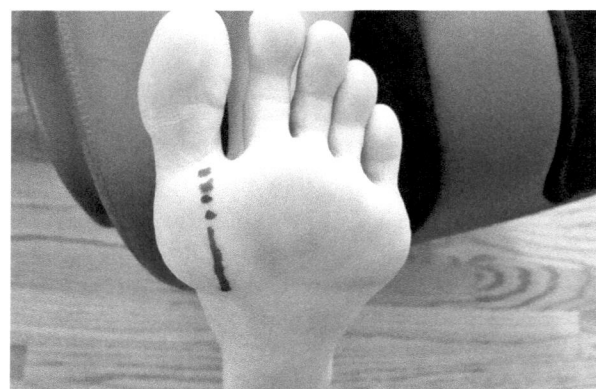

a medial approach to access the tibial sesamoid and a plantar longitudinal central incision for access to the lateral sesamoid[9] (Figs. 1.3 and 1.4). Specifically related to sesamoidectomy, if a partial tibial sesamoid excision is required, then a medial approach is recommended. For total tibial sesamoidectomy, a dorsomedial approach can be utilized if a concomitant bunionectomy is performed; otherwise, a medial or plantar-central incisional approach may be utilized. If a partial or total fibular or total tibial and fibular sesamoidectomy is to be performed, then a plantar longitudinal central approach is recommended. A plantar-central approach is recommended for a total tibial sesamoidectomy (without bunionectomy) because after the sesamoid is removed, a repair of the medial slip of the FHB to the intersesamoidal ligament is recommended (to prevent post-op lateral translation of the fibular sesamoid) and

Fig. 1.5 Several year post-op plantar incision in a triathlete with fibular sesamoidectomy (Photo courtesy of Amol Saxena, DPM)

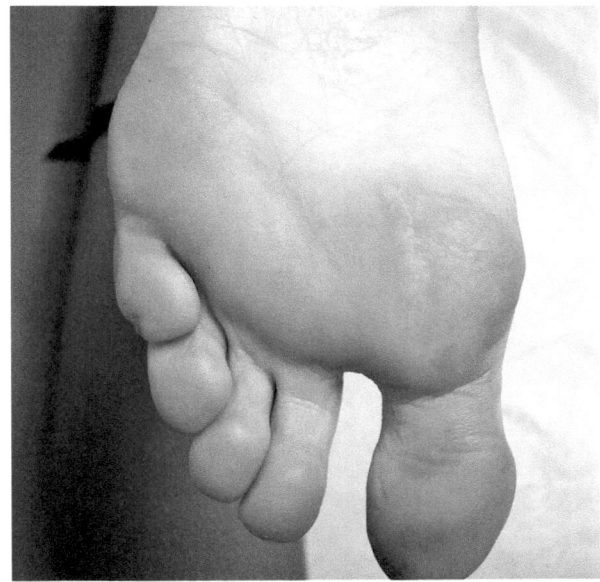

may not be easily be performed through a medial incision. The plantar incision heals well if patients adhere to the recommendation of 3 weeks non-weight bearing post surgery (Fig. 1.5).

Newer and different sesamoid surgery techniques have been described[19,20] and though interesting more studies would be needed to rationalize their use. As an example, if a high-level athlete presents with an acute tibial sesamoid fracture, open or percutaneous reduction with internal fixation has been suggested[19] but would require a period of time NWB postoperatively followed by a period in a walking boot or cast and potential for another surgery to remove the fixation. The author has performed 3 partial tibial sesamoidectomies in the acute situation through a medial incision requiring 3 weeks NWB followed by 1–3 weeks in a SLW boot (Fig. 1.6). Partial sesamoidectomies result in minimal-to-no functional deficit as long as the FHB tendon slip is preserved, then this is a rational and viable choice allowing a predictable earlier return to sports activity for the athlete. Likewise, in the case of a chronic sesamoid nonunion, open curettement with bone grafting has been suggested[20] but partial sesamoidectomy is also another viable option that would likely be more predictable and would allow an earlier return to activities of daily living and sports activities. Further future studies will be needed to validate which surgical technique would be the best and most functional.

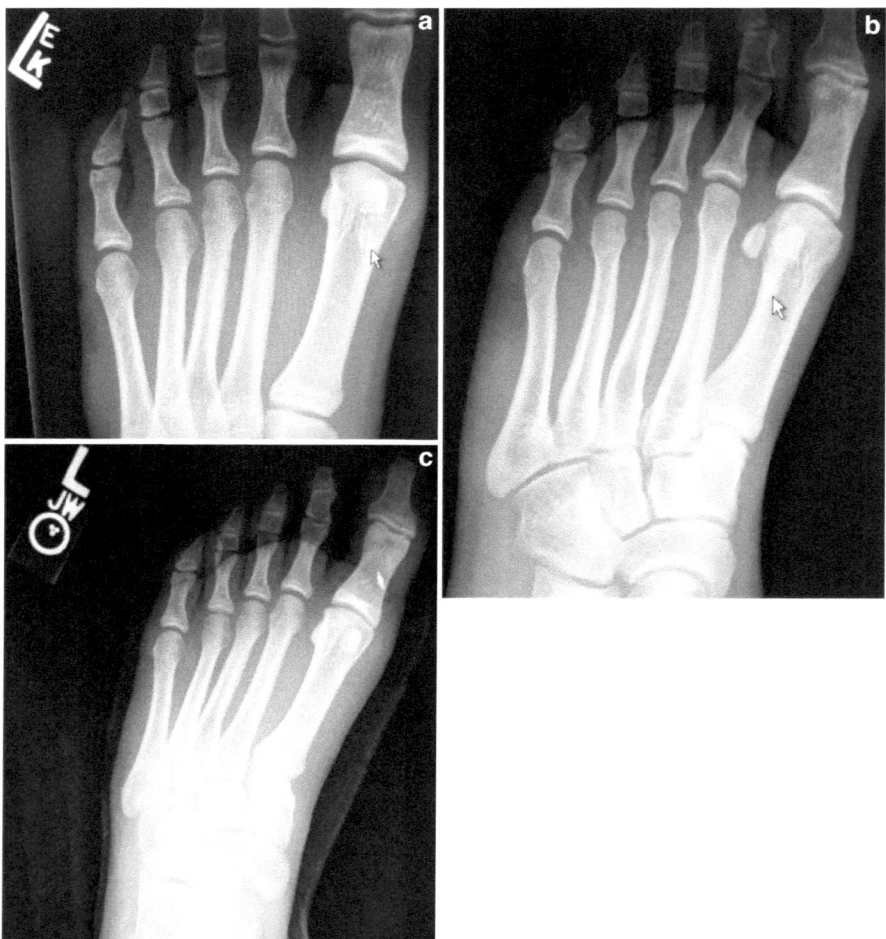

Fig. 1.6 (**a**, **b**) Pre- and (**c**) post-op partial tibial sesamoidectomy in a patient with a proximal avulsion (Photo courtesy of Amol Saxena, DPM)

References

1. Helal B. The great toe sesamoid bones – the lus or lost souls of Ushaia. Clin Orthop Relat Res. 1981;157:82–7.
2. Richardson EG. Injuries to the hallucal sesamoids in the athlete. Foot Ankle Int. 1987;7:229–44.
3. Richardson EG. Hallucal sesamoid pain: causes and surgical treatment. J Am Acad Orthop Surg. 1999;7:270–8.
4. Dedmond BT, Cory JW, McBride A. The hallucal sesamoid complex. J Am Acad Orthop Surg. 2006;14:745–53.

5. Stainsby GD. Pathological anatomy and dynamic effect of the displaced plantar plate and the importance of the integrity of the plantar plate-deep transverse metatarsal ligament tie-bar. Ann R Coll Surg Engl. 1997;79:58–68.
6. Sarrafian SK. Anatomy of the Foot and Ankle. 2nd ed. Philadelphia: JB Lippincott Company; 1993.
7. Pretterklieber ML, Wanivenhaus A. The arterial supply of the sesamoid bones of the hallux: the course and source of the nutrient arteries as an anatomical basis for surgical approaches to the great toe. Foot Ankle. 1992;13:27–31.
8. McBryde AM, Anderson RB. Sesamoid foot problems in the athlete. Clin Sports Med. 1988;7:51–60.
9. Bouché RT, Heit E. Surgical approaches for hallucal sesamoid excision. J Foot Ankle Surg. 2002;41(3):192–6.
10. Saxena A, Krisdakumtorn T. Return to activity after sesamoidectomy in athletically active individuals. Foot Ankle. 2003;24(5):415–9.
11. Inge GAL, Ferguson AB. Surgery of the sesamoid bones of the great toe. Arch Surg. 1933;27:466–88.
12. Mann RA, Coughlin MJ. Hallux valgus- etiology, anatomy, treatment and surgical considerations. Clin Orthop Relat Res. 1981;151:31–41.
13. Mann RA, Coughlin MJ, Baxter D. Sesamoidectomy of the great toe. In: Mann RA, Coughlin MJ, editors. Surgery of the Foot. St. Louis: CV Mosby; 1993. p.494.
14. Brodsky J. Sesamoid excision for chronic non-union. In: Mann RA, Coughlin MJ, editors. Surgery of the Foot. St. Louis: CV Mosby; 1993. p.498.
15. Bouché RT. Letter to the editor. J Foot Ankle Surg. 1997;36:393–4.
16. Aper RL, Saltzman CL, et al. The effect of hallux sesamoid resection on the windlass moment of the flexor hallucis brevis. Foot Ankle. 1994;15:462–70.
17. Aper RL, Saltzman CL, et al. The effect of hallux sesamoid excision on the flexor hallucis longus moment arm. Clin Orthop Relat Res. 1996;325:209–17.
18. Biedert R, Hintermann B. Stress fractures of the medial great toe sesamoids in athletes. Foot Ankle. 2003;24(2):137–41.
19. Blundell CM, Nicholson P, Blackney MW. Percutaneous screw fixation for fractures of the sesamoid bones of the hallux. J Bone Joint Surg Br. 2002;84(8):1138–41.
20. Anderson RB, McBride AM. Autogenous bone grafting of hallux sesamoid nonunions. Foot Ankle Int. 1997;18(5):293–6.

Chapter 2
Turf Toe Injuries

Michael D. VanPelt, Amol Saxena, and Marque A. Allen

In 1976, Bowers and Martin coined the term "turf toe" in the literature in response to the increasing injuries to the great toe joint being seen by athletes playing on new artificial surfaces and playing in lighter and more flexible shoes.[1,2] The term classically describes a first metatarsophalangeal joint (MTPJ) ligament sprain, commonly seen in field-related sports.[1-8] This malady can be an undertreated and oversimplified athletic injury of the great toe joint. Unfortunately, many times, any injury to the great toe joint that occurs during a sporting event is erroneously termed turf toe. Often a complete and systematic evaluation of all the structures of the great toe joint is not performed. A differential exam may be performed and injuries other than to the ligamentous supports may be appreciated but all are still coined turf toe. Some authors recommend reserving the term only when injuries to other structures (i.e., muscle, tendon, metatarsal, cartilage, sesamoids, etc.) are not involved and the injury to the great toe joint is purely ligamentous.[1]

In 1978, Coker et al. correlated the increased incidence with a debilitating effect on return to play among college football players.[3] This injury continues to be seen despite advances in artificial turf and shoe interface.[9,10] Long-term sequelae has been noted to many different anatomical structures of the first MPTJ, including the cartilage and sesamoids. We feel involvement to these additional anatomical structures each have a spectrum of injury to themselves or in combination that, if not

M.D. VanPelt, D.P.M. (✉)
Department of Orthopaedic Surgery, University of Texas Southwestern Medical Center, 1801 Inwood Road, Dallas 75390-8883, TX, USA
e-mail: michael.vanpelt@utsouthwestwern.edu

A. Saxena, D.P.M.
Department of Sports Medicine, PAFMG-Palo Alto Division, Palo Alto, CA, USA

M.A. Allen, D.P.M.
Texas Center for Athletes,
San Antonio, TX, USA

A. Saxena (ed.), *Sports Medicine and Arthroscopic Surgery of the Foot and Ankle*,
DOI 10.1007/978-1-4471-4106-8_2, © Springer-Verlag London 2013

appreciated and treated appropriately, will increase the misunderstanding and morbidity of this injury. Proper diagnosis of the structures involved in turf toe injuries should lead to better treatment outcomes.

2.1 Pathophysiology

The severity of the injury will be a summation of the amount of energy imparted to the great toe joint and the extent and direction of abnormal or excessive range of motion at the time of force. This is known as the mechanism of injury. The mechanism of injury will predictably place various anatomical structures at risk. Among the various mechanisms described for turf toe injuries, hyperextension force to the first MTPJ is the most commonly accepted and reported (Fig. 2.1). In a study by Rodeo et al., 80 professional football players were surveyed, 45% experienced a turf toe injury.[4] In this study, 83% of these players reported their initial turf toe injury occurring on artificial turf and 85% of injuries occurring secondary to a hyperextension injury. The hyper-dorsiflexion force to the MTPJ will occur when the forefoot is in a flexed position to the ground and a concurrent axial load is applied to the heel. This will result in a change of the joint kinematics. As the great toe joint continues to dorsiflex or hyperextend, a compression force is applied between the base of the proximal phalanx and the dorsal central articular surface of the first metatarsal head and base of the phalanx which could result in articular injury (Fig. 2.1). Simultaneously, a distraction force occurs to the plantar plate, the sesamoid apparatus, and/or short flexors to the point of possible rupture or fracture. This hyperextension motion will commonly involve varus or valgus moments around the joint that will also place the collateral ligaments at risk. Conversely, a hyper-plantarflexion injury can cause injury to the dorsal ligaments of the great toe joint as well to extensor tendons joint producing pain and inflammation. This injury is more commonly seen in sand sports such as volleyball and this injury has been coined "sand toe." This injury is usually self-limiting and, unlike turf toe, is not plagued with long-term morbidity.[7,11]

2.2 Etiology

A flexible shoe in combination with a hard artificial surface was considered the source of the turf toe injury in the 1970s.[3,9,10] Even with the return to natural grass from artificial surfaces and third-generation artificial surfaces, this injury is still present. Risk factors for turf toe that have been investigated include: increased shoe sole to surface friction with a fixed forefoot, increased shoe flexibility, reduction in artificial turf's ability to absorb force with wear.[4,9] Valgus and varus stress mechanisms have also been theorized as causative factors of turf toe injuries.[5] One possible risk factor that has not been investigated is chronic, repetitive, low-grade stress across the first MTPJ with physical activity of pushing, pulling, and jumping.

Fig. 2.1 (**a**) Hyperextension injury; (**b**) clinical presentation of acute turf toe

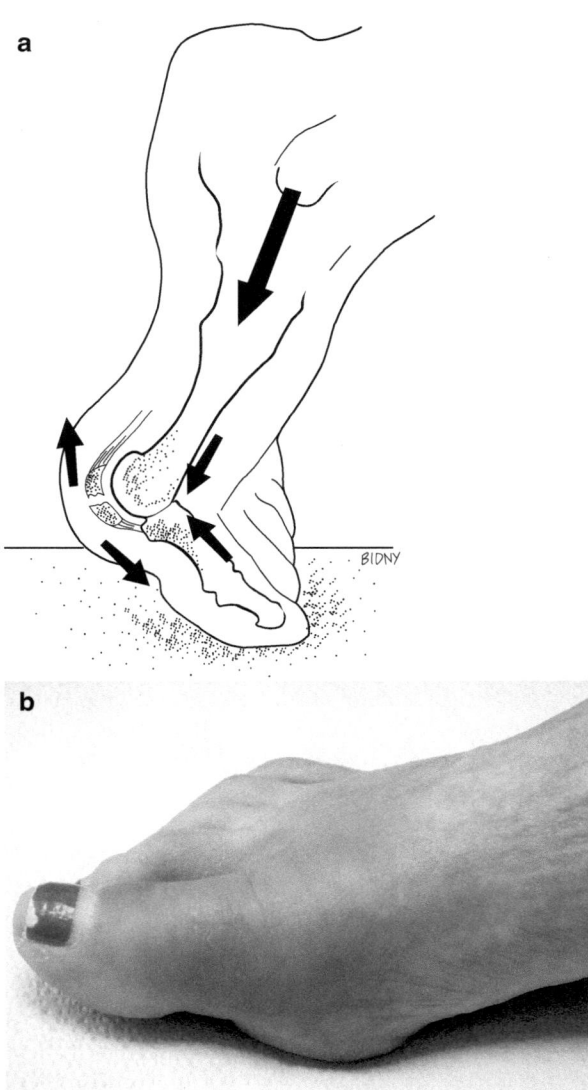

These ballistic movements may contribute to inflammation of the first MTPJ causing a low-grade sprain on surfaces of varying rigidity. With repeated practices and games throughout a season including off-season workouts, overuse and breakdown of the joint tissue may occur. If 90% of the body's weight is translated through the forefoot and 40–60% of the weight being placed across the great toe joint, overuse due to repetitive stretching or excessive tension on the plantar capsule ligaments could cause breakdown and disruption. An additional factor would include the increased physical ability of the modern athlete, being faster and stronger, intensifying the speed and velocity of ballistic movements.

2.3   Clinical Evaluation

Evaluation of the acute or subacute injured great toe joint needs to occur in a systematic, concise, and accurate manner. Initial exam may be thwarted by pain and splinting and thus, serial examination as acute symptoms resolve is mandatory. Each anatomical structure of the joint should be considered injured until proven otherwise. Identifying all structures that are potentially involved and determining the severity or lack thereof will allow the specialist to accurately grade the initial injury(s), outline an appropriate treatment program, determine a return to sports timeline, and to predict long-term morbidity. These goals are the cornerstone to the treatment of athletes.

The initial assessment includes ascertaining the mechanism and timing of the injury. Observe for any generalized deformity of the toe, the extent of joint effusion, the soft tissues around the distal first ray, and the possible presence and location of ecchymosis and swelling. Neurovascular compromise is not common except for extreme examples as seen with nonreduced dislocations. The author believes that ecchymosis is a hallmark clinical indicator of either a fracture or rupture of ligamentous or tendon structures. Ecchymosis plantarly increases the suspicion for sesamoid fracture and disruption of the plantar capsule-ligamentous structures or tear of the flexor hallucis brevis (FHB) muscle belly. Observation of ecchymosis dorsally may indicate dorsal tearing of the joint capsule, dorsal articular injury, or dorsal cortical fracture of the metatarsal. Palpation of the dorsal metatarsal head and neck along with the dorsal aspect of the base of the proximal phalanx provide suspicion for periarticular fracture. Further, palpation of the sesamoids and the long and short flexor and extensor tendons will provide information in regard to possible injury or fracture. Following palpation of the joint structures, manual manipulation of the joint should be performed. Specifically the medial and lateral collateral ligaments along with the phalangeal sesamoid ligaments provide controlled range of motion, proprioception and structural stability of the joint. Each ligament can and should be evaluated for the presence of pain and varying degrees of instability. A universal grading system should be applied to each ligament as increasing degree of injury will prolong return to sport and increase morbidity. A circumferential examination of the MTPJ should be performed beginning dorsal, medial then lateral and finally, plantar. The dorsal ligaments are assessed with plantar flexion of the joint, while the collaterals are evaluated with varus and valgus force with the hallux in a rectus position. Valgus stress can result in a ruptured medial joint capsule including the medial collateral ligament, abductor hallucis insertion and sesamoid apparatus (Fig. 2.2). The plantar ligaments are assessed by performing a Lachman-type maneuver. Again, while each ligament is evaluated (stressed), the presence or absence of pain as well as the amount of instability should be noted. Comparing stress evaluation of the noninjured side will at times be helpful. Tendonous injuries to the great toe will primarily involve the three main tendons of the great toe joint, the extensor hallusis longus (EHL), flexor hallusis longus (FHL), and FHB. Each tendon should be assessed for integrity and strength. In the authors' experience,

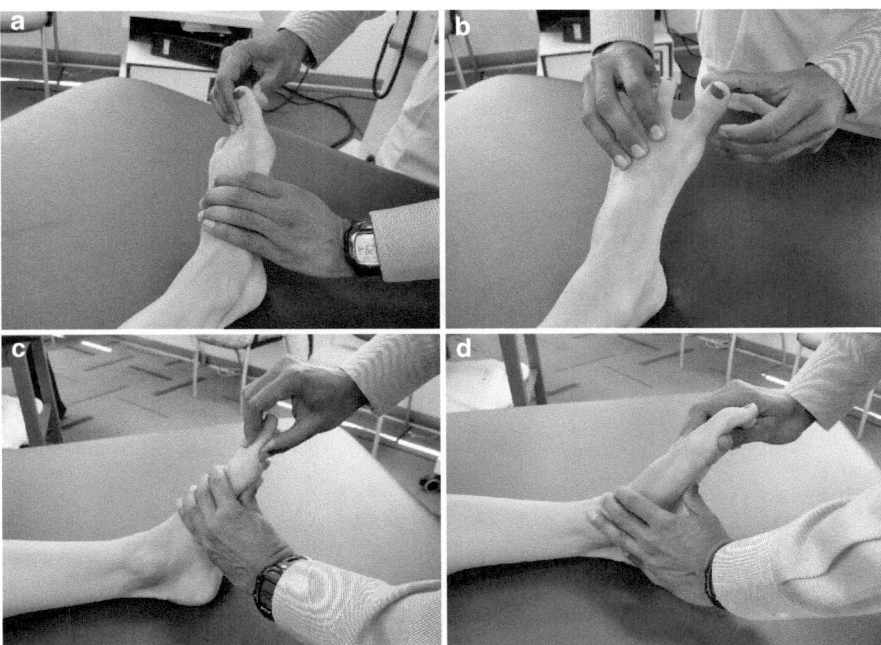

Fig. 2.2 (**a**) Abduction stress test to assess medial collateral ligament/medial capsule/abductor hallucis; (**b**) Adduction stress test to assess lateral collateral ligament/lateral capsule/adductor hallucis; (**c**) "Lachman" of first MPJ to assess plantar plate; (**d**) FHB strength/integrity assessment

injury to tendons other than the FHB has not been encountered. As the exam is carried out, a clinical scorecard of the noninjured and injured structures and severity should be kept. The clinical exam will be prognostic for further imaging modalities.

2.4   Imaging of Turf Toe Injuries

When imaging turf toe injuries, a protocol is necessary for accurate diagnosis. These radiographs should be evaluated for overt or small avulsion fractures of the distal first ray as well as mal-alignment, chondral injury, and sesamoid position. Radiographs of the contralateral foot should be performed for comparison. Initial imaging of the injured foot begins with plain radiographs taken in a standard anteroposterior (AP) projection, lateral oblique projection, and lateral views of the foot in weight bearing. Sesamoid position on an AP radiograph can provide information regarding the presence of sesamoid injury such as dislocation, retraction of the sesamoids (Fig. 2.3), disruption of the inter-sesamoid ligament, or fracture of the sesamoids. An additional image is the axial sesamoid view, with the foot weight bearing,

Fig. 2.3 X-ray of dislocation
with sesamoid retraction

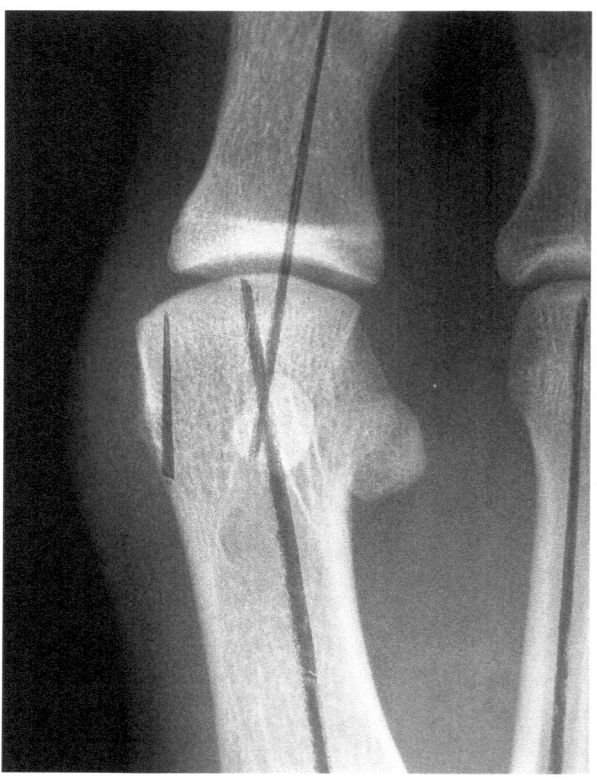

the heel raised with the toe dorsiflexed and the radiographic beam being introduced from posterior 90° to the foot.

Additional radiographs can be taken performing provocative maneuvers to the first MTPJ, stressing the plantar joint capsule and surrounding ligamentous attachments. A Lachman's type maneuver or dorsiflexion stress maneuver can be performed at the joint to accentuate instability. Performing dorsiflexion stress maneuvers can reveal retraction of the sesamoids or disruption of the plantar plate on the metatarsal showing evidence of metatarsal sesamoid ligament disruption. In addition, fluoroscopic imaging can be used to evaluate range of motion of the first MTPJ and demonstrate instability.

There is very little information defining the indications of magnetic resonance imaging (MRI) for turf toe injuries. But clearly, this advanced imaging modality will allow the clinician to appreciate the full spectrum of the injury and serve as an adjunct to the clinical exam. MRI will allow for each potentially injured structure to be evaluated for the presence or absence of injury and severity (Fig. 2.4). MRI imaging of the MTPJ complex using a non-fat-suppressed T1-weighted or proton density–weighted sequence in three standard planes is recommended.[6] In addition, according to Crain et al.,[6] a proton density–weighted fat-suppressed or short tau inversion recovery

Fig. 2.4 (**a**) MRI showing plantar first MTPJ plate rupture without sesamoid fracture; (**b**) Repaired plantar plate

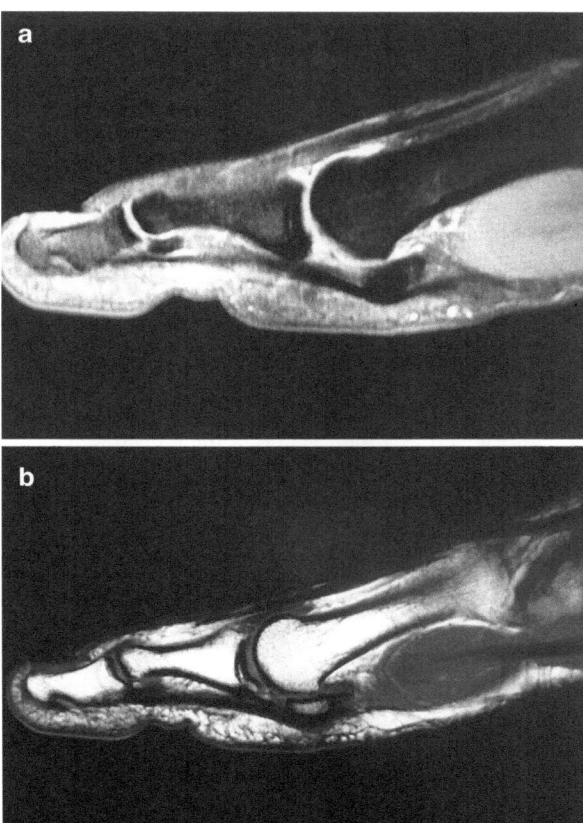

(STIR) sequence in all three planes is recommended for optimal evaluation of the turf toe pathology. A STIR sequence should be used to evaluate acute pathology. Proton density–weighted fat-suppressed images provide better resolution than STIR with shorter imaging time and also provide more detail of the anatomy than heavily fat-suppressed T2-weighted images and STIR sequences. To optimize the resolution with lower field MRI scanners, that field of view should range from 13 to 15 cm with a slice thickness of no less than 3.5 mm of STIR images.[6] Higher field MRI scanners such as 3.0 T magnet provide better definition and detail. Injury of the metatarsal sesamoid ligament and phalangeal sesamoid ligament is best visualized on sagittal slices. The inner sesamoid ligamentous anatomy is best visualized on axial images. The most common injured soft tissue structures along the plantar first MTPJ capsule are the phalangeal sesamoid ligamentous attachments. In MRI, evaluation of the injured plantar phalangeal sesamoid ligamentous structures will reveal incontinuity or edema. Once the clinical exam is correlated with radiographic and possible advanced imaging, the clinician can now truly understand the full spectrum of the injury.

2.5   Classification of Turf Toe

Turf toe injuries are classified on the basis of severity. To date, there is no grading system that is truly comprehensive and takes into consideration injuries to structures other than the ligaments. As can be appreciated, if there is injury to osseous, articular, or tendonous structures, each will have its own spectrum of injury, treatment protocol, and morbidity. A general assumption can be made that with increasing degrees and involvement of ligamentous structures, there is a greater chance of associated injuries to occur. It is often the lack of appreciation of these associated injuries that will lead to an inaccurate initial diagnosis and prognosis. In treating athletes, the specialist is tasked with working with a small margin of error. This margin will decrease as the level of the athlete increases. Establishing the grade of turf toe injury from clinical evaluation and imaging protocol will provide the most accurate initial diagnosis and treatment, shorten the convalescent period, reduce the time to return to play, and predict possible morbidity that may affect long-term performance.

Grade 1 injuries are the least severe. These injuries typically are a minor stretch or strain without compromise to the soft tissue restraints. Clinically, patients with Grade 1 injuries present with localized plantar or medial tenderness, mild edema, and no visible ecchymosis. The patient is able to bear weight and there is little change in the range of motion or strength. Radiographs are normal, and MRI demonstrates intact capsular integrity with mild soft tissue edema.

Grade 2 injuries are moderate in severity. They represent partial tears of the capsuloligamentous structures, most often the sesamoid phalangeal and metatarsal phalangeal ligaments. But, the medial collateral ligament is commonly involved (Fig. 2.5). Clinically, patients present with more diffuse and intense tenderness, mild to moderate edema with ecchymosis on the plantar and medial surface of the first MTPJ. These injuries typically have varying levels of disability. The MTPJ has a restricted range of motion with severe pain and antalgic gait with weight bearing. Symptoms are typically progressive. Radiographs may appear normal with the sesamoid bones lying in the normal position. MRI demonstrates moderate soft tissue edema extending through the plantar plate indicating a partial thickness disruption. This can be seen plantarly at the level of the sesamoid phalangeal or metatarsal phalangeal ligaments.

Grade 3 injuries are the most severe type of turf toe injury. This stage describes severe acute injuries with plantar capsuloligamentous disruption or the lasting chronic effects of a capsuloligamentous injury. Clinically, patients present with severe and diffuse tenderness. There is often marked swelling accompanied with moderate to severe ecchymosis to the MTPJ with an acute injury. Pain is often so severe that patients are unable to bear weight. Radiographs may demonstrate proximal migration of sesamoids, compression fractures, asymmetric lateral, medial or dorsal subluxation, or capsular avulsion fragments or capsular avulsion. Joint subluxation or deviation may also be apparent on radiographs or stress views. MRI typically demonstrates complete disruption of the plantar plate as well as any other associated injuries to the capsuloligamentous structures.[2,5]

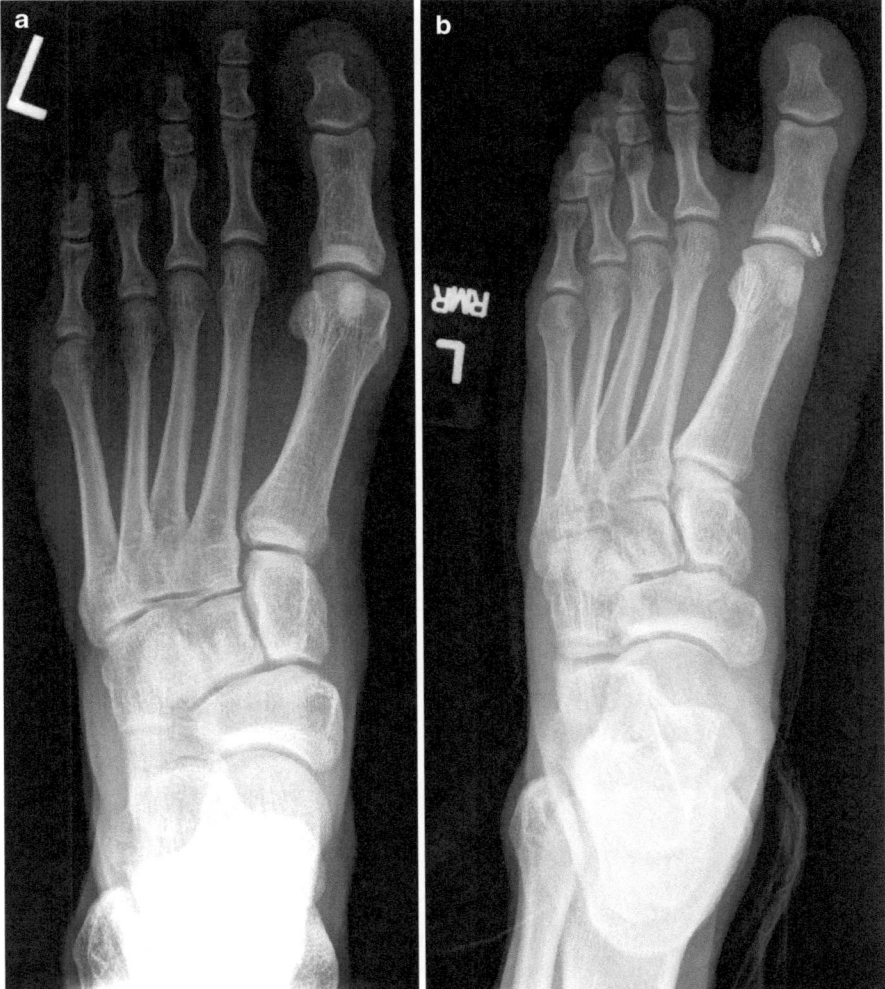

Fig. 2.5 (a) Valgus stress injury resulting in medial collateral first MPTJ rupture ("traumatic bunion") Patient felt a "pop" while running 10 days post-injection for 1st MP synovitis and notice acute lateral deviation of his hallux; (b) Post-op X-ray of repair of medial collateral ligament with a soft tissue anchor

MRI can also delineate osteochondral injury (Fig. 2.6). Imaging is helpful to stage these lesions and determine if surgery is needed for displaced fragments or significant bony defects. Ascertaining the entire spectrum of injury and potential need for treatment via MRI is helpful and strongly recommended for athletic patients.

Fig. 2.6 (**a**, **b**) MRIs showing osteochondral injuries of the first metatarsal head after hyperextension injuries

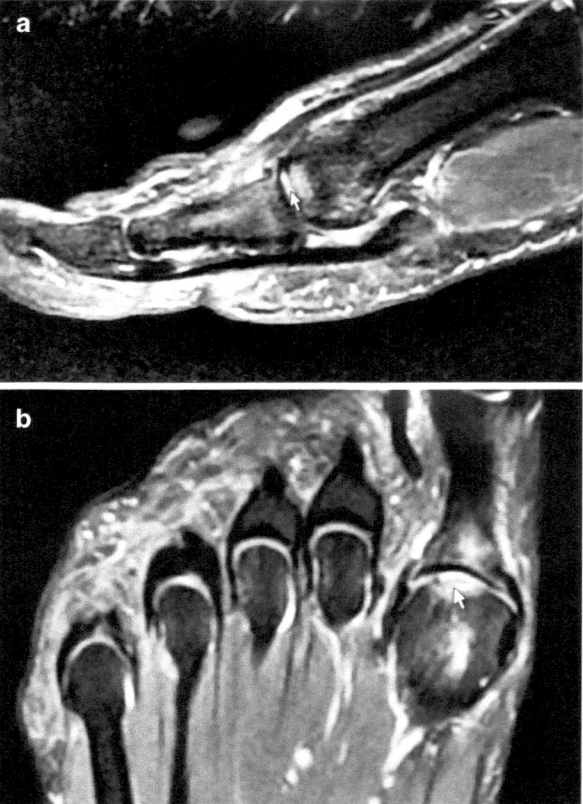

2.6   Treatment of Turf Toe Injuries

Grade 1 injuries require immobilization, nonsteroidal anti-inflammatories (NSAIDs), and cryotherapy. Functional immobilization with taping of the joint provides adequate stability for the athlete to return to play with minimal discomfort. Functional immobilization with a short leg weight-bearing cast with toe spica for 3–5 days can be helpful in patients that do not tolerate taping. A postoperative shoe or short leg walking boot can be used when not playing or practicing to allow the soft tissues of the plantar aspect of the MTPJ to rest by reducing dorsiflexion stress across the joint. The athlete may return to activity with spica taping (Fig. 2.7) or even a turf toe plate (Fig. 2.8) temporarily in the shoe. This plate can be removed later as the athlete gains more confidence and function in the great toe joint.

Grade 2 injuries require immediate immobilization, NSAIDs, and cryotherapy. The athlete should be placed in a short leg cast boot with strict non-weight bearing on crutches for approximately 2 weeks. After healing of the partial plantar

Fig. 2.7 Toe spica taping

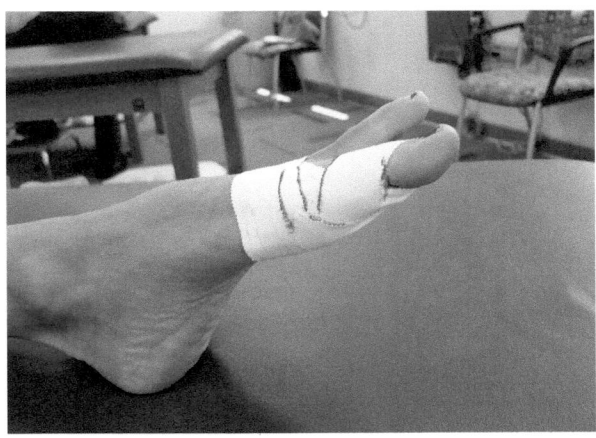

capsule-ligamentous structures, the athlete must complete a rehabilitation program in order to safely return to play. A custom orthotic with Morton's extension (Fig. 2.9) can be placed in a shoe; changing to a shoe with a stiffer forefoot construction may help reduce re-injury rate. A turf toe plate is the alternative to an orthotic with Morton's extension and can provide the necessary rigidity in the forefoot to allow comfortable play. An orthotic with Morton's extension can also be used until the patient transitions to pre-injury performance level.

Grade 3 injuries are the most severe and usually involve dislocation or subluxation of the first MTPJ due to disruption of the plantar capsular ligamentous structures of the first MTPJ. Grade 3 injuries can require immediate closed reduction if dislocation is present followed by immobilization, cryotherapy, NSAIDs, and short leg cast with toe plate or toe spica to the hallux non-weight bearing for 4–6 weeks. Physical therapy and rehabilitation will be required for an additional 4–6 weeks. The athlete should have rehabilitation to restore function to the first MTPJ and restoration of strength to the EHL and FHL muscles also strengthen to the FHL and EHL muscles for safe return to play at pre-injury strength, mobility, and pain-free function. Generalized de-conditioning of the musculature may require 8–16 weeks of additional rehabilitation for the athlete to return to ballistic maneuvers of running, jumping, and cutting. The athlete will have to be able to tolerate a significant amount of dorsiflexion at the first MTPJ when considering stance positions in football where the dorsiflexed position is needed for propulsion and push-off. The athlete needs to be able to perform this activity with a minimal amount of pain and discomfort in order to return to the game at full speed. Steroid injections should not be performed in the area of the injury and can be detrimental to healing of the soft tissues. Steroid injections can mask pain which would be an important indicator whether an athlete is ready to return to pre-injury performance. If there is no improvement with conservative management, surgical repair of the plantar capsular ligamentous structures may be required. Table 2.1 highlights these recommendations.

Fig. 2.8 Turf toe plate/insole

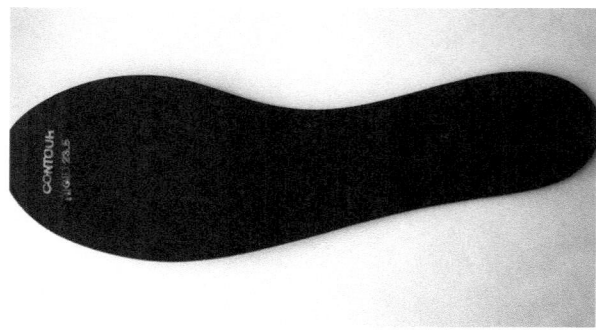

Fig. 2.9 Morton's extension insole with more rigid material, in this case cork, under 1st MPTJ

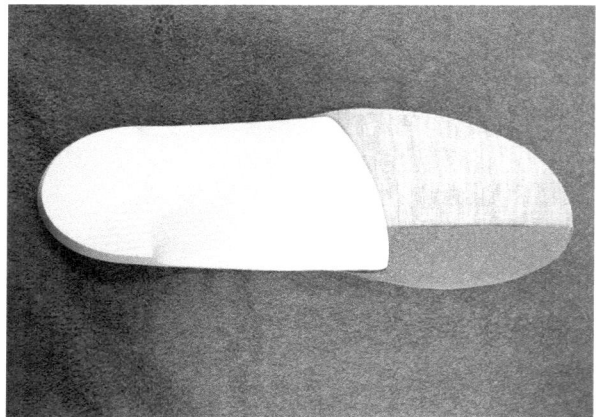

2.6.1 Surgical Treatment

Sesamoid avulsion fractures and sesamoid fractures may occur with turf toe injuries. Sesamoid fractures have a low occurrence rate, but a high incidence of nonunion due to avascularity to the surrounding fibro-cartilaginous structures. If the sesamoid fractures are not healed and symptomatic after 3–4 months, surgical excision of the sesamoid is advised. Dislocation and subluxation injuries of the MTPJ often have a dislocation of the FHL tendon present. Immediate reduction is necessary, to prevent loss of plantar flexion function, nonanatomic scar, and fibrosis. Severe turf toe injuries with first MTPJ instability or dislocation as a result of complete disruption of the plantar capsular ligamentous structures, surgical repair is indicated. The approach to this should include a plantar or plantar medial incision to help with direct visualization of the plantar capsular ligamentous structures and repair (Fig. 2.10). Chapter 21 gives good insight to plantar approaches and repair of the anatomical structures.

The postoperative course includes short leg cast immobilization with toe spica for 2–3 weeks followed by physical therapy which would progressively return the

Table 2.1 Treatment recommendations for turf toe injuries

	Grade 1	Grade 2	Grade 3
Description	Attenuation of the plantar joint capsule	Partial tear of the plantar joint capsule	Complete tear of the plantar joint capsule
Clinical findings	Mild swelling no ecchymosis tenderness with palpation	Moderate swelling, ecchymosis, limited motion with pain, moderate pain	Swelling, ecchymosis, limited motion with pain, severe pain, positive Lachman's
Treatment	Taping and continued play	Immobilization in walking boot or cast, NSAIDs, and physical therapy	• Immobilization in cast or surgical repair. • Dislocation with instability after reduction requires surgical repair of plantar plate. • Symptomatic sesamoid fracture nonunion requires surgical excision.

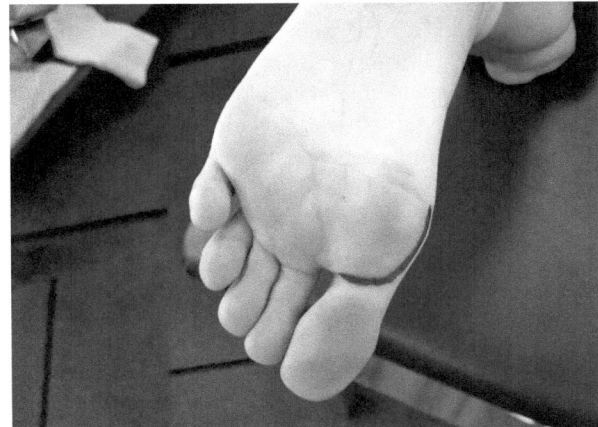

Fig. 2.10 Incisional approach as an option for plantar first MPTJ capsule and plate repair

athlete back to pre-injury performance. Protected weight bearing would begin at 3 weeks after surgery in a walking boot.

The indications for surgical repair are the following[8]:

- Large capsular avulsion with unstable joint
- Diastasis of partite sesamoid
- Diastasis of sesamoid fracture
- Retraction of sesamoids
- Traumatic hallux valgus deformity
- Vertical instability with Lachman's test
- Loose body
- Chondral injury
- Failed nonsurgical treatment

Osteochondral defects sustained from turf toe injuries deserve special mention. Chondral lesions require treatment with microfracture techniques treated with microfracture techniques after débridement of loose cartilage flaps. Some of these isolated lesions may be amenable to arthroscopic treatment. Osteochondral defects sustained during the injury may need to be treated with bone grafting. An osteochondral autograft transfer (OATS) procedure of the first metatarsal head can be performed with autograft from the medial talar head, or in cases with hypertrophic dorsal exostoses, a portion of the resected bone can be harvested and placed into the defect (Fig. 2.11). Postoperative management will be dictated by the performance of additional procedures such as capsular or plantar plate repair. Generally, a period of 3 or more weeks non-weight bearing is required for chondral and osteochondral injuries.

Hallux malleus, hallux varus, hallux valgus, and hallux rigidus deformities may be secondary deformities as a result of turf toe injuries, these late sequelae of turf toe injuries may be addressed with various procedures. If these sequelae are asymptomatic, they should be addressed at the end of the athlete's career to restore normal function. If these deformities are symptomatic while the athlete is still active, the hallux rigidus can be addressed with cheilectomy (dorsal exostectomy) in the off-season. The hallux valgus deformity can be addressed with a bunionectomy. The hallux malleus should be addressed at the end of an athlete's professional career because of tendon transfers required to restore function and anatomic alignment. Transfer of tendons may result in a loss of strength and power in regard to an athlete, but the hallux malleus deformity should be addressed with shoe accommodations, orthotics, and proper foot care.

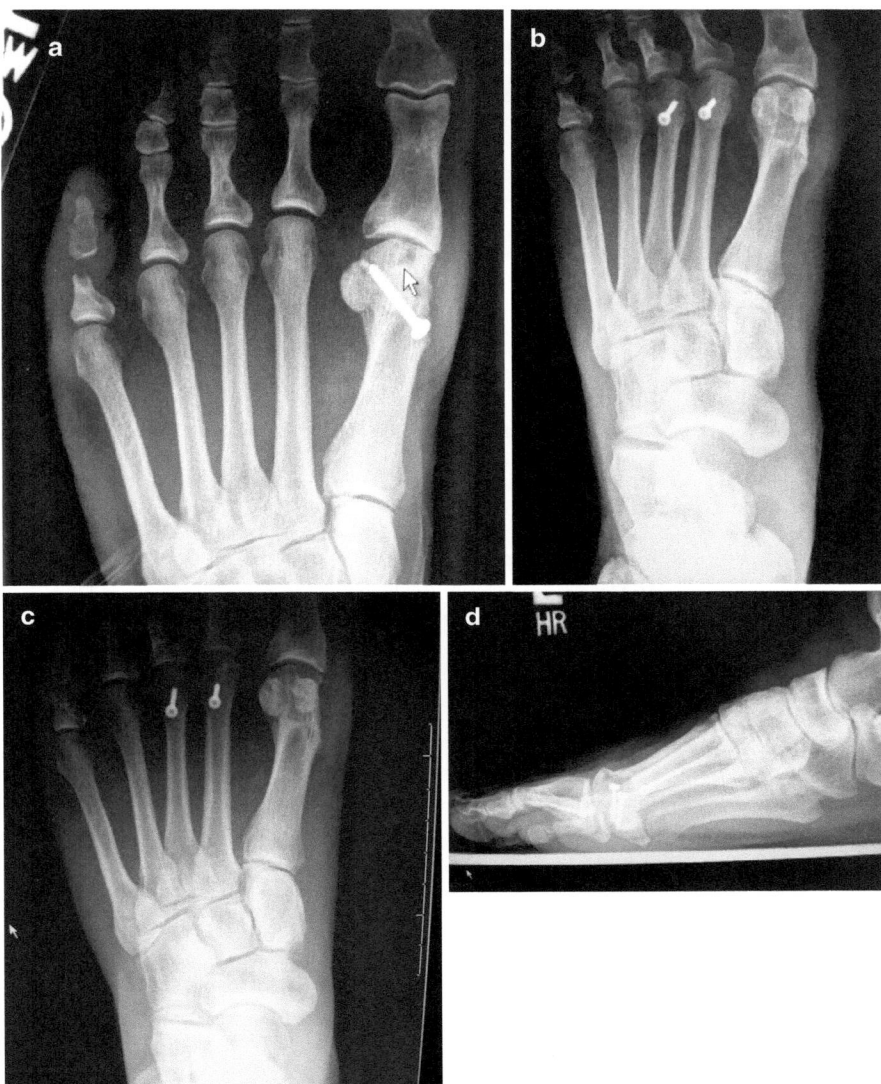

Fig. 2.11 (**a–d**) Pre-operative (**a**), immediate (**b**) and one year post-operative (**c** & **d**) X-rays of autogenous "OATS" repair of 1st metatarsal head (donor graft from medial talar head). Note normal appearing talo-navicular joint

References

1. Brophy RH, Gamradt SC, Ellis SJ, et al. Effect of turf toe on foot contact pressures in professional American football players. Foot Ankle Int. 2009;30:405–9.
2. Clanton TO, Ford JJ. Turf toe injury. Clin Sports Med. 1994;13:731–41.
3. Coker TP, Arnold JA, Weber DL. Traumatic lesions of the metarsophalangeal joint of the great toe in athletes. Am J Sports Med. 1978;6:326–34.
4. Rodeo SA, O'Brien S, Warren RF, et al. Turf-toe: an analysis of metatarsophalangeal joint sprains in professional football players. Am J Sports Med. 1990;18:280–5.
5. Clanton TO, Butler JE, Eggert A. Injuries to the metatarsophalangeal joints in athletes. Foot Ankle Int. 1986;7(3):162–76.
6. Crain JM, Phancao J, Stidham K. MR imaging of turf toe. Magn Reson Imaging Clin N Am. 2008;16:93–103.
7. Nihal A, Trepman E, Nag D. First ray disorders in athletes. Sports Med Arthrosc. 2009;17:160–6.
8. McCormick JJ, Anderson RB. The great toe: failed turf toe, chronic turf toe, and complicated sesamoid injuries. Foot Ankle Clin. 2009;14:135–50.
9. Nigg BM, Segesser B. The influence of playing surfaces on the load on the locomotor system and on football and tennis injuries. Sports Med. 1988;5:375–85.
10. Torg JS, Stilwell G, Rogers K. The effect of ambient temperature on the shoe-surface interface release coefficient. Am J Sports Med. 1996;24:79–82.
11. Frey C, Andersen GD, Feder KS. Plantarflexion injury to the metatarsophalangeal joint ("sand toe"). Foot Ankle Int. 1996;17(9):576–81.

Chapter 3
Hallux Rigidus: The Valenti Arthroplasty

John F. Grady, Audra M. Smith, Yelena Boumendjel, and Amol Saxena

3.1 Background

Surgical treatments reported in literature for the treatment of hallux rigidus include implant arthroplasty, cheilectomy, various osteotomies (i.e., Hohmann, Regnauld/enclavement, plantarflexory), non-implant arthroplasty (i.e., Keller-Brandes, Mayo-Hueter), and arthrodesis.[1-15] The original Valenti procedure, described at the Hershey, Pennsylvania Surgical Seminar in 1987, was a dorsally biased joint resection arthroplasty of the first metatarsophalangeal joint in a V-type fashion. Valente Valenti (personal communication) had performed his procedure on more than 600 patients since 1976, with great success. More than 90% demonstrated improved and pain-free range of motion. A modification of the Valenti procedure for treatment of hallux rigidus is presented, which preserves the joint for greater stability, and allows future revision to arthrodesis or implant arthroplasty if necessary.

3.2 Indications

Patients with Grade II, III, and possibly IV hallux rigidus who do not respond to nonsurgical care, that is, change in foot gear, orthoses, injections, or oral anti-inflammatory medication (which research has shown that more than half do), are

J.F. Grady, D.P.M. (✉)
Department of Surgery, Foot and Ankle Institute of Illinois,
4650 Southwest Highway, Oak Lawn 60453, IL, USA
e-mail: grady@footandankleinstitute.com

A.M. Smith, D.P.M. • Y. Boumendjel, D.P.M.
Department of Podiatry, Jesse Brown VA Medical Center, Chicago, IL, USA

A. Saxena, D.P.M.
Department of Sports Medicine, PAFMG-Palo Alto Division,
Palo Alto, CA, USA

A. Saxena (ed.), *Sports Medicine and Arthroscopic Surgery of the Foot and Ankle*, 29
DOI 10.1007/978-1-4471-4106-8_3, © Springer-Verlag London 2013

candidates for surgery.[7] Typical patients' preoperative radiographs show dorsal hypertrophic exostoses (Fig. 3.1) The decision is whether the surgery should be arthroplasty, arthrodesis, or joint replacement. It is our experience (JFG, AS) that arthroplasty gives better performance, better postoperative pain relief, and a less difficult postoperative course than arthrodesis or joint replacement.[6,13] It also has better long-term results with less related morbidity (alternative foot problems, knee and hip problems, or lower-back problems).

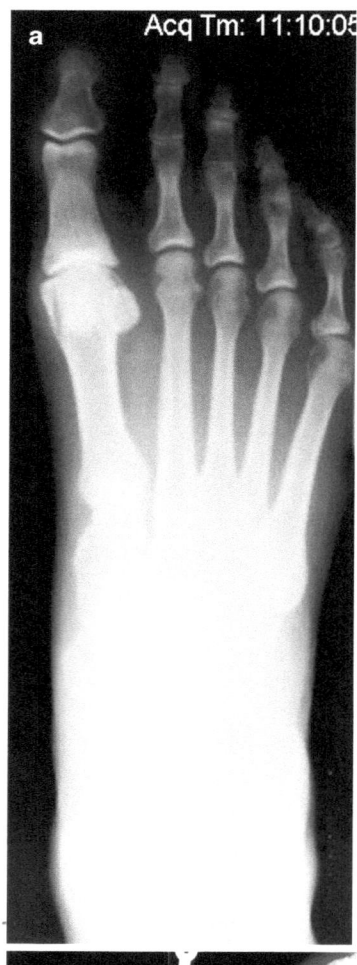

Fig. 3.1 (**a**) AP X-ray. (**b**) Lateral X-ray. Preoperative X-rays of typical Valenti candidate

Fig. 3.2 Incisional approach

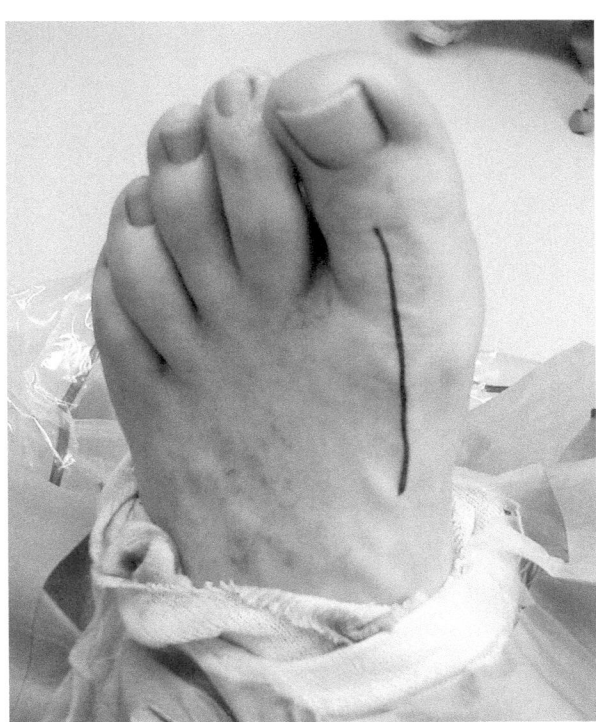

3.3 Author's Preferred Technique: The Valenti Arthroplasty

A linear incision is made approximately 5 cm over the first metatarsophalangeal joint (Fig. 3.2). It is deepened and great care is taken to dissect the capsule off the proximal phalanx first in the medial aspect. Next was coming up in the "student" hole and dissecting the capsule off the medial aspect of the first metatarsal (Fig. 3.3). Then, the periosteum is gently removed underneath the extensor hallucis longus tendon along with capsule to expose the entire head of the joint and base of the proximal phalanx (Fig. 3.4).

Great care is taken not to resect the flexor hallucis brevis tendon plantarly nor the extensor hallucis longus dorsally. Next, our attention is focused on the degenerative bone around the first metatarsal. First we use a power saw to resect the medial hypertrophic bone and cartilage (Fig. 3.5). We then resect the hypertrophic bone laterally. The dorsal resection is via a cut at an oblique angle from the inferior aspect of the typical central chondral defect (Fig. 3.6), usually midline in the central aspect of the defect, terminating at the proximal aspect of the metatarsal neck dorsally on a very oblique angle (Fig. 3.7) avoiding invading the medullary canal of the first metatarsal. After this is removed, we then use a rongeur to resect the hypertrophic bone off the base of the proximal phalanx leaving the standard normal contour of the base of the proximal phalanx and taking what is hypertrophic dorsally, medially, and laterally

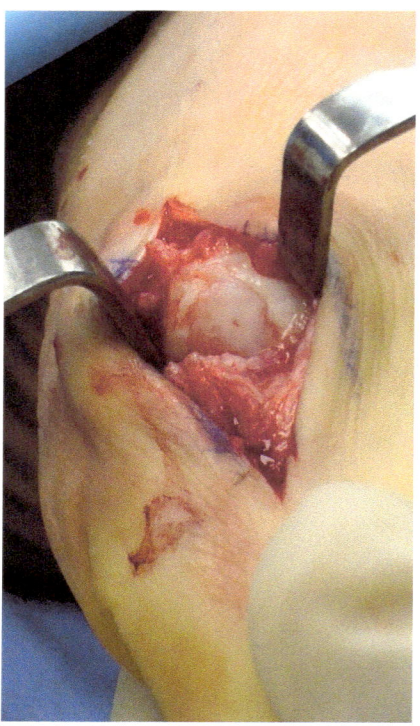

(the latter which is known as the "Valenti spur") (Fig. 3.8). Great care is taken to leave
the plantar aspect of the joint totally intact (Fig. 3.9). The next focus is on determining
the amount of dorsiflexion present. At this point, if the toe is able to be dorsiflexed
passively without much pressure to get to 90° of dorsiflexion, everything is left alone.
If one is not able to get 90° of dorsiflexion, we then gently free up the tibial and fibular
sesamoids from within the joint with a #15 blade eccentrically (from the center medially and from the center laterally). Great care is taken not to disrupt the arterial supply
between the sesamoids or below the sesamoids. We just separate the adhesed tissue
from the tibial sesamoid medially and the fibular sesamoid laterally, staying between
the sesamoids and periosteum as well as bone. After this is performed, we close by
hour-glassing the medial and lateral capsule to each other with absorbable suture (2-0
Vicryl™), draped dorsally but not directly interposed between the distal portions of
the joint. Hypertrophic synovium that will impede dorsiflexion is resected.

Next, attention is focused on closure, and we leave the toe in dorsiflexion when
we close (usually about 60° of dorsiflexion) the periosteum and superficial tissue
still using 2-0 Vicryl. This is done so that remodeled scar will favor dorsiflexion of
the joint. It should be noted that passive dorsiflexion is ideally in the 60–90° range
at this point, even after closure (Fig. 3.10). Plantarflexion should also be more than
10° for normal function. Deep closure is performed often with 3-0 Vicryl™ subcutaneous sutures. Skin is closed with a subcuticular suture of 4-0 Monocryl™ or

Fig. 3.4 (**a**) Medial view. (**b**) Dorsal view. Dissection exposes the entire dorsal first

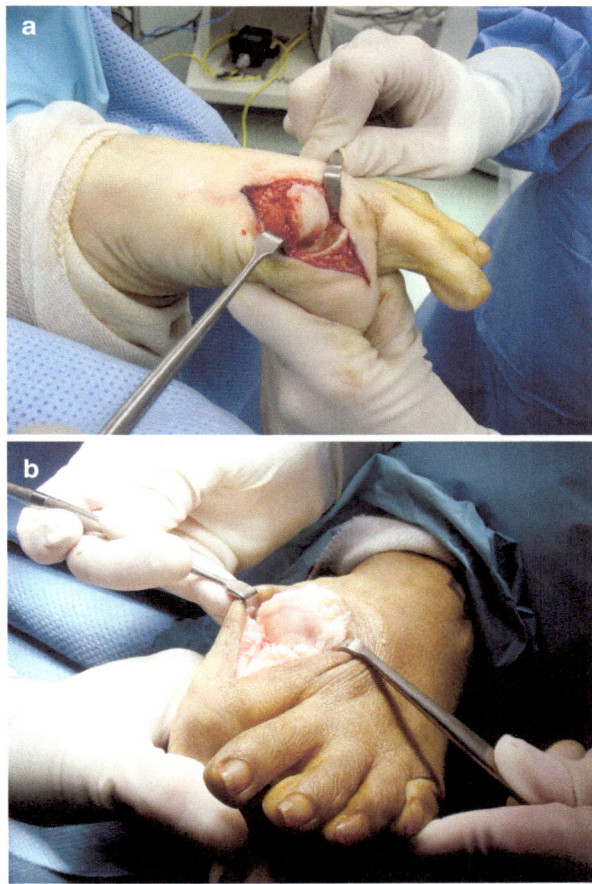

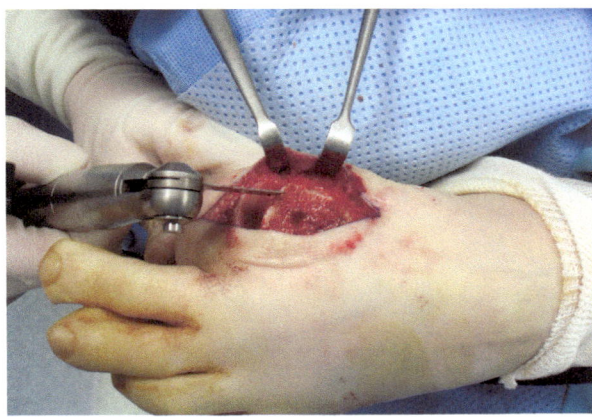

Fig. 3.5 Medial exostosis resection

Fig. 3.6 Dorsal resection
of dorsal hyperostosis (**a**).
Note: resection is below the
osteochondral defect but is
angled to avoid invading the
medullary canal (**b**)

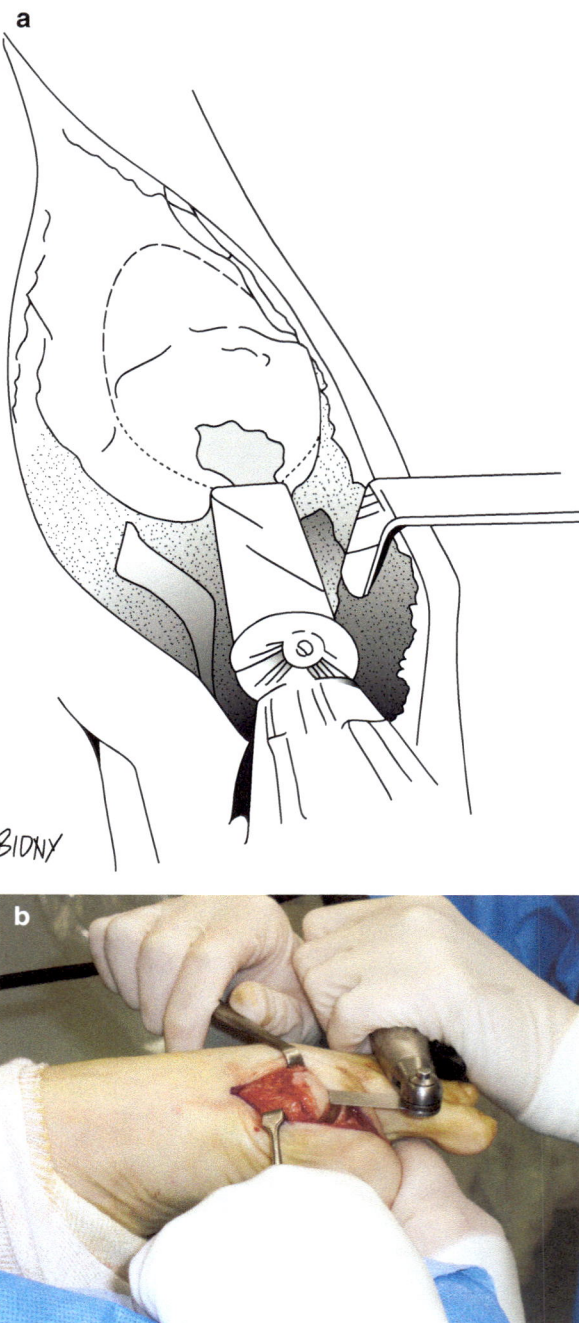

Fig. 3.7 Dorsal resection
completed

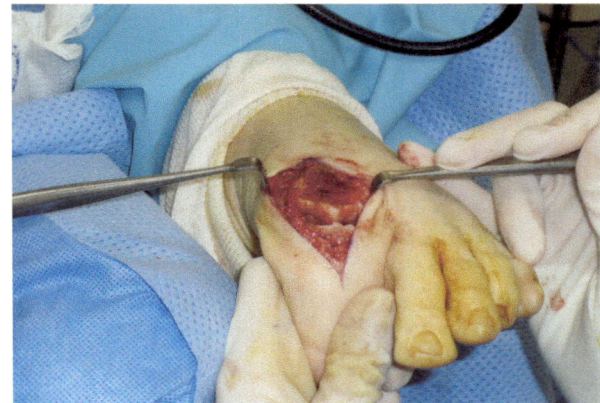

Fig. 3.8 Lateral spur from
base of proximal phalanx
resected with a rongeur

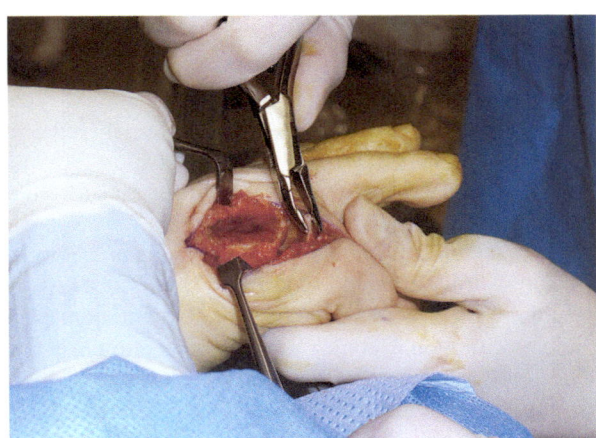

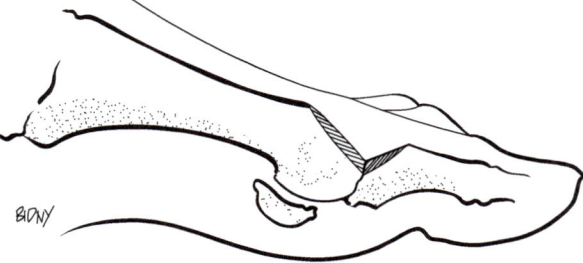

Fig. 3.9 Diagram showing
appropriate resection on both
sides of the first MPTJ

nylon. Postoperative bandaging can consist of steri-strips, Adaptic or Xeroform™,
4 × 4 gauze sponges, and Webril™. Postoperatively, these arthroplasties sometimes
swell significantly, especially if the medullary canal was entered with the dorsal
resection of bone. If that is the case, swelling will be intolerable if a restrictive,

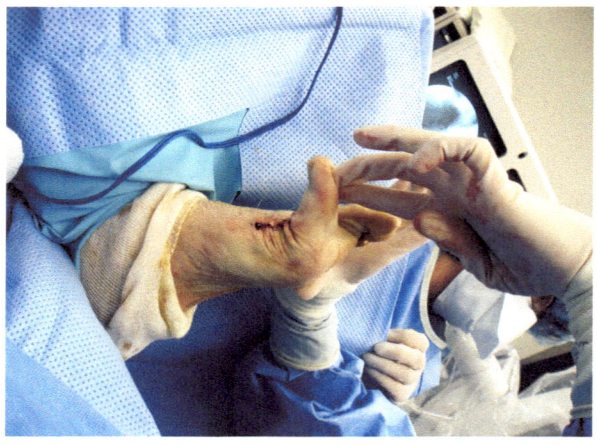

Fig. 3.10 Immediate postoperative motion achieved

nonelastic dressing is used. The patient will have resultant stiffness from excessive scarring and possible hematoma. To avoid this, we cover the wound with 4 × 4s and Webril® only. Elevation and icing is extremely important in the initial postoperative period (see Chap. 18).

Initially, passive range of motion is engaged from day 1. Active range of motion is engaged after day 2. Then for the first 2 weeks, edema control is maintained by elevation and ice. Ambulation is able to occur, but for a maximum of 10 min an hour. The rest of the time the foot has to be elevated. After the first 2 weeks, we get the patient into active and passive range of motion, physical therapy, and aggressive range-of-motion exercises and proprioception exercises. It is important to maintain these proprioception exercises for the next year, spending 10 min at least per day doing proprioceptive exercises and passive range of motion. Usually, there is dorsiflexion after 2 weeks of approximately 30°, and it can improve up to double over the ensuing year if exercises are maintained in an aggressive fashion (Fig. 3.11).

3.4 Discussion

Historically, the Valenti procedure for hallux rigidus was first described in American literature by Grady and Axe.[6] This procedure is considered a resectional arthroplasty but leaves the instrinsics of the flexor apparatus intact. Many authors present good to excellent results in large series with medium to long-term follow-up.[6,10,13,16] Olms et al. presented their results of the largest series of the Valenti arthroplasty (162 patients) with an average increase in dorsiflexion of 27°. Twelve patients had progression of their osteoarthritis after surgery. Ten patients underwent implant arthroplasty, while two had an arthrodesis. In their series, 80% of their patients had experienced some form of sesamoiditis. They performed sesamoid mobilization and "hour-glassing" of the joint capsule.[16]

Sesamoiditis continues to be the most common complication after Valenti arthro-plasty, affecting almost 80% of postoperative patients.[16] We attribute this to the fact that we are mobilizing a joint which has not moved for so long. The sesamoids are adhered, and mobilizing them is actually somewhat of a painful endeavor. Offloading this region with an accommodative pad (i.e., "reverse Morton's") for up to 6 months usually is enough to make this pain-free. Injection with corticosteroid may be indicated. Another option is to avoid aggressive mobilization of the sesamoids. Furthermore, one author (AS) does not "hour-glass" the capsule. This may decrease the postoperative synovitis.

There has been concern about the Valenti resectional arthoplasty potentially destabilizing the joint, leading to arthrosis. These patients already have arthrosis, and often hallux rigidus is a progressive deformity whether or not patients have

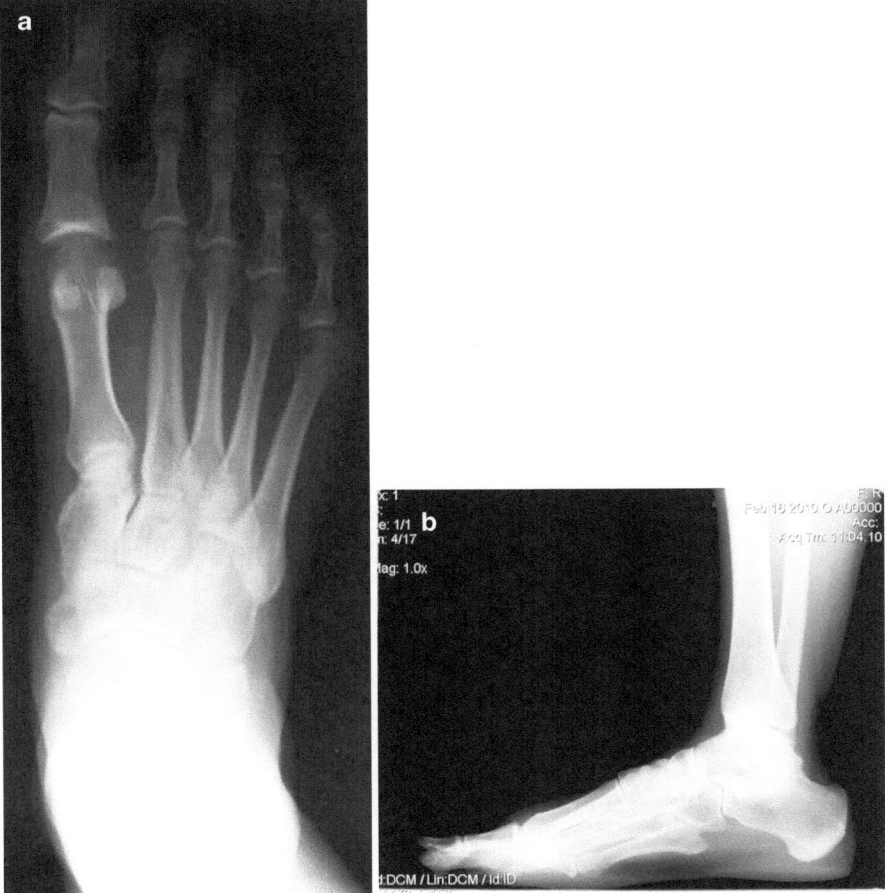

Fig. 3.11 (**a**) X-rays (AP), (**b**) Lateral, (**c**) oblique, (**d**) stress lateral at one year postoperative of same patient shown in Fig. 3.1

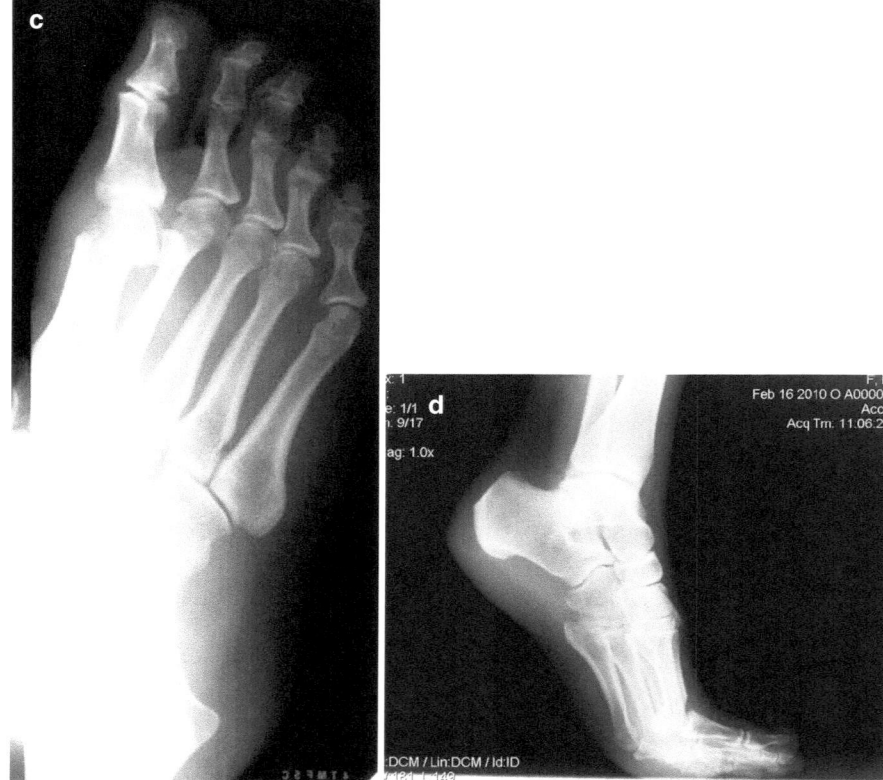

Fig. 3.11 (continued)

surgery. A Valenti arthoplasty can be easily converted to an arthrodesis or implant procedure, often without any additional bone graft.[11,14,16]

3.5 Conclusions

The authors describe the Valenti resectional arthroplasty surgical procedure that provides excellent symptomatic relief for patients suffering from painful hallux rigidus. This should be the first option for recalcitrant hallux rigidus unresponsive to nonsurgical care in most cases because if it fails it is revisable to arthrodesis or implant arthroplasty. The procedure should be technically easy to perform and allows for a rapid return to activity. Resection of the degenerated articular dorsal surfaces on both sides of the first metatarsophalangeal joint without violating the medullary canal is critical. Postoperative mobilization is required. Sesamoiditis is noticed transiently in most patients. The procedure does not address the biomechanical etiology of hallux rigidus such as structural elevatus, thus, mechanical accommodation is recommended as needed.

References

1. Coughlin MJ, Shurnas PS. Hallux rigidus: grading and long-term results of operative treatment. J Bone Joint Surg Am. 2003;85:2072–88.
2. Easley ME, Davis WH, Anderson RB. Intermediate to long-term follow-up of medial-approach dorsal cheilectomy for hallux rigidus. Foot Ankle Int. 1999;20:147–52.
3. Ess P, Hamalainen M, Leppilahti J. Non-constrained titanium-polyethylene total endoprosthesis in the treatment of hallux rigidus. A prospective clinical 2-year follow-up study. Scand J Surg. 2002;91:202–7.
4. Fellman J, Zollinger H. Resektionsarthroplastik des ersten Metatarsophalangealgelenkes nach Keller-Brandes. Oper Orthop Traumatol. 1998;10:143–51.
5. Geldwert JJ, Rock GD, McGrath MP. Cheilectomy: still a useful technique for grade I and grade II hallux limitus/rigidus. J Foot Surg. 1992;31:154–9.
6. Grady JF, Axe TM. The modified Valenti procedure for the treatment of hallux limitus. J Foot Ankle Surg. 1994;33:365–7.
7. Grady JF, Axe TM, Zager EJ. A retrospective analysis of 772 patients with hallux limitus. J Am Podiatr Med Assoc. 2002;92:102–8.
8. Haddad SL. The use of osteotomies in the treatment of hallux limitus and hallux rigidus. Foot Ankle Clin. 2000;5:629–61.
9. Hanft JR, Mason ET, Landsman AS. A new radiographic classification for hallux limitus. J Foot Ankle Surg. 1993;32:397–404.
10. Kurtz DH, Harrill JC, Kaczander BI. The Valenti procedure for hallux limitus; a long-term follow-up and analysis. J Foot Ankle Surg. 1999;38:123–30.
11. Oloff L. The Valenti procedure for hallux limitus/rigidus. J Foot Ankle Surg. 1996;35:178–9, author reply 180–1.
12. Root ML. An approach to foot orthopedics. J Am Podiatr Med Assoc. 1964;54:115–8.
13. Saxena A. The Valenti procedure for hallux limitus/rigidus. J Foot Ankle Surg. 1995;34:485–8; discussion 511.
14. Vanore J, O'Keefe R, Bidny M. Hallux rigidus. In: Marcinko D, editor. APMA textbook of podiatric medical and surgical practice. Baltimore: Williams & Wilkins; 1990. p. 93–5.
15. Weil LS. The Valenti procedure for hallux limitus/rigidus. J Foot Ankle Surg. 1996;35:179–80, author reply 180–1.
16. Olms K, Grady J, Schulz A. The Valenti resection arthroplasty in the treatment of advanced hallux rigidus. Oper Orthop Traumatol. 2008;20(6):492–9.

Chapter 4
Hallux Rigidus: Distal First Metatarsal Osteotomy/Hohmann Procedure

Amol Saxena

4.1 Introduction

Treatment of hallux rigidus with distal first metatarsal osteotomy has been advocated for many years.[1-7] In clinical situations when there is a significantly long and elevated first metatarsal, along with dorsal hyperostosis, decreased hallux dorsiflexion, and pain, a surgical solution is to shorten and plantarflex the first metatarsal. This can be achieved by many techniques. These include distal, mid, and proximal first metatarsal osteotomies, Lapidus-type procedures and Cotton (dorsal opening-wedge) osteotomy of the first cuneiform.[1,4] The results of these types of procedures are currently evidence Level IV. Randomized study of various procedures including comparing osteotomy for hallux rigidus to other techniques, such as arthrodesis, has not been performed. The results of reasonably sized case series in the short and medium term appear promising; there is only one study with more than 10 years average postsurgery follow-up.[1,3,5]

4.2 Indications

The indications to consider a distal first metatarsal osteotomy ("modified Hohmann") for a patient with hallux rigidus is pain with daily and recreational activities despite nonsurgical therapies including shoe modification, insoles/orthoses, anti-inflammatories, and injections.[1,2,5] Clinically, the patient will have pain with hallux dorsiflexion and possibly crepitus. Dorsiflexion is often decreased to <10°. One must differentiate plantar sesamoid pain. Typical patients are classified as Grade II or III hallux rigidus (on the Grade I–IV scale).[1-5] Radiographically, the first

A. Saxena, D.P.M.
Department of Sports Medicine, PAFMG-Palo Alto Division,
Clark Bldg., 3rd Flr, 795 El Camino Real, Palo Alto, CA 94301, USA
e-mail: heysax@aol.com

A. Saxena (ed.), *Sports Medicine and Arthroscopic Surgery of the Foot and Ankle*,
DOI 10.1007/978-1-4471-4106-8_4, © Springer-Verlag London 2013

Fig. 4.1 Preoperative anteroposterior (**a**) and lateral (**b**) X-ray

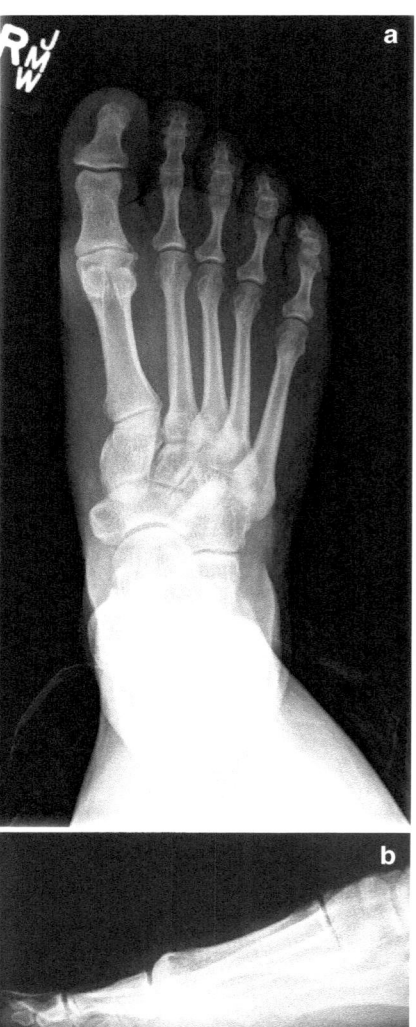

metatarsal-phalangeal (MP) joint space is narrowed, possibly have juxtapositioned loose bodies and fractured exostoses, but should not be ankylosed (Grade IV), and have minimal sesamoid hypertrophy. (A relative contraindication would be severe sesamoid disease, since plantarflexion of the distal first metatarsal would aggravate sesamoiditis.) The first metatarsal should be longer than the second metatarsal (Fig. 4.1a). Elevation of the first metatarsal on the weight-bearing lateral X-ray is noted (Fig. 4.1b). If these three radiographic criteria are noted, that is, dorsal exostoses, elongated first metatarsal, and elevated first metatarsal, the indications to perform a distal first metatarsal osteotomy are met.

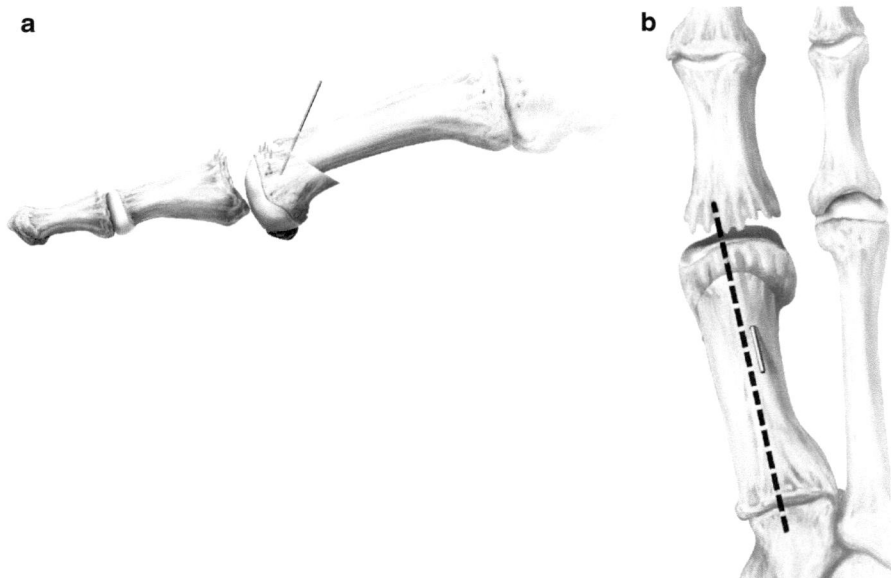

Fig. 4.2 (a, b) Intraoperative temporary fixation after realignment (plantarflexion) of the distal first metatarsal head (Courtesy Arthrex, Inc., used with permission)

4.3   Author's Preferred Technique

The modified Hohmann procedure is often performed with regional anesthesia and an ankle tourniquet. A dorsomedial incision is performed at the level of the first MP, medial to the long extensor tendon and course proximally more medial to the first metatarsal shaft-neck region. After first MP capsulotomy, dorsal exostoses from both sides of the first MP are removed along with any loose bodies, fractured exostoses, and synovitis. Chondral lesions can be drilled. A pear-shaped burr is used to remodel the first MP. Next, a power saw is used to create an osteotomy at the first metatarsal neck, biased dorsal distal, to proximal plantar, avoiding the sesamoid complex (Fig. 4.2). Often at this point, the capital fragment will "fall" into plantarflexion, reducing the elevatus and excessive length. Usually, the first metatarsal capital fragment is plantarflexed about 5 mm, and shortened to be the same length as the second metatarsal. The osteotomy is temporarily pinned from the proximal first metatarsal into the capital fragment in the desired position. There will be a "dorsal overhang" (that will be removed later).

Permanent fixation can be achieved with additional pins or a screw from the proximal first metatarsal shaft into the capital fragment. A counter-sinking pilot hole should be created on the medial surface of the first metatarsal. Often, a 3.5–4.0 mm bioresorbable or metal screw is utilized (Fig. 4.3). The temporary fixation pin can also be replaced with a bioresorbable 1.5–2.0 mm pin to counter any rotation. Any bony overhang is reduced, particularly dorsally (Fig. 4.4). Capsule and skin is

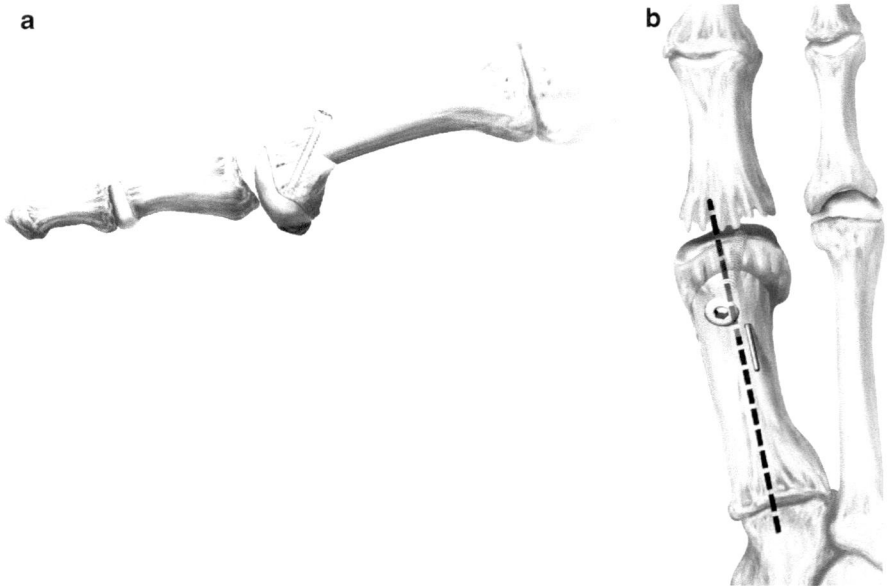

Fig. 4.3 (**a, b**) Use of bioabsorbable screw to fixate osteotomy (Courtesy Arthrex, Inc., used with permission)

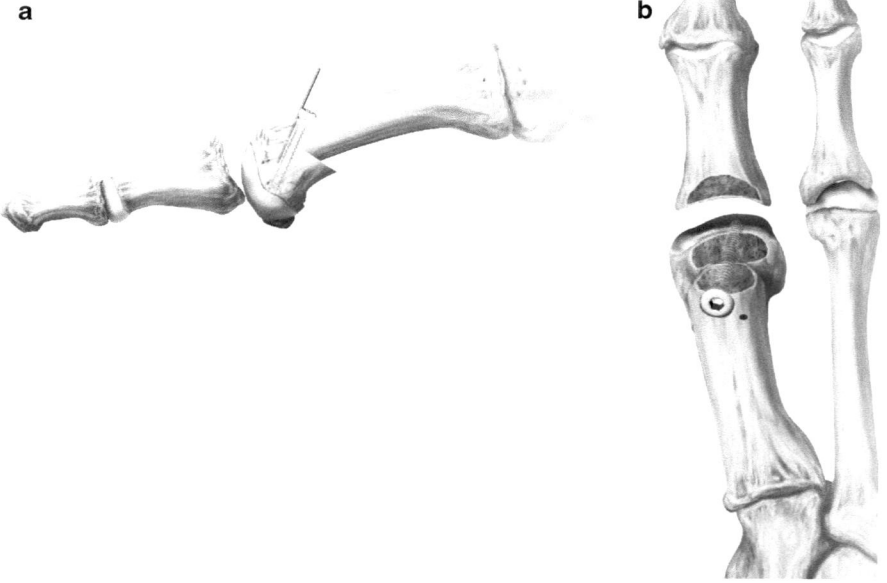

Fig. 4.4 (**a**) The temporary wire is removed and replaced with a resorbable pin. (**b**) The dorsal overhang is removed on both sides of the joint. Reduction of dorsal overhang (Courtesy Arthrex, Inc., used with permission)

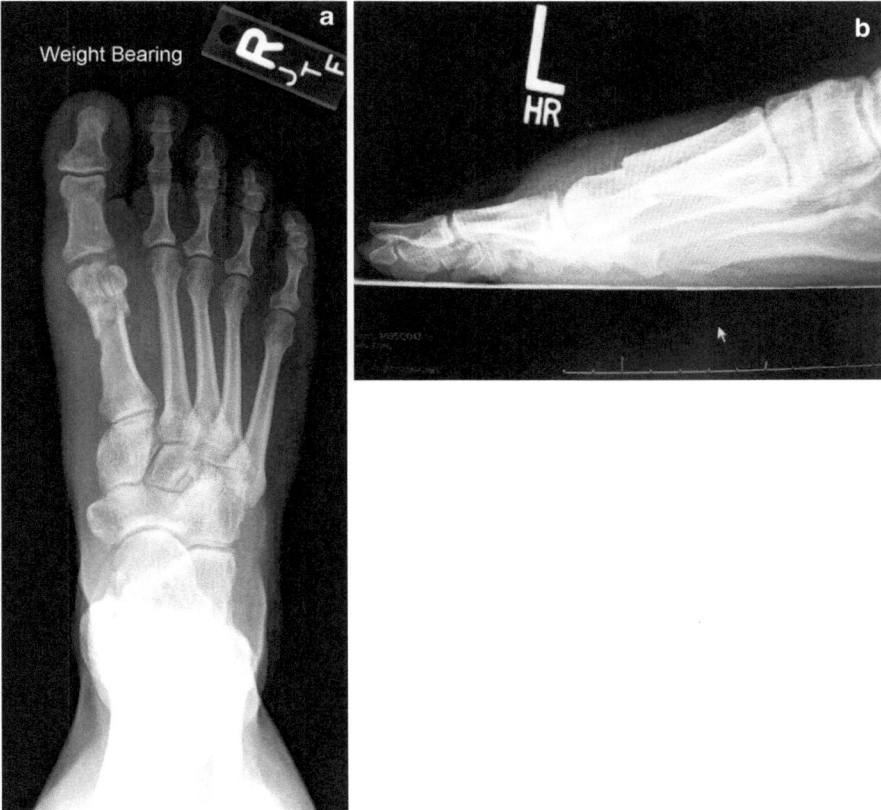

Fig. 4.5 (**a**) AP X-ray. (**b**) Lateral X-ray postoperative

closed in standard fashion. Patients are kept non-weight-bearing for 3 weeks in a below-knee cast or cast boot, and weight-bear an additional 2 weeks in the boot. Though it may lag radiographically, X-rays should confirm bony healing (Fig. 4.5). Often patients are clinically healed at 5 weeks post-op. Alternatively, K-wire fixation can be employed; wire removal is performed typically between 4 and 12 weeks when union is achieved (Fig. 4.6). Physical therapy with home exercises begins at 3 weeks. Formal therapy begins at 6 weeks. Return to impact sports is variable but can occur as soon as 8 weeks postsurgery.[1]

4.4 Discussion

Malerba et al. have the longest postoperative study on distal first metatarsal osteotomies for hallux rigidus. They retrospectively reviewed 20 patients at an average of 11 years postsurgery. One had lateral (transfer) metatarsal pain. Postoperative

Fig. 4.6 K-wire fixation used often in Europe for similar osteotomies (Courtesy of Nicola Maffulli, MD, PhD)

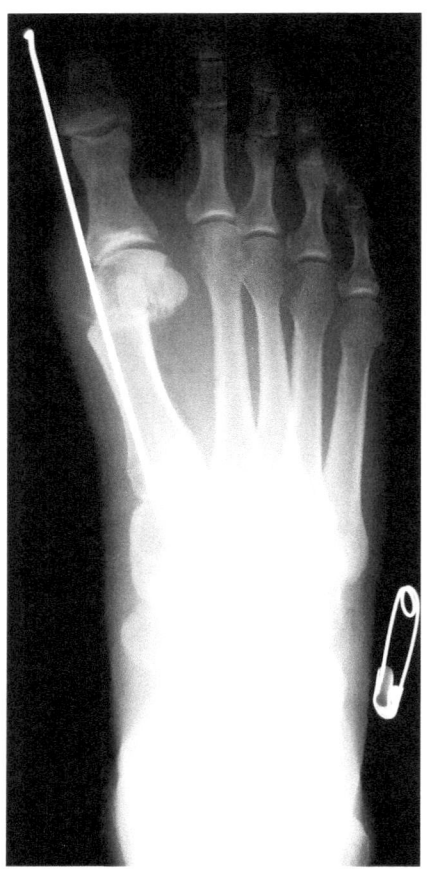

dorsiflexion improved from 8° to 44°. No patient in their series needed subsequent surgery and all were classified as Type III hallux rigidus.[4] One set of authors recommend decompression osteotomy even for more severe, Type IV (end-stage) hallux rigidus,[4] though most others do not.[1,6,7] Another slightly larger series also had patients with lateral metatarsal pain (4 out of 26), one whom necessitated a lesser metatarsal osteotomy. Patients should be cautioned on the potential of developing lateral metatarsal pain after first metatarsal osteotomy and possibly needing a second metatarsal osteotomy. In fact, lesser metatarsal osteotomy should be considered at the time of first MP surgery if the second metatarsal is also significantly longer as compared to the third metatarsal.

Improving hallux dorsiflexion is one of the goals of first metatarsal osteotomy. Gonzalez et al's study showed improved dorsiflexion from pre-op average of 18–41° postsurgery with a loss in plantarflexion of 17°, ending at 4° post-op (pre-op was 21°). Patients should be advised that improved dorsiflexion will decrease plantarflexion with this procedure.[1] Most studies show significant improvement in dorsiflexion and functional scores, though one fairly large series in the short term did not.[6] Some of the differences in results may be due to lack of standard measurement, assessment, and classification techniques. There is also variability with intra-operative fixation and postoperative care. Assessment of postoperative activity is often lacking, though one study documented light jogging was allowed by 8 weeks but did not reveal in their results how many patients actually achieved this.[1] In this study, they utilized 3.0 mm cannulated metallic screws to fixate their Hohmann osteotomies, some necessitating hardware removal.[1]

More study is needed comparing various osteotomy techniques for hallux rigidus. Kilmartin compared 49 patients who had phalangeal osteotomy to 59 who had distal first metatarsal osteotomy for hallux rigidus. Both groups had a significant number of satisfied patients and improved dorsiflexion. He noted more patients had lateral foot complaints with the first metatarsal osteotomy, 18 versus 4 with phalangeal osteotomy. He concluded neither procedure was definitive for hallux rigidus.[7]

4.5 Conclusion

Distal first metatarsal osteotomy with the modified Hohmann procedure is a viable option for hallux rigidus patients with a long and elevated first metatarsal. It is useful in situations of hallux rigidus in which arthroplasty is not sufficient in reducing structural deformity and more dorsiflexion needs to be achieved. In current studies, the short- and medium-term results show improved patient activity levels and range-of-motion. Potential complications include lateral metatarsal pain, nonunion/malunion, sesamoiditis, and decreased toe purchase. The procedure does allow for additional surgical intervention to occur, should it be needed. Long-term study is needed to see how the modified Hohmann procedure compares to arthrodesis and other techniques for hallux rigidus.

References

1. Gonzalez J, Garrett P, Jordan J, Reilly C. The modified Hohmann osteotomy: an alternative joint salvage procedure for hallux rigidus. J Foot Ankle Surg. 2004;43(6):380–8.
2. Derner R, Goss K, Postowski H, Parsley N. A plantarflexory-shortening osteotomy for hallux rigidus: a retrospective analysis. J Foot Ankle Surg. 2005;44(5):377–89.
3. Ronconi P, Monachino P, Baleanu PM, Favilli G. Distal oblique osteotomy of the first metatarsal for the correction of hallux limitus and rigidus deformity. J Foot Ankle Surg. 2000;39(3):154–60.
4. Oloff L, Jhala-Patel G. A retrospective analysis of joint salvage procedures for grades III and IV hallux rigidus. J Foot Ankle Surg. 2008;47(3):230–6.

5. Malerba F, Milani R, Sartorelli E, Haddo O. Distal oblique first metatarsal osteotomy in grade 3 hallux rigidus: a long-term follow-up. Foot Ankle Int. 2008;29(7):677–82.
6. Roukis T, Jacobs P, Dawson D, Erdmann B, Ringstrom J. A prospective comparison of clinical, radiographic, and intra-operative features of hallux rigidus: a short-term follow-up and analysis. J Foot Ankle Surg. 2002;41(3):158–65.
7. Kilmartin T. Phalangeal osteotomy versus first metatarsal decompression osteotomy for the surgical treatment of hallux rigidus: a prospective study of age-matched and condition-matched patients. J Foot Ankle Surg. 2005;44(1):2–12.

Chapter 5
Lisfranc's and Midfoot Injuries

Amol Saxena

Injuries to the Lisfranc's (tarso-metatarsal) and midfoot (Chopart's and naviculo-cuneiform) joints are being more recognized with sports injuries.[1-4] Historically, these injuries occurred with higher energy trauma such as equestrian accidents and motor vehicle accidents.[5-8] Overt traumatic loading and plantarflexion of the forefoot can cause fracture-dislocation of the midfoot, but often subtle sprains and diastasis may not be noted unless weight-bearing films and another diagnostics such as computed tomography (CT) and magnetic resonance imaging (MRI) scans are performed.[6] Soccer players and dancers are among the most vulnerable in sports (Fig. 5.1). Other sports where the forefoot is fixed such as wind surfing and when patients get the foot stepped on (i.e., football, baseball and basketball) are also commonly associated with these injuries.[1-4]

5.1 Anatomy, Biomechanics, and Evaluation

Axial loading of the metatarsals can cause fracture and diastasis/dislocation, particularly in regards to the second metatarsal base and medial cuneiform. Normally the second metatarsal base is the "keystone" to the midfoot arch in the frontal plane and should be the "high point". The relationship of each metatarsal to their respective tarsal bone they articulate with is critical as is the distance between the second metatarsal and the first (medial) cuneiform. After midfoot injury, weight-bearing and oblique radiographs should show off-set (mal-alignment) of no more than 1 mm with the metatarsals to their respective tarsals. Ideally, though the region of the main Lisfranc's ligaments (spanning between the second metatarsal and the first cuneiform) can have an acceptable difference to the asymptomatic foot of 2 mm.

A. Saxena, D.P.M
Department of Sports Medicine, PAFMG-Palo Alto Division,
Clark Bldg., 3rd Flr, 795 El Camino Real, Palo Alto, CA 94301, USA
e-mail: heysax@aol.com

A. Saxena (ed.), *Sports Medicine and Arthroscopic Surgery of the Foot and Ankle*,
DOI 10.1007/978-1-4471-4106-8_5, © Springer-Verlag London 2013

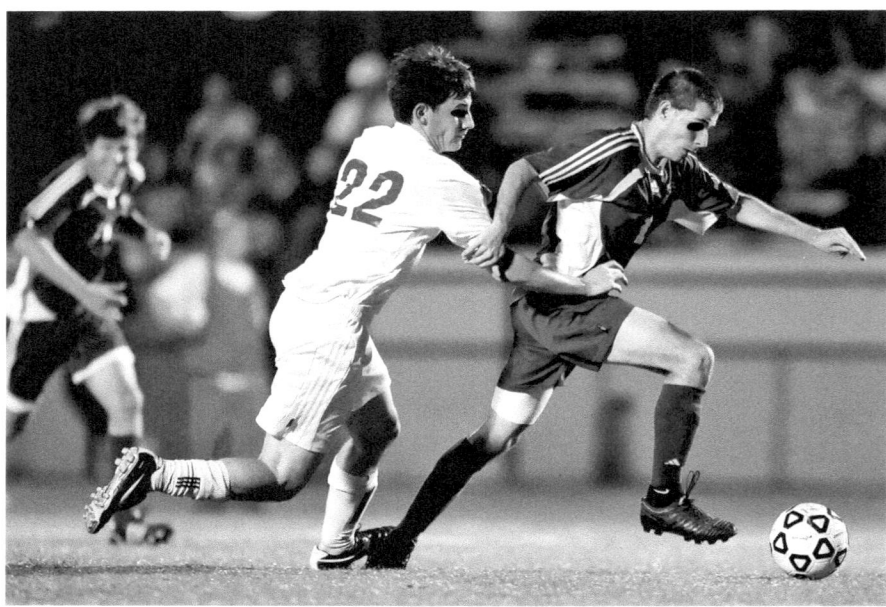

Fig. 5.1 Common mechanism of injury in sports

These dislocations are best seen with weight-bearing X-rays. A "fleck" sign is often seen with the Lisfranc's ligament avulsion (Fig. 5.2). CT/MRI may be warranted.[6] Nunley and Vertullo described a classification system where Stage I was a sprain with no diastasis and is treated nonsurgically, Stage II diastasis of 2–5 mm with no loss of arch height while Stage III exhibits loss of arch height along with abnormal diastasis, both of which are treated surgically.[3]

5.2 Clinical Presentation

The typical presentation in sports is an athlete complaining of pain on top of the foot after a forefoot twist, loading injury, or a fall. Patients may have felt or heard a "pop". Edema and ecchymosis maybe be present, especially with fracture. Compartment syndrome can occur with severe injuries and should be addressed acutely. Subtle Lisfranc's injuries such as milder sprains may have minimal edema and no ecchymosis. Provocative maneuvers include frontal plane stress of the metatarsals against the tarsals, or between the midfoot bones. A good test for Lisfranc's ligament involvement is moving the first and second metatarsals in opposite directions to provoke pain (Fig. 5.3). This is indicative of a Lisfranc's injury. Weight-bearing (unshod) examination for symmetry especially of arch height is performed

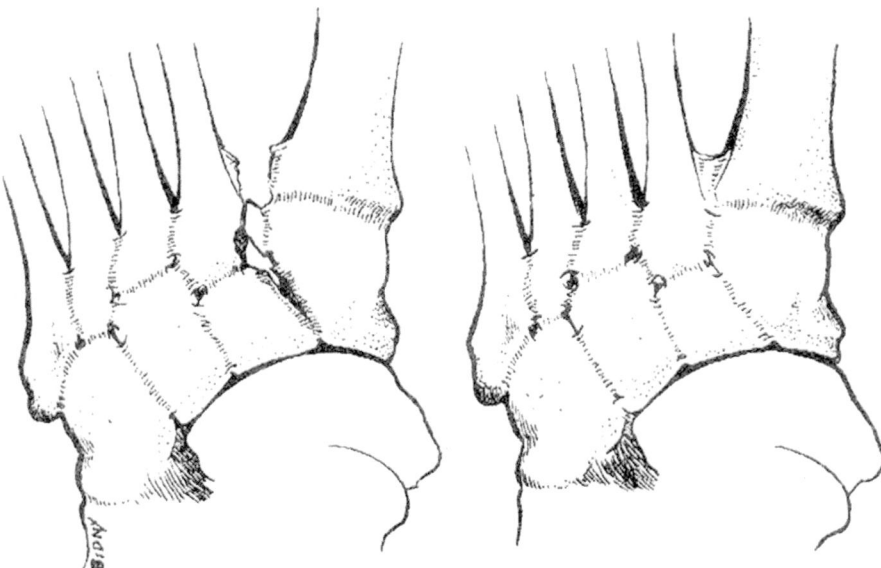

Fig. 5.2 "Fleck" sign from lateral Lisfranc's ligament attachment

Fig. 5.3 Stress maneuver of
Lisfranc's joint

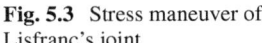

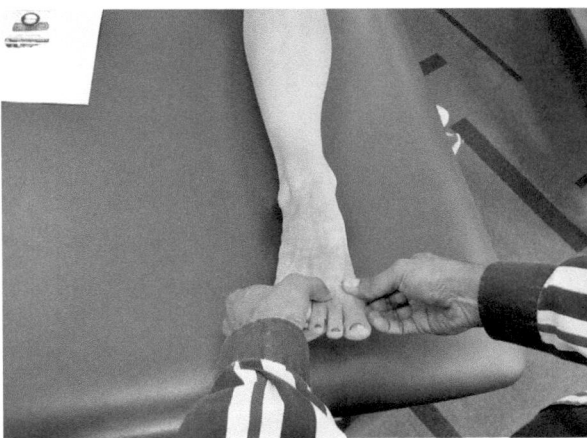

if possible. If pain and edema does not allow for comparison weightbearing examination and X-rays, patients should have careful inspection of their non-weight-bearing films; if fracture or dislocation is suspected, a CT should be performed (Figs. 5.4 and 5.5). Initial treatment consists of non-weight bearing, compression dressing, posterior splint or cast boot, and ice packs behind the knee or ice bucket submersion for 15 min four times/day.

Fig. 5.4 Preoperative
weight-bearing
anteroposterior (AP) X-ray
showing widening

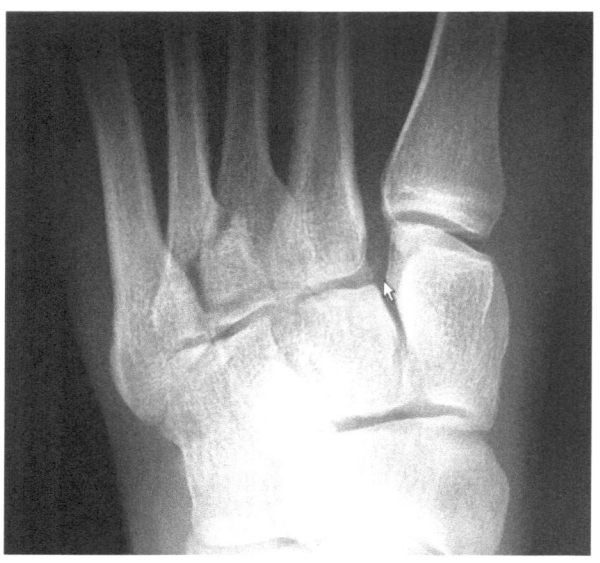

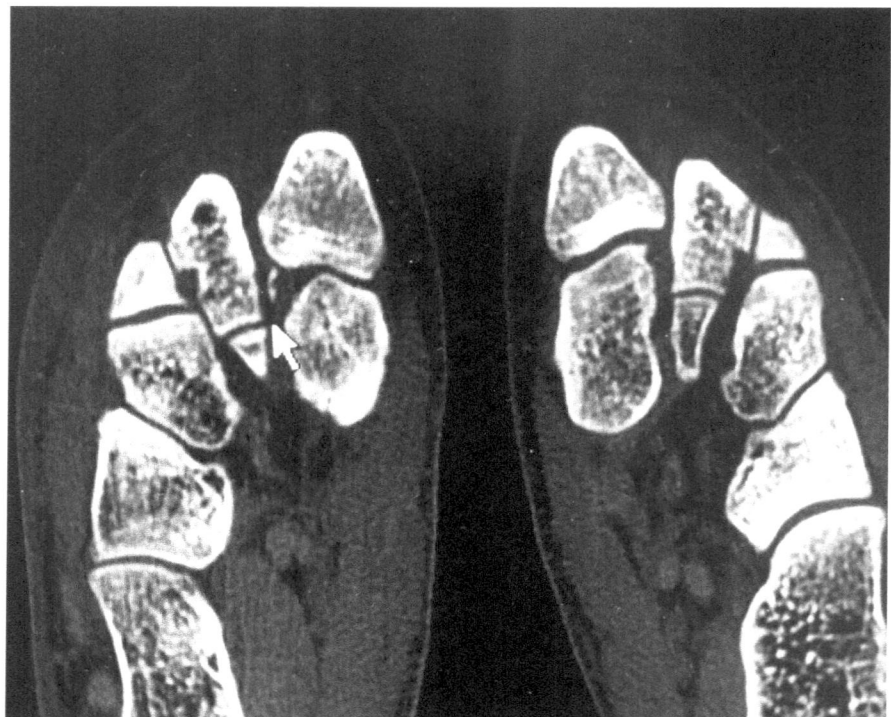

Fig. 5.5 Preoperative CT

Fig. 5.6 Postoperative
weight-bearing AP X-ray

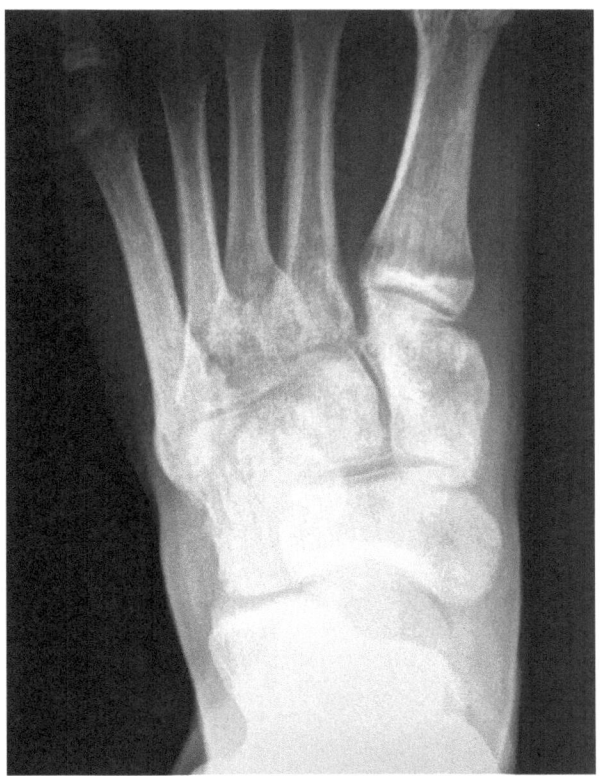

5.3 Treatment

Lisfranc's and midfoot sprains can be treated nonsurgically when the corresponding
articulations are not disrupted more than 2 mm with weight-bearing images.[1-5] If
there is widening of more than 4 mm of Lisfranc's ligament or off-set of 2 mm or
more, surgery should be considered (Fig. 5.4). Stabilization is achieved, often with
screw fixation. With severely comminuted intra-articular injuries, primary arthrodesis, particularly in the medial three Lisfranc's articulations, can be considered.
Bioabsorbable screws can be utilized for open-reduction internal fixation (ORIF) as
they may decrease the need for hardware removal at a later date.[4,5] (Fig. 5.6) In
chronic cases where arthrodesis is not preferred (such as in athletes), a "soft" fusion
with bioabsorbable or metallic screws may be needed. An incision to expose the
first and second tarso-metatarsal articulations may be needed to remove fibrotic tissue so that realignment can be achieved. As with any surgery in this region, great
care should be taken to avoid traumatizing the neurovascular structures.

Newer fixation options exist for stabilization of Lisfranc's ligament, including
suture button techniques such as a Tightrope or Tightrope FT™ (Arthrex Inc,
Naples, FL USA) (Fig. 5.7). Primary fusion can be active with screws and/or plates.

Fig. 5.7 Tightrope fixation for Lisfranc's:
(**a**) Image-guided tapping, (**b**) placement with
suture button being tied, (**c**) image confirmation
of reduction

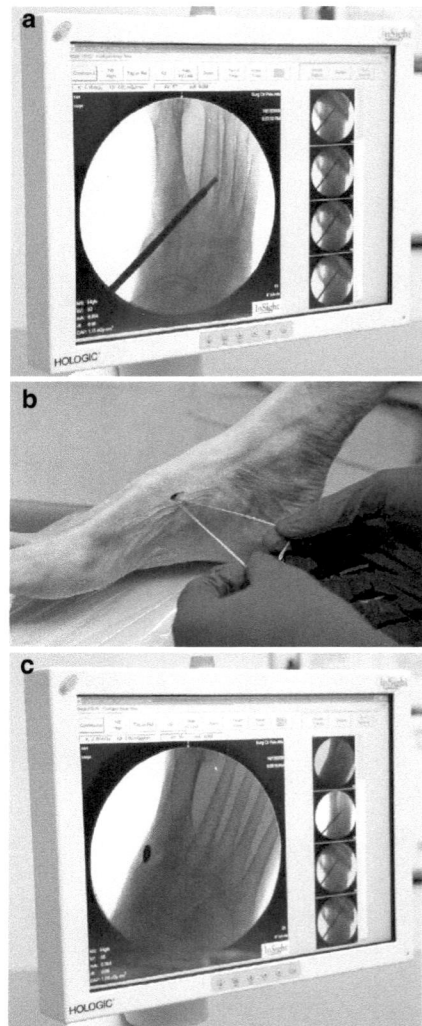

Displaced avulsion fragments of Chopart's region (such as dorsal talo-navicular and
the anterior calcaneal process) can be excised or fixated as needed.

5.4   Author's Preferred Surgical Technique

Generally ORIF is performed within the first 2 weeks after injury. Confirmation of
dislocated joints and intra-articular fractures is generally performed preoperatively,
though with patients who have suspected Lisfranc's diastasis and questionable
widening, stress view under anesthesia can be done. Patients with isolated Lisfranc's
injury can often have the procedure performed without tourniquet, percutaneously.

Fig. 5.8 Additional screw fixation for Lisfranc's

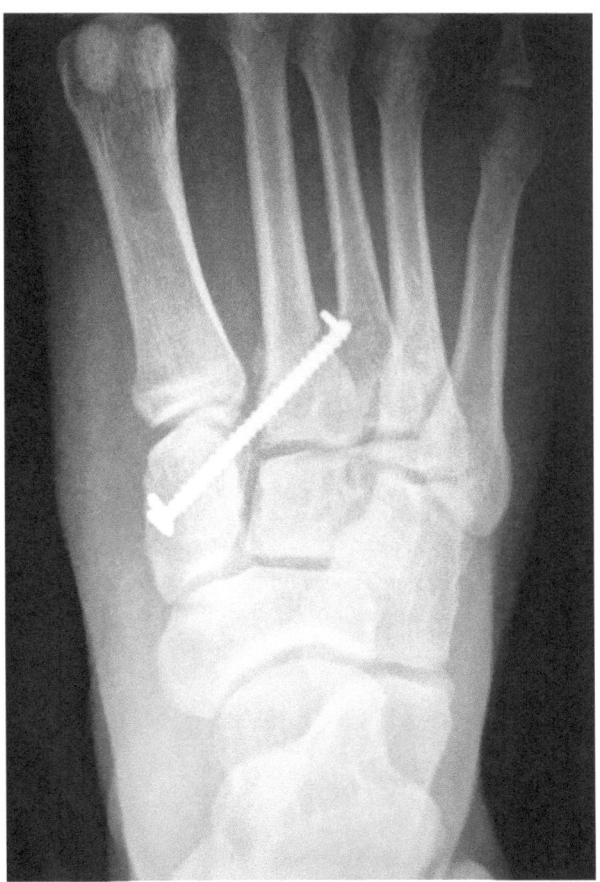

Neuro-vascular structures are indentified. A large (pelvic) reduction forceps is placed after manual reduction with the tips on the medial cuneiform and lateral second or even third metatarsal base. Imaging can be used to help guide placement of an approximately 2.6-mm drill, which will course from the medial cuneiform and exit the lateral aspect of the second metatarsal base. One should avoid drilling into the first metatarsal cuneiform joint for placement of this particular fixation. In cases with isolated Lisfranc's injury in this region, a Tight Rope FT™ can be utilized. After proper placement, the foot is stressed to see if it is stable and secure. If widening still occurs, a 3.5–4.5-mm bioresorbable or metallic screw can be placed more proximally (Fig. 5.8). It is critical to stress the patient "on the table" to ensure that fixation sufficiently stabilizes the dislocation and instability is reduced.

In cases where there is also first or second tarso-metatarsal disruption, the clamp and drill bit are maintained in place; however, stabilization screws for these joints are placed first from distal to proximal, then the final "Lisfranc's" fixation is placed. In situations where there is significant comminution of the medial aspect of the second metatarsal base, the "Lisfranc's" fixation can be placed from the second or even third metatarsal base proximally into the first cuneiform. In situations where the first tarso-metatarsal joint is disrupted, the diastasis should be reduced first. However, when using a Tight Rope FT™, the temporary drill bit can be left in place until other screw fixation is performed elsewhere so that the suture does not inadvertently get "drilled-out". If displaced as well, inter-cuneiform and naviculo-cuneiform screws should be placed as needed.[8] In patients over 50 years who have significant comminution, primary fusion with screws and plates are a serious consideration, as this may save them a second surgery.[7] Ligamentous laxity in patients may be an indication for fusion or at least longer maintenance of screw fixation. Hardware removal typically occurs after 12 weeks; generally removal of the metallic "Lisfranc's" screw is recommended. During screw removal if recurrent instability is revealed, one may require additional stabilization with a Tightrope™ which can be placed within the prior screw's drill hole.

Typical postoperative care is cast/boot immobilization for 4–6 weeks. Generally partial weight bearing is allowed after 4 weeks if weight-bearing X-rays show good alignment and reduction. The midfoot is not mobilized in physical therapy, which typically begins around 8 weeks. Patients often wear a walking boot until 8–12 weeks postoperative. Return to sports typically takes more than 4 months and athletes who sustain these injuries "in-season" will miss at least one season as full return can take 1 year.[3,4,8] Chronic cases both with and without prior surgery may still necessitate arthrodesis which has not been well-studied in the athletic population. Anecdotally the author has performed midfoot fusions both in the acute and chronic setting on patients who have been able to do some running and jumping sports.

5.5   Discussion

Lisfranc's and midfoot sprains often result in a loss of one sports session. Average return to sports for sprains is 4 or more months. One study on athletes showed that a delay in diagnosis and treatment of more than 6 weeks resulted in statistically decreased likelihood of full return to activity.[4] Arthrosis can still occur despite anatomic reduction.[8] Follow-up with arch supports or inserts is often recommended.[3] Chronic instability and pain after these injuries may require arthrodesis of the affected joints.[3,8] Patients with Lisfranc's and midfoot injuries should be counseled on the potential debilitation and rehabilitation involved with their injury.

References

1. Curtis M, Myerson M, Szura B. Tarsometatarsal joint injuries in the athlete. Am J Sports Med. 1993;21(4):497–502.
2. Harwood M, Raikin S. A Lisfranc fracture dislocation in a football player. J Am Board Fam Pract. 2003;16(1):69–72.
3. Nunley J, Vertullo C. Classification, investigation and management of midfoot sprains: Lisfranc injuries in the athlete. Am J Sports Med. 2002;30(6):871–8.

4. Saxena A. Bioabsorbable screws for reduction of Lisfranc's diastasis in athletes. J Foot Ankle Surg. 2005;44(6):445–9.
5. Thordarson DB, Hurvitz G. PLA screw fixation of Lisfranc injuries. Foot Ankle Int. 2002;23:1003–7.
6. Peicha G, Preidler KW, Lajtai G, Seibert FJ, Grechenig W. Diagnostic value of conventional roentgen image, computerized and magnetic resonance tomography in acute sprains of the foot. A prospective clinical study. Unfallchirurg. 2001;104(12):1134–9.
7. Mulier T, Reynders P, Dereymacker G, Broos P. Severe Lisfrancs injuries: primary arthrodesis or ORIF? Foot Ankle Int. 2002;23(10):902–5.
8. DeOrio M, Erickson M, Usuelli F, Easley M. Lisfranc injuries in sport. Foot Ankle Clin. 2009;14(2):169–86.

Chapter 6
Stress Fractures of the Foot and Ankle in Athletes

Amol Saxena, George Tye Liu, Brian W. Fullem, and Marque A. Allen

Stress fractures of the foot and ankle can be a source of significant disability and rapid deconditioning of the high-performance athlete, resulting in lost time in competitive play and training. Additionally, complications such as nonunions or delayed unions prolong the time for healing and can be a career-altering event. Certain anatomical regions in the foot and ankle are prone to fracture, delayed union and nonunion, along with re-fracture. Due to the high-demand of athletic and active patients, surgery is often recommended for specific injuries. The most well-known and notorious injuries involved are "Jones" fractures, proximal fifth metatarsal stress fractures, Navicular stress fractures; less common but equally debilating are medial malleolar stress fractures.

A. Saxena, D.P.M. (✉)
Department of Sports Medicine, PAFMG-Palo Alto Division,
Clark Bldg., 3rd Flr, 795 El Camino Real, Palo Alto, CA 94301, USA
e-mail: heysax@aol.com

G.T. Liu, D.P.M.
Department of Orthopaedic Surgery, University of Texas Southwestern Medical Center,
Dallas, TX, USA

B.W. Fullem, D.P.M.
Tampa, FL, USA

M.A. Allen, D.P.M.
Texas Center for Athletes,
San Antonio, TX, USA

A. Saxena (ed.), *Sports Medicine and Arthroscopic Surgery of the Foot and Ankle*,
DOI 10.1007/978-1-4471-4106-8_6, © Springer-Verlag London 2013

6.1   Proximal Fifth Metatarsal Injuries: Jones and Stress Fractures

6.1.1   Epidemiology

Metatarsal fractures are common foot injuries in the adult population with an estimated prevalence of 6.7 per 10,000. The fifth metatarsal is the most frequently fractured metatarsal of the five metatarsals with an incidence of 68.0%.[1] Stress fractures of the foot yield an incidence of 126 per 100,000 person-years. Metatarsals comprise 35.7% of all stress fractures of the foot of which 13.7% of all metatarsal stress fractures involve the fifth metatarsal.[2]

6.1.2   Anatomy

The proximal aspect of the fifth metatarsal consists of the shaft, base, and tuberosity. The posterior medial aspect of the fifth metatarsal base articulates with the cuboid posteriorly and fourth metatarsal medially. The styloid process protrudes posteriorly from the fifth metatarsal base and provides an insertion for the lateral band of the plantar aponeurosis. The peroneus brevis tendon inserts broadly over the dorsal lateral aspect of the fifth metatarsal tuberosity.[3]

Fractures of the fifth metatarsal are particularly problematic due to higher risk of delayed unions and nonunions.[4-8] This increased risk has been attributed to the anatomy of blood supply to the fifth metatarsal. Two distinct arteries supply blood flow to the fifth metatarsal. The nutrient vessel which enters at the medial fifth metatarsal diaphysis supplies the distal blood flow where a series of small perforators provide blood supply proximally to the metaphysis. The absence of central blood supply leaves a watershed zone approximately 1.5 cm from the tuberosity at the metaphyseal–diaphyseal junction.[9,10]

6.1.3   Fracture Type, Classification, and Mechanism

According to Torg, three types of fifth metatarsal base fractures are categorized by location.[11] Location of injury provides prognosis for healing based on anatomic blood supply relative to zone of dysvascularity (Fig. 6.1). The poorer the blood supply, the worse the prognosis.

Type I describes a lateral fracture of the fifth metatarsal tuberosity which extends into the metatarsocuboid joint. Fractures of this area are typically avulsion type injuries resulting from tension from the peroneus brevis tendon and lateral band of the plantar aponeurosis from inversion of the foot.

Type II injuries, known as Jones fractures, involve the metaphyseal–diaphyseal junction of the fifth metatarsal and are a result of indirect adduction mechanism.

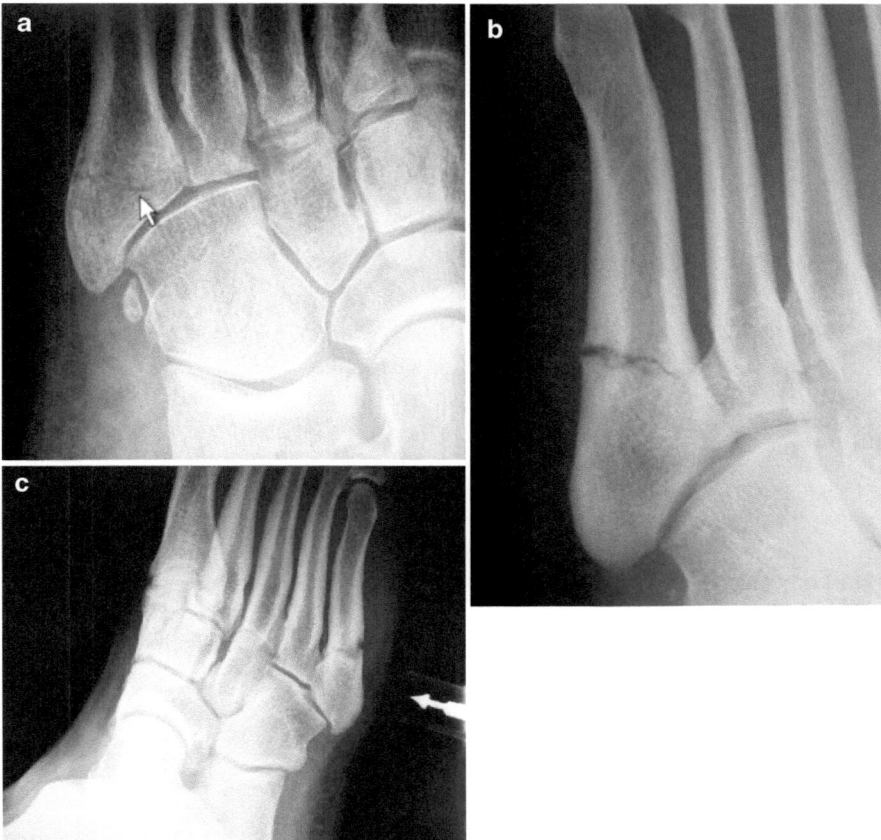

Fig. 6.1 (**a**) Type I denotes fracture of the fifth metatarsal tuberosity extending into the metatarso-cuboid joint. (**b**) Type II describes fracture at the diaphyseal–metaphyseal junction of the fifth metatarsal commonly known as the "Jones fracture." (**c**) Type III fractures, also referred to as "proximal diaphyseal stress fractures," are fifth metatarsal fractures at the diaphysis which is distal to the fourth and fifth intermetatarsal articulation

Type III injuries describe fractures of the diaphyseal section of the fifth metatarsal which are commonly referred to as proximal diaphyseal stress fractures caused by overuse and repetitive loading.

6.1.4   Distinguishing Between Metaphyseal–Diaphyseal (Jones) and Proximal Diaphyseal Fractures

Fractures of the metaphyseal–diaphyseal junction and proximal diaphysis are common in the athletic population. Because the distinction between the two fractures is not always clear, the term "Jones fracture" has been used interchangeably to describe any fractures proximal to the tuberosity. This is misleading and incorrect. Previous reported series of Jones fractures have revealed inclusion of proximal diaphyseal fractures.[6,12-14] Though the anatomic distinction between the two fractures may not always be obvious due to the close proximity of both fractures, differentiation of the two fracture types has been recommended to help guide best possible treatment.

6.1.5   Jones Fractures

In 1902, Sir Robert Jones described a small case series of patients with fifth metatarsal fractures of which the transverse fracture anterior to the metatarsal base bears his name.[15] In 1960, Stewart[13] later identified a difference in mechanism of injury and prognosis for healing for fractures at the shaft-base junction and fractures of the styloid process. He defined the Jones fracture as a transverse fracture at the diaphyseal–metaphyseal junction that may not extend distal, but through the fourth and fifth metatarsal articulation. The mechanism has been described as adduction to a plantarflexed foot with sufficient force to produce a transverse fracture at the metaphyseal–diaphyseal junction entering the lateral intermetatarsal articulation.[12,13] Patients often report pain and mild swelling to the lateral foot and difficulty bearing weight. Since Jones fractures are defined as acute injuries, no prodromal symptoms are reported.[8]

6.1.6   Proximal Diaphyseal Stress Fractures

Proximal fifth metatarsal fractures, also known as proximal diaphyseal stress fractures, are fatigue injuries primarily seen in the athletic population. The fracture occurs approximately 1.5 cm distal to the tuberosity and is commonly seen as the result of repetitive cyclic stress from high-performance athletic activities.[16] This continuous bending stress eventually exceeds the fatigue failure threshold of the metatarsal, leading to microcracks in the bone.[17] Prodromal symptoms have been reported in 41% of cases of proximal diaphyseal fifth metatarsal fractures supporting fatigue fracture etiology in these patients.[6,7] Criteria for stress fracture of the proximal fifth metatarsal diaphysis has been established by Delee et al.[7] to include prodromal symptoms to the lateral foot, radiographic signs of stress fracture, and no prior history of fracture to the fifth metatarsal.

6.1.7   Management of Metaphyseal–Diaphyseal (Jones) and Proximal Diaphyseal Fractures

Recommended treatment for a nondisplaced Jones fracture is immobilization in a non-weight-bearing short leg cast for 6–8 weeks. Surgical intervention is considered for displaced fractures, fractures that demonstrate intramedullary sclerosis or fracture that show little-to-no healing in 3 months. Torg et al.[11] reported a 93% healing rate of 15 acute Jones fractures treated in short leg cast non-weight-bearing in an average 6.5 weeks. Clapper et al.[8] evaluated 25 Jones fractures treated nonoperatively in a short leg cast non-weight-bearing. They reported 72% healing in an average of 21.2 week with this method. The remaining cohort underwent surgical treatment, 28% achieving healing 12.1 weeks after intramedullary screw placement. Chuckpaiwong et al.[18] reported 82.4% healing rate of Jones fractures with nonoperative management in short leg non-weight-bearing cast in 12 weeks and 17.6% developing delayed or nonunion requiring surgical intervention. Porter et al.[19] reported 100% clinical healing and 98.9% radiographic healing in 24 surgically treated Jones fractures with a 4.5 mm cannulated screw with return to sports in an average 7.5 weeks.

In contrast, prior reports have suggested prolonged healing periods of up to 21 months and 25% rate of nonunions with proximal diaphyseal stress fractures of the fifth metatarsal with nonoperative treatment.[6,20] Therefore, operative management is often recommended for proximal diaphyseal stress fractures. Average radiographic healing rates for operatively managed proximal diaphyseal stress fractures with intramedullary screw range from 6.5 to 9.8 weeks.[5,7,18]

Chuckpaiwong et al.[18] retrospectively compared healing rate of Jones and proximal diaphyseal stress fractures to determine whether distinguishing between the two fractures was necessary to guide treatment. They identified that the overall clinical outcomes of 32 Jones and 29 proximal diaphyseal stress fractures of the fifth metatarsal were not significantly different to warrant differentiating the two fractures. Non-operative care with a short leg cast for at least 4 weeks followed by a short leg cast boot resulted in healing by 12 weeks for up to 87.5% of fractures; however re-fracture and delayed healing was common.

6.1.8   Operative Versus Nonoperative Management of Metaphyseal–Diaphyseal (Jones) and Proximal Diaphyseal Fractures

Though few studies have compared healing rates between operatively versus nonoperatively treated Jones and proximal diaphyseal fractures, operative intervention has shown to have a predictable endpoint of healing in acute and chronic fractures.[3,5-8,11-13,16,18,21,22] While little difference is seen in radiographic union rates between operative and nonoperative managed Jones and proximal diaphyseal fractures, operative management offers quicker return to weight-bearing activities and improved patient satisfaction.[18] Therefore, operative intervention is recommended for high-performance athletes, recreational athletes, high-demand workers, and displaced fractures to decrease the time to return to sport and high-demand activities. Jones fractures averaged 14.7 weeks quicker return to sport with operative versus nonoperative care (15.3 weeks versus 30.0 weeks). This was a trend also seen in proximal diaphyseal stress fractures which averaged 11.1 weeks quicker return to sports (15.2 weeks versus 26.3 weeks).[18]

6.1.9 Surgical Technique

Intramedullary screw technique is a minimally invasive method of providing needed compression and stability to these higher risk fractures. The patient is usually positioned in the lateral recumbent position and secured with bean bag positioner (Fig. 6.2). Pillows and blankets are used to pad and position the lower extremity. Fluoroscopic C-arm can then be positioned orthogonal to the operative table

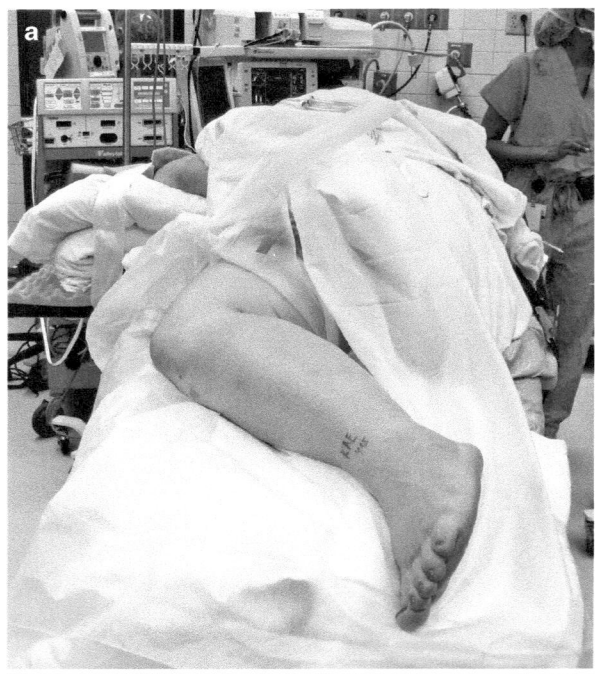

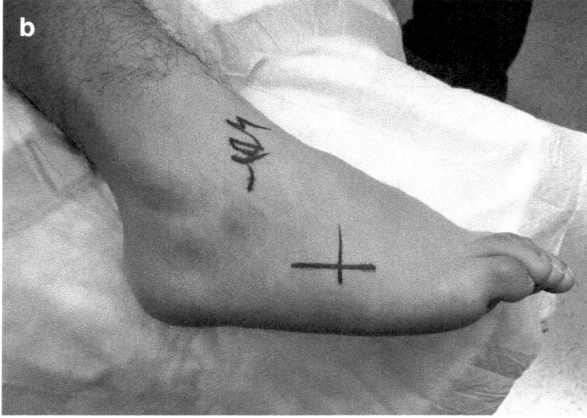

Fig. 6.2 (**a, b**) Patient is positioned in the lateral recumbent position and secured with bean bag positioner. This position facilitates both surgical access to the fifth metatarsal and ease of fluoroscopic imaging

Fig. 6.3 The medial
endosteal border of the fifth
metatarsal (denoted with a
line) may serve as a guide for
axial screw placement into
the metatarsal shaft

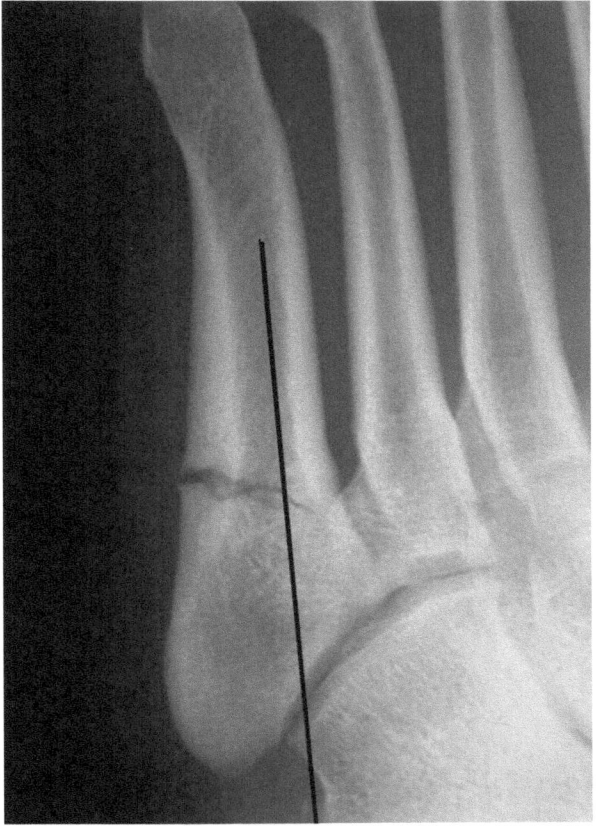

facilitating imaging without obstructing the surgical field. A Kirschner wire is
placed over the fifth metatarsal to guide axial alignment of the medullary canal and
line is drawn with marking pen. The medial border of the fifth metatarsal endosteal
cortex or lateral border of the cuboid may be used as guides for axial alignment to
the metatarsal (Fig. 6.3). A 2- to 3-cm incision is made proximal to the fifth metatarsal base in line with the skin marking. The sural nerve is often in the proximity of
this incision; therefore, due care is exercised to gently retract and avoid nerve injury.
Blunt dissection is performed to the fifth metatarsal base. Guide wire for an appropriately diameter cannulated screw (4.0, 4.5, 5.5, or 6.5 mm) and 45–55 mm in
length may be used. Alternatively, guide wires may be placed for cannulated drilling; however, often a solid screw is utilized (Fig. 6.4). Starting position of the guide
wire is "high and inside" position to ensure axial positioning of the screw[23] (Fig.
6.4). Cadaveric study describes the starting position of the guide wire as 1 cm
superior to the inferior margin of the tuberosity medial to the peroneus brevis
insertion site directed 7° plantarly.[24] A more lateral starting position on the fifth

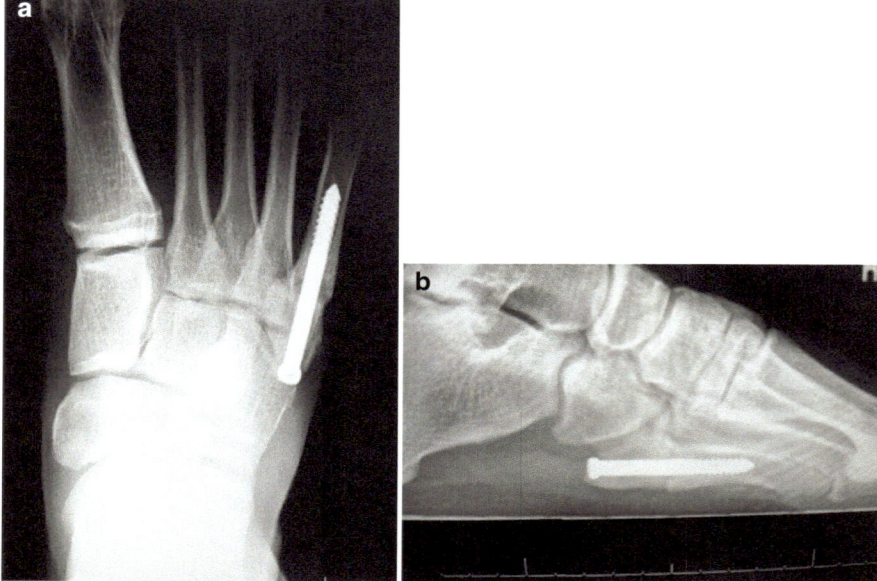

Fig. 6.4 (**a**, **b**) Solid 5.5-mm Jones fracture screw for a Jones fracture

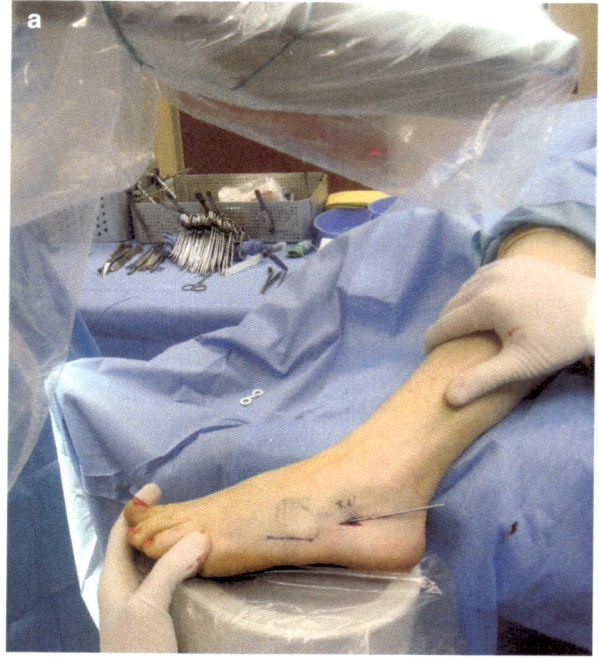

Fig. 6.5 The "high and inside" position on the styloid process of the fifth metatarsal is shown with guide pin (**a**) and subsequent screw placement (**b**)

Fig. 6.5 (continued)

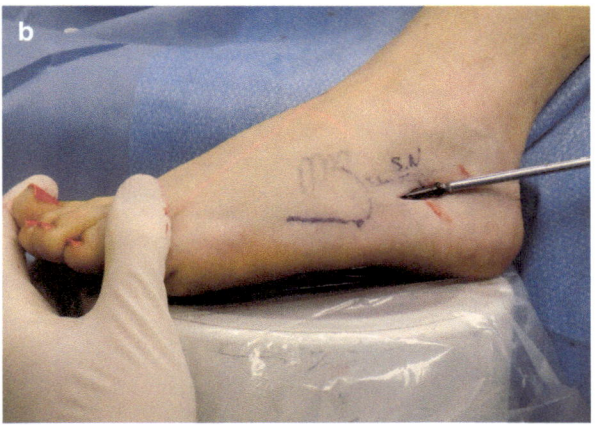

metatarsal tuberosity may engage the bow of the metatarsal shaft resulting in gapping of the fracture (Fig. 6.5). Once the guide is past the fracture, appropriately sized cannulated drill is used to drill through the medullary canal. Depth gauge is used to determine appropriate screw length with screw threads passing the fracture site to achieve compression and stability (Figs. 6.6 and 6.7).

6.1.10   Biomechanical Comparisons of Intramedullary Screws

Evaluating the strength of a solid versus cannulated screw, Pietropaoli et al.[25] performed three-point bending testing on simulated Jones fractures fixed with intramedullary 4.5 mm malleolar or 4.5 mm partially threaded, cancellous, cannulated screws. Though force at complete displacement was higher for cannulated screw (608.4 N) versus solid screw (519.3 N), there was no significant difference seen between the two screw types in forces at initial or complete displacement.

Sides et al.[26] compared bending and pull-out strengths of a 6.5-mm partially threaded lag screw to a variable pitch compression screw with a 4-mm lead thread diameter and 5-mm trailing thread diameter (Acutrak 4/5) screw in simulated Jones fractures. They reported no significant difference in bending stiffness between the two screws but a significant higher resistance to pull-out with 6.5-mm partially threaded lag screw.

Nunley et al.[27] compared fatigue resistance of a 4.5-mm thread diameter 3.2-mm core diameter Charlotte Carolina™, Acutrak 4/5, 4.5-mm malleolar, and 4.5-mm cannulated screw to cyclic three-point bending testing. The solid large core diameter Charlotte Carolina™ screw demonstrated significantly higher fatigue resistance in three-point bending compared to the contemporary screws. A limitation of this

Fig. 6.6 (**a**) Pre-op proximal fifth stress fracture. (**b**) A guide wire with a more lateral starting position on the styloid process may be acceptable granted the screw length does not exceed the curvature of the fifth metatarsal which will cause the gapping of the fracture site

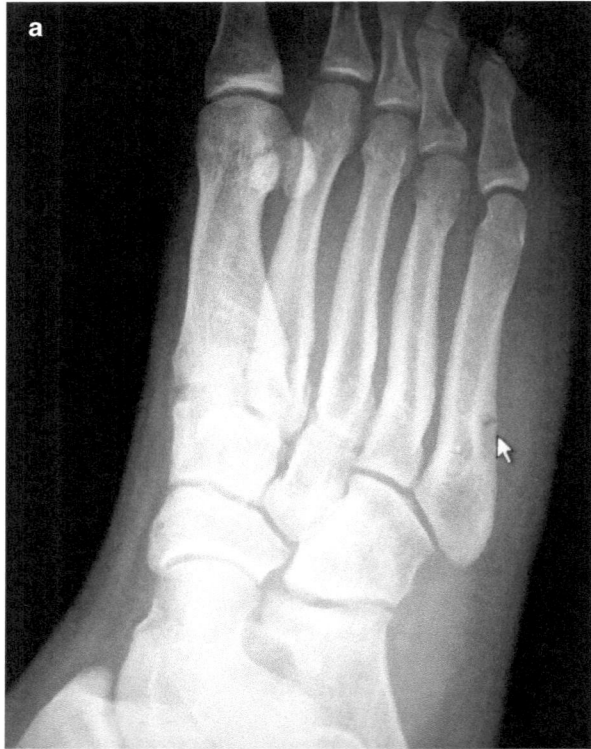

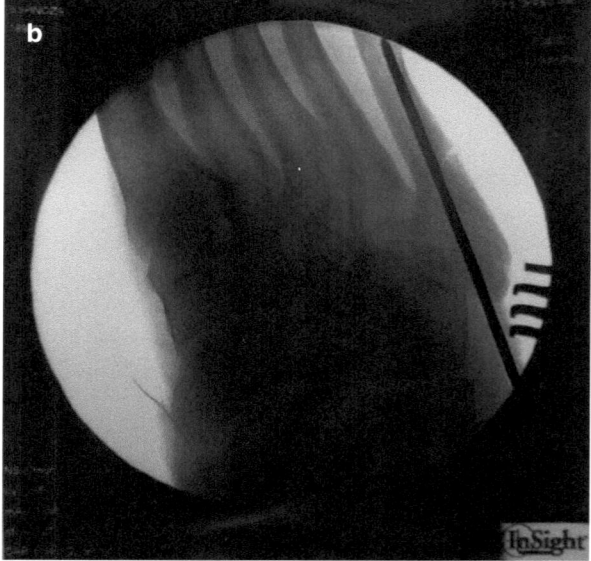

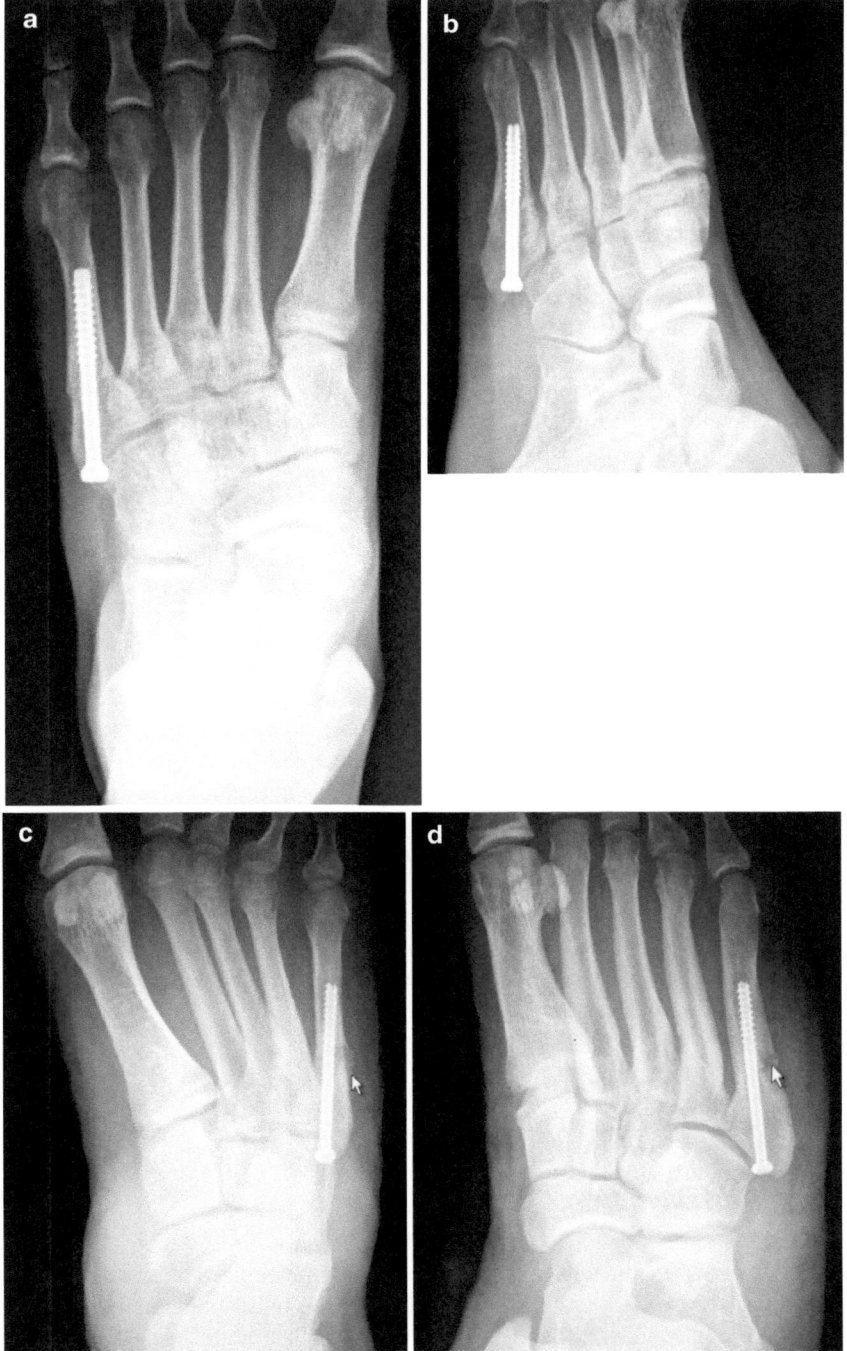

Fig. 6.7 Appropriate placement of a well-sized screw will achieve compression and stability of a Jones fracture (**a**, **b**) and proximal fifth metatarsal stress fracture (**c**, **d**)

study was that the method of testing did not replicate physiologic loads that would cause the intramedullary screws to fail.

6.1.11   Postoperative Care

There is little consensus on the postoperative weight-bearing status of surgically treated fifth metatarsal fractures. Management is often conservative non-weight-bearing in a short leg cast for 4–6 weeks. Taking into consideration, high-performance athletes need to return to activities as quickly as possible, most patients are allowed to partial weight-bear as tolerated in a short leg cast in 10–14 days after sutures are removed. Progression into sports-specific training is allowed once pain has resolved and radiographic union is seen. Most athletes return to competitive sports between 7 and 15 weeks after surgery.

6.1.12   Re-fracture

Re-fracture of Jones and proximal diaphyseal fifth metatarsals has been reported in operatively and nonoperatively managed fractures.[6,28-30] Re-fracture of proximal diaphyseal fifth metatarsals has been estimated to be less than 5% of these surgically treated fractures.[30] The primary risk factor associated with re-fracture of fifth metatarsals was premature return to activity, particularly in elite athletes, prior to radiographic union.[29,30] Because re-fracture of the fifth metatarsal is a significant though rare complication, the recommendation is to not remove hardware until the athlete's professional career is completed. Chronic nonunions (generally from failed nonsurgical treatment) with sclerosis of the fracture margins should be treated surgically.[28-30] These can be treated via a rectangular window, curettement of sclerotic bone, autogenous bone graft insertion, and intramedullary screw placement (Fig. 6.8). The bony window is replaced. Patients are kept in non-weight-bearing status for 6 weeks in a below-knee cast, and then allowed to ambulate with a cast boot for an additional 6 weeks until radiographic union.

6.2   Navicular Stress Fractures

6.2.1   Introduction

Navicular stress fractures have recently been more recognized as an athletic injury. First described in the literature in 1970 by Towne, these fractures often have an insidious onset and are difficult to diagnose without a high index of suspicion.[31] There appears to be a higher incidence in track and field athletes. Bruckner et al.

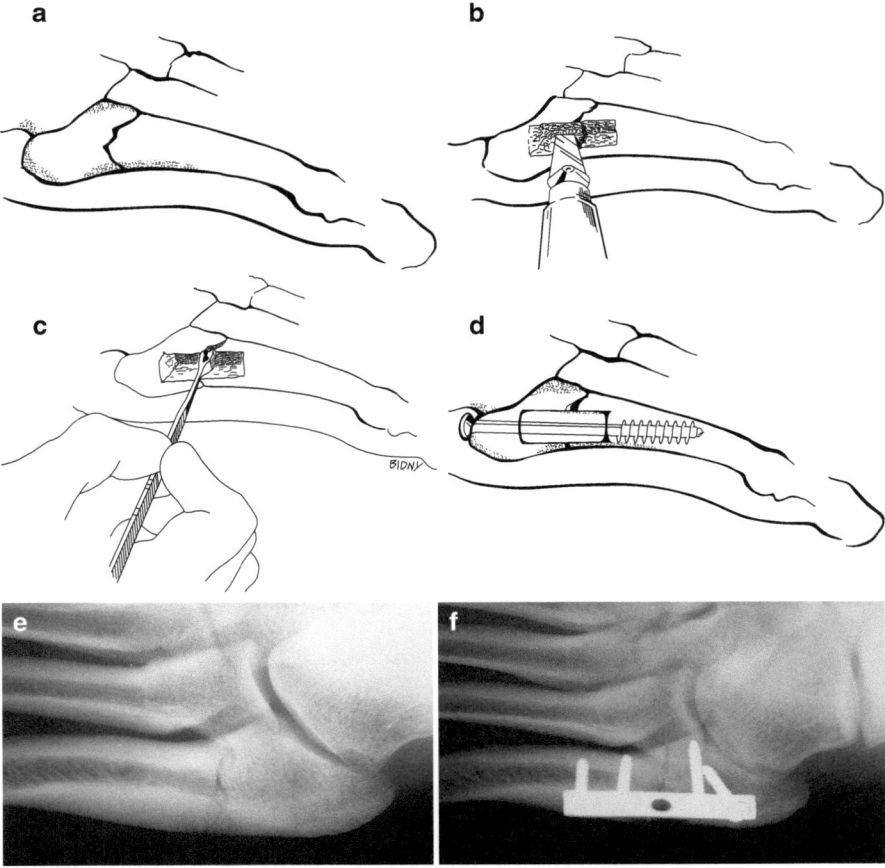

Fig. 6.8 (**a–d**) Jones fracture non-union treated by windowing technique, currettement, autograft and screw placement. (Drawings by Maria Bidny, DPM). (**e**) Pre-operative X-ray of Jones fracture non-union (Courtesy of Richard Bouche, DPM) (**f**) Post-operative treatment with dowel-trephine graft from calcaneus with plating (Courtesy of Richard Bouche, DPM)

examined 180 stress fractures in athletes and found that 26 were of the navicular, a rate of 14%.[32] The navicular is disk shaped and it is theorized by Torg that the central portion of the bone has poor vascular supply.[33] This central portion may be subject to greater stress from a "nutcracker" type effect of impingement between the talus and the medial cuneiform. Clinical suspicion should be raised when an athlete presents with vague midfoot pain and palpable pain over the dorsal aspect of the midportion of the bone, sometimes referred to as the "N" spot[31] (Fig. 6.9). Unless the fracture line is significant, it is often not visualized on radiographs. A bone scan followed by a computed tomography (CT) scan are the best diagnostic tests to properly diagnose this injury. Saxena et al. proposed a classification system to help guide treatment which ranges from non-weight-bearing immobilization to surgical intervention.[34]

Fig. 6.9 "N" spot location of
pain in a suspected navicular
stress fracture

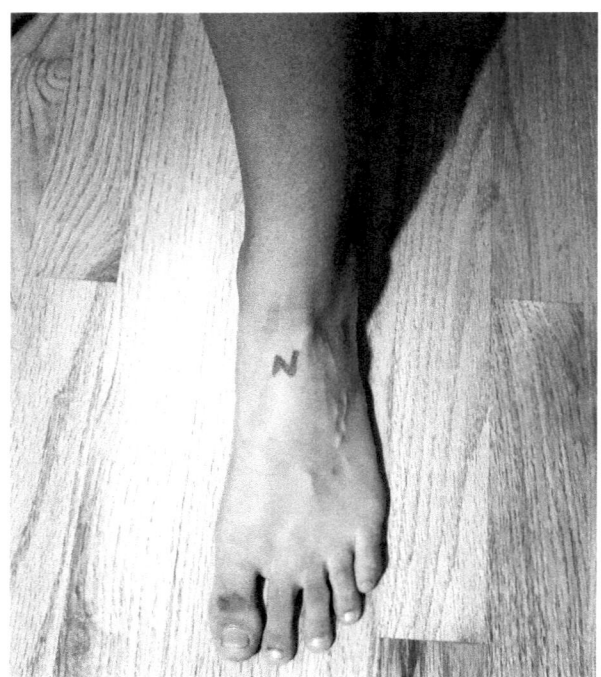

6.2.2 Navicular Anatomy

The navicular has a concave proximal portion that articulates with the head of the talus and the distal aspect articulates with the medial, middle, and lateral cuneiforms. Fitch proposed a sheer effect on the lateral portion of the navicular bone from a long second metatarsal with the resulting fracture line being midportion.[35] Torg studied the microangiography in cadavers and found arteries supplying the medial and lateral portions leaving the middle aspect lacking a direct blood supply.[33] Midfoot sprains may also lead to a fracture of the dorsal cortex due to the various ligamentous attachments to the bone.

6.2.3 Clinical Findings

Patients with navicular stress fractures often present with pain across the dorsal midfoot that is difficult to define. Pain with palpation of the "N" spot should lead the clinician to follow up the physical examination with further diagnostic testing.

Athletes will rarely recall any specific injury or event leading to this injury. Early intervention is paramount to successful conservative nonsurgical treatment. Khan et al. studied the outcome of 86 navicular stress fractures and concluded that

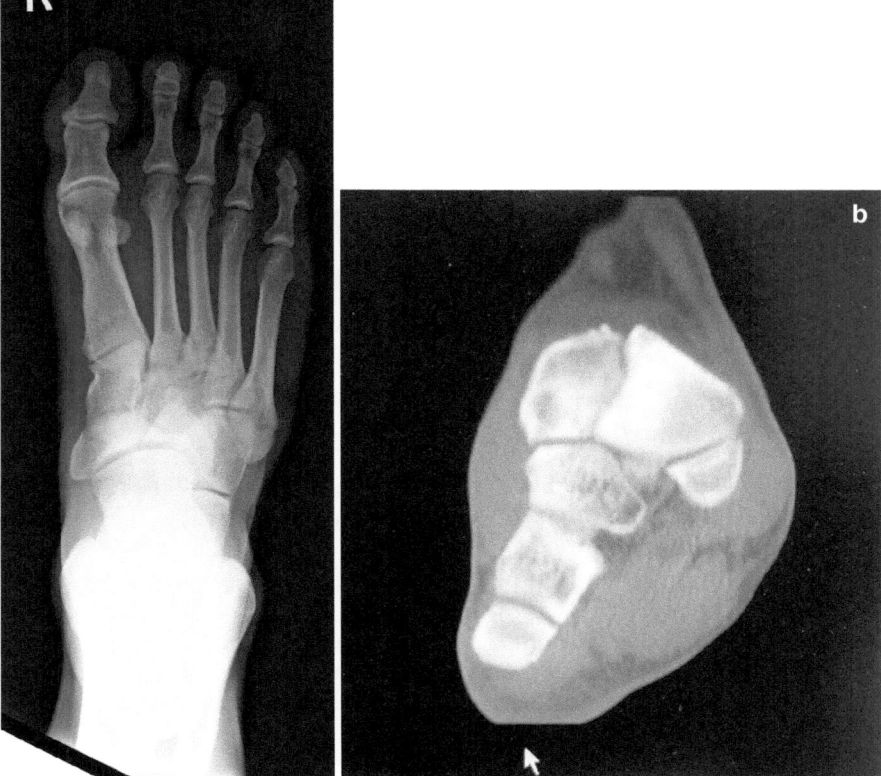

Fig. 6.10 (**a**) Plain X-ray showing a Type III (complete) navicular stress fracture. (**b**) CT of same patient

non-weight-bearing cast immobilization is the standard of care treatment.[36] Saxena et al. further classified this injury in different types with type I being a fracture only in the dorsal cortex, type II extending in the body of the bone, and type III involving more than one cortex or a complete fracture line.[34] Type III injuries can be visualized on plain X-ray, though CT is confirmatory (Fig. 6.10). In theory, the fracture line progresses the longer the injury is left untreated. The smaller the fracture line, the greater the chance that conservative treatment will be successful.[34] Other findings effecting healing were presence of cysts, sclerosis, and avascular necrosis, which often required surgery as nonsurgical treatment often failed.[34] Saxena et al. showed longer healing periods occurred with more severe fractures in their original series. In their subsequent series, because approximately half of their patients with Type II and III injuries already had nonsurgical treatment and/or a delay in diagnosis, they recommended surgical treatment (open reduction, internal fixation [ORIF]) and bone graft with fractures showing sclerosis.[37]

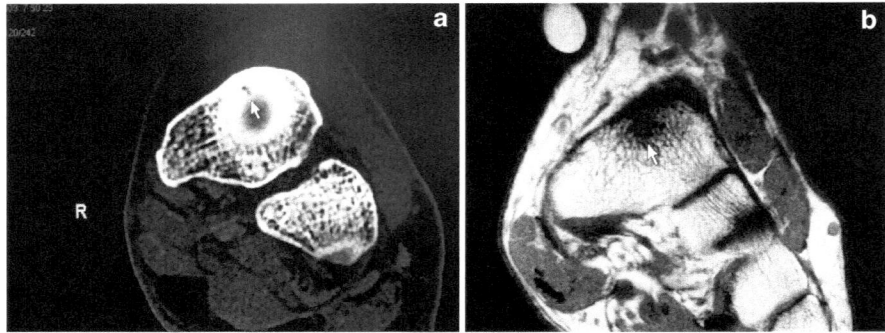

Fig. 6.11 (**a**) CT of Type II navicular stress fracture. (**b**) MRI of same patient failing to demonstrate actual fracture

Radiographs will only show signs of the fracture line in advanced cases. The best diagnostic test following an initial radiograph is a Tc99 bone scan. A positive bone scan should then be followed by a CT scan to assess the extent of the fracture line. The Saxena et al. classification system can then be used as a treatment guide as Type I fractures are often successfully treated with non-weight-bearing cast immobilization. Type III fractures are best treated with surgical management while Type II fractures may or may not be successfully treated with conservative care.

It is important to note that while magnetic resonance imaging (MRI) offers more convenient options and no radiation exposure to the patient, it may not accurately depict the actual fracture. Navicular stress fractures may therefore be undertreated based on MRI findings (Fig. 6.11).

6.2.4   Treatment of Navicular Stress Fractures

Conservative treatment consists of non-weight-bearing immobilization for a period of 6–8 weeks in a below-knee cast boot. At least three separate studies show that appropriate nonsurgical protocols are often not adhered to and this subsequently can impair healing and successful return to activity. Athletes should be encouraged to not perform any activity out of the boot that will increase stress on the navicular, including pool running as plantarflexion places dorsal tension on the fracture, and motion of the tendon insertions around the navicular may hinder healing.

Khan showed a statistically significant difference in healing when the patients are allowed to weight-bear with 19/22 (86%) patients returning to their previous sporting activities in an average of 5.6 months when treated with complete non-weight-bearing versus 9/34 (26%) who continued weight-bearing with limited activity. Saxena et al. and Fitch et al. both found that surgically treated athletes returned faster to activity than those treated conservatively.[34,35,37] Current literature supports ORIF for athletic and active patients as many otherwise fail to return to their prior sports level.[38,39]

In one study, Saxena et al. also reported a faster return to activity (RTA) in conservatively treated athletes that used bone stimulation with pulsed electromagnetic fields (PEMF). The PEMF group had a RTA of 3.85 months for the 10 patients in the study that used a bone stimulator versus 4.14 months for the 11 patients treated without PEMF. Those treated surgically with ORIF had a much faster RTA: Khan had 6/7 RTA at an average time of 3.8 months, Fitch et al. had 12/15 RTA between 5 and 12 months (no average was noted), and Saxena et al. had all 9 ORIF's return to prior sports with average RTA of 2.67 months.

6.2.5   Surgical Technique of Navicular Stress Fractures

Surgical technique involves a dorsal incision generally lateral to the neurovascular bundle starting dorsally over the talonavicular joint and extending to the navicular-medial cuneiform articulation. (The initial dissection can be performed without a tourniquet in order to ascertain hemostasis.) The fracture line is identified with guidance from the CT scan and disarticulation of the talonavicular joint. Any sclerotic margins should be resected and the margins should be carefully burred or drilled. Autogenous grafting can be implanted from the ipsilateral calcaneus. A 3.5-mm bi-cortical or 4.0-mm cancellous screw should be placed across the fracture. The wound is closed in layers (Fig. 6.12). In larger athletes, two 3.5-mm screws may be needed (Fig. 6.13).

Healing should be assessed clinically as diagnostic studies often lag behind actual healing time. CT can be helpful in persistently painful patients, though asymptomatic individuals may have false-positives.[38] Healing in general should be expected to take at least 3 months with Type I navicular stress fractures. Type II and III injuries take 4 or more months. This generally means that one sports season will be lost. We typically allow cross-training on a stationary bike with the heel on the pedal, even when the patient is in a cast or boot during the first 6 weeks post-surgery or injury. Patients involved in jumping and kicking sports should be carefully monitored for aggravation of symptoms. Foot support with a custom insert may be needed but is individualized, as limiting motion in a cavus foot or even a very flexible flatfoot using a rigid device could be detrimental. Furthermore Saxena et al. showed no difference as to prevalence of navicular stress fractures in cavus versus planus foot types.[37]

Navicular stress fractures are significant injuries that often are categorized synonymously and therefore may be treated similarly. Based on the significant findings of more severe fractures taking longer to heal and fail with nonsurgical treatment, this is not appropriate. As other authors have noted, these injuries are susceptible to misdiagnosis, undertreatment, and re-fracture.[38,40,41] We feel it is important to differentiate fracture type and base treatment accordingly.

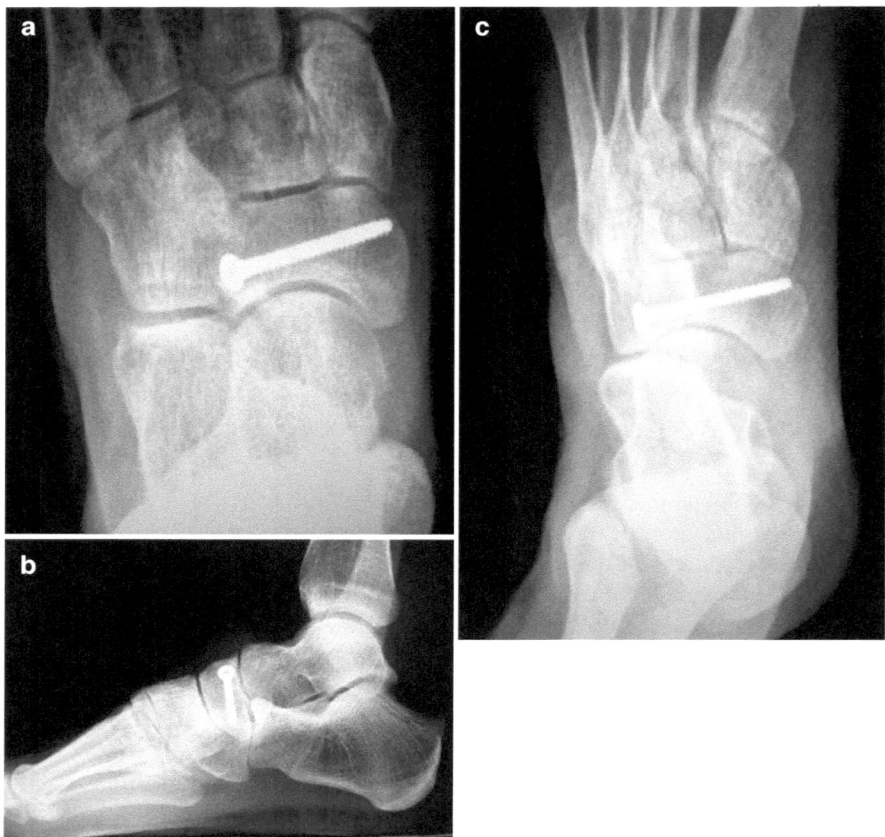

Fig. 6.12 (**a–c**) Post-op ORIF of a Type III navicular stress fracture. Note on oblique view screw avoid the joint and tendon insertion

6.3   Medial Malleolar Stress Fractures

Medial malleolar stress fractures are considered extremely rare.[41-43] The etiology is considered to be a supination-adduction injury resulting in an incomplete fracture often propagating from the notch of Hardy (Fig. 6.14). Similar to navicular stress fractures, minimal edema and ecchymosis maybe present though patients are point tender on the medial malleolus and have a positive "hop" test (i.e., pain with hopping on one limb is the region of symptoms). X-rays are often negative particularly in early cases. Patients often have an insidious onset. MRI and CT exams are often definitive.[42,43]

Treatment of medial malleolar stress fractures is somewhat controversial; though similar to Jones fractures, surgical treatment is recommended for athletes.[42,43] Nonsurgical treatment is similar to navicular stress fractures, i.e., 6 weeks non-weight-bearing in a below-knee cast/boot, followed by additional weight-bearing until pain-free.

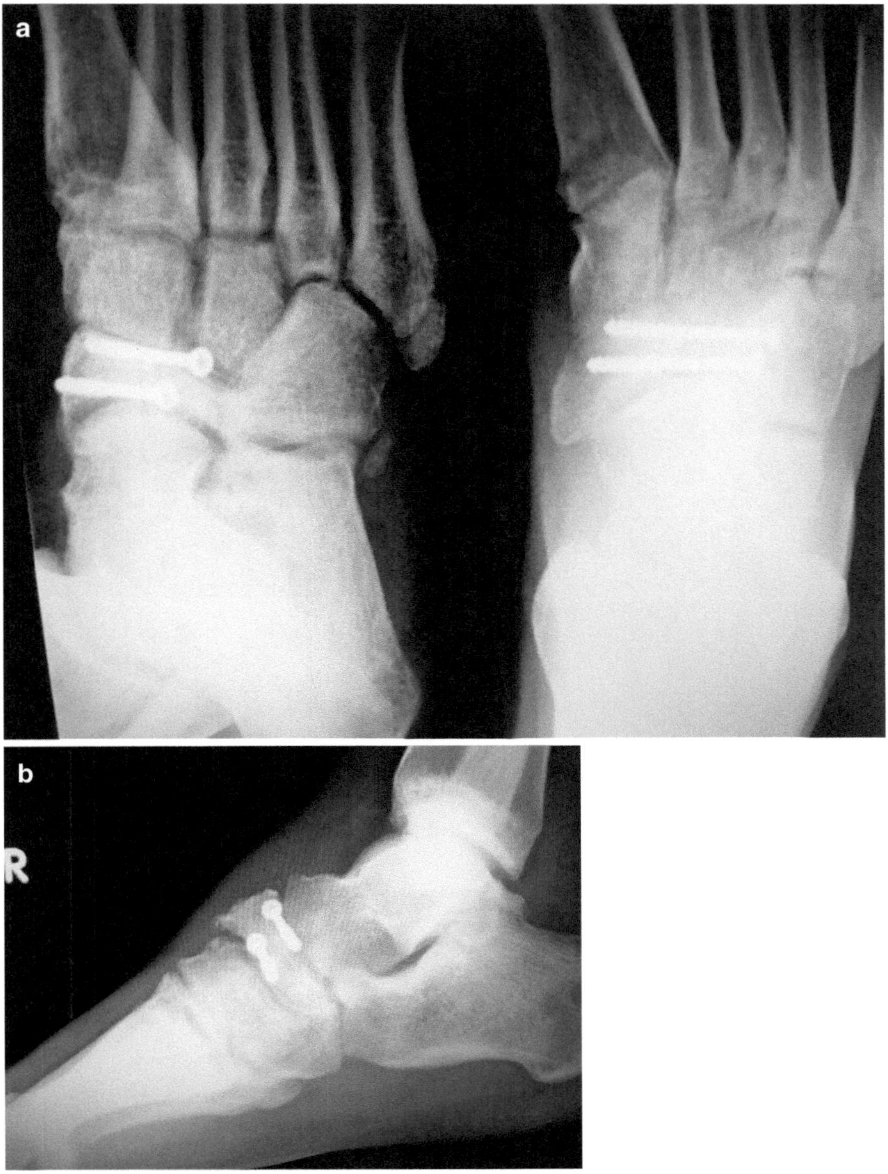

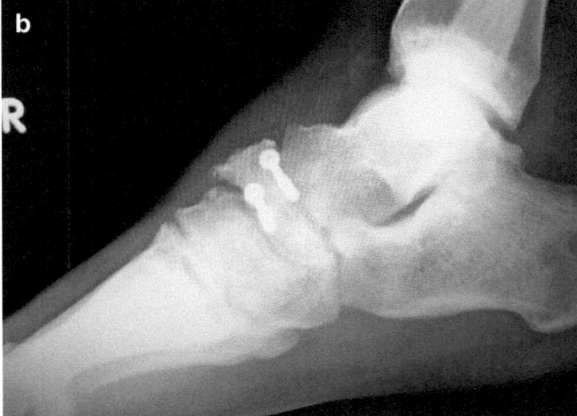

Fig. 6.13 (**a–c**) Post-op ORIF of a severe Type III navicular stress fracture that showed AVN and had already been treated with two rounds of 8 weeks non-weight-bearing. A mini-external fixator was used intraoperatively to help realign the fragments and verify screw placement was extra-articular

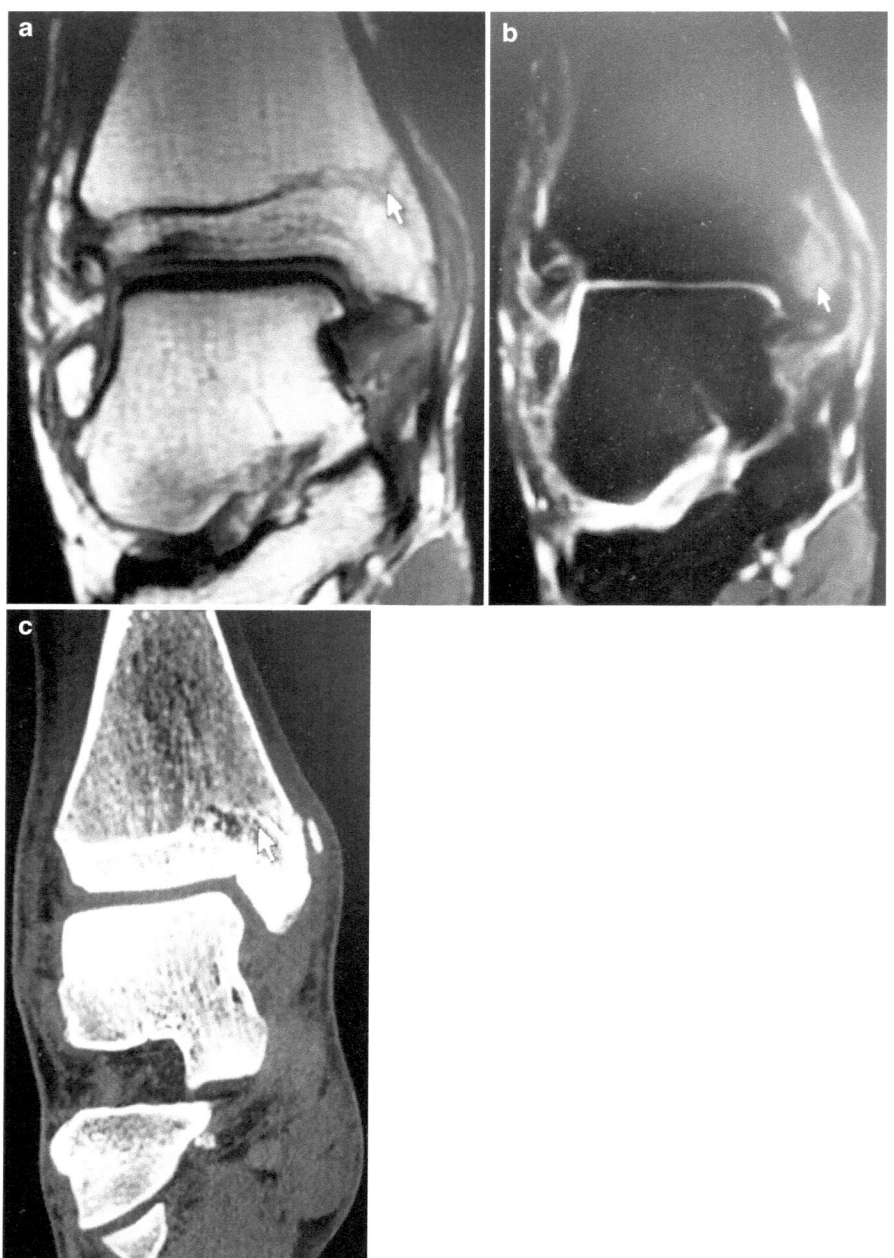

Fig. 6.14 MRI T1 (**a**) and T2 (**b**) and (**c**) CT showing a medial malleolar stress fracture

6.3.1   Surgical Treatment of Medial Malleolar Stress Fractures

Surgical treatment is definitely indicated for complete fractures, displaced fractures, and nonunited fractures with sclerosis. Typically ORIF with either a 4.0-, 4.5- or 5.0-mm screw is placed obliquely and perpendicular across the fracture to stabilize and compress it (Fig. 6.15). A 6.5-mm screw may be needed in larger athletes. Care should be taken when using a percutaneous approach to avoid impinging the posterior tibial tendon and other neurovascular structures. Generally, the safe zone at the anterior colliculus is used to place the screw and sufficient counter-sinking should be performed. Autogenous bone graft is used for nonunions after curettage of the sclerotic bone.

Postoperative treatment after ORIF of medial malleolar stress fractures consists of 3 weeks non-weight-bearing in a below-knee cast/boot and an additional 3 weeks in a cast boot, though one group of authors was able to return an athlete to basketball in less than 4 weeks. Generally running and jumping sports are resumed after 6–8 weeks unless bone graft supplementation is used for nonunions. In those cases, impact sports are delayed for at least 12 weeks post-surgery.

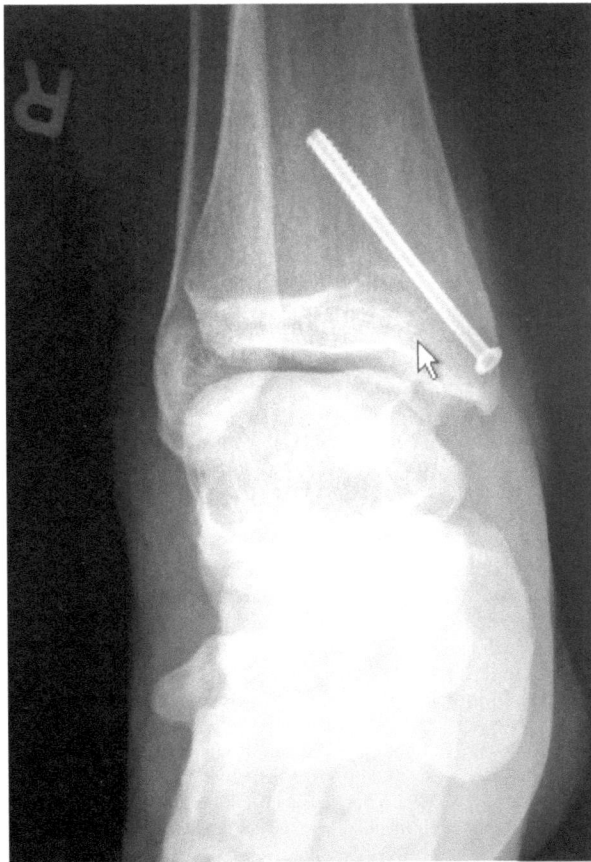

Fig. 6.15 Post-op ORIF of medial malleolar stress fracture

References

1. Petrisor BA, Ekrol I, Court-Brown C. The epidemiology of metatarsal fractures. Foot Ankle Int. 2006;27(3):172–4.
2. Niva MH, Sormaala MJ, Kiuru MJ, et al. Bone stress injuries of the ankle and foot: an 86-month magnetic resonance imaging-based study of physically active young adults. Am J Sports Med. 2007;35(4):643–9.
3. Sarrafian S. Anatomy of the foot and ankle. Philadelphia: Lippincott; 1993.
4. Carp L. Fracture of the fifth metatarsal bone: with special reference to delayed union. Ann Surg. 1927;86(2):308–20.
5. Quill GE Jr. Fractures of the proximal fifth metatarsal. Orthop Clin North Am. 1995;26(2):353–61.
6. Kavanaugh JH, Brower TD, Mann RV. The Jones fracture revisited. J Bone Joint Surg Am. 1978;60(6):776–82.
7. DeLee JC, Evans JP, Julian J. Stress fracture of the fifth metatarsal. Am J Sports Med. 1983;11(5):349–53.
8. Clapper MF, O'Brien TJ, Lyons PM. Fractures of the fifth metatarsal. Analysis of a fracture registry. Clin Orthop Relat Res. 1995;315:238–41.
9. Smith JW, Arnoczky SP, Hersh A. The intraosseous blood supply of the fifth metatarsal: implications for proximal fracture healing. Foot Ankle. 1992;13(3):143–52.
10. Shereff MJ, Yang QM, Kummer FJ, et al. Vascular anatomy of the fifth metatarsal. Foot Ankle. 1991;11(6):350–3.
11. Torg JS, Balduini FC, Zelko RR, et al. Fractures of the base of the fifth metatarsal distal to the tuberosity. Classification and guidelines for non-surgical and surgical management. J Bone Joint Surg Am. 1984;66(2):209–14.
12. Dameron TB Jr. Fractures and anatomical variations of the proximal portion of the fifth metatarsal. J Bone Joint Surg Am. 1975;57(6):788–92.
13. Stewart IM. Jones's fracture: fracture of base of fifth metatarsal. Clin Orthop. 1960;16:190–8.
14. Rosenberg GA, Sferra JJ. Treatment strategies for acute fractures and nonunions of the proximal fifth metatarsal. J Am Acad Orthop Surg. 2000;8(5):332–8.
15. Jones R. Fractures of the base of the 5th metatarsal bone. Ann Surg. 1902;35:697–702.
16. Zelko RR, Torg JS, Rachun A. Proximal diaphyseal fractures of the fifth metatarsal—treatment of the fractures and their complications in athletes. Am J Sports Med. 1979;7(2):95–101.
17. Donahue SW, Sharkey NA, Modanlou KA, et al. Bone strain and microcracks at stress fracture sites in human metatarsals. Bone. 2000;27(6):827–33.
18. Chuckpaiwong B, Queen RM, Easley ME, et al. Distinguishing Jones and proximal diaphyseal fractures of the fifth metatarsal. Clin Orthop Relat Res. 2008;466(8):1966–70.
19. Porter DA, Duncan M, Meyer SJ. Fifth metatarsal Jones fracture fixation with a 4.5-mm cannulated stainless steel screw in the competitive and recreational athlete: a clinical and radiographic evaluation. Am J Sports Med. 2005;33(5):726–33.
20. Dameron TB Jr. Fractures of the proximal fifth metatarsal: selecting the best treatment option. J Am Acad Orthop Surg. 1995;3(2):110–4.
21. Landorf KB. Clarifying proximal diaphyseal fifth metatarsal fractures. The acute fracture versus the stress fracture. J Am Podiatr Med Assoc. 1999;89(8):398–404.
22. Roca J, Roure F, Fernandez Fairen M, et al. Stress fractures of the fifth metatarsal. Acta Orthop Belg. 1980;46(5):630–6.
23. Den Hartog BD. Fracture of the proximal fifth metatarsal. J Am Acad Orthop Surg. 2009;17(7):458–64.
24. Johnson JT, Labib SA, Fowler R. Intramedullary screw fixation of the fifth metatarsal: an anatomic study and improved technique. Foot Ankle Int. 2004;25(4):274–7.
25. Pietropaoli MP, Wnorowski DC, Werner FW, et al. Intramedullary screw fixation of Jones fractures: a biomechanical study. Foot Ankle Int. 1999;20(9):560–3.

26. Sides SD, Fetter NL, Glisson R, et al. Bending stiffness and pull-out strength of tapered, variable pitch screws, and 6.5-mm cancellous screws in acute Jones fractures. Foot Ankle Int. 2006;27(10):821–5.
27. Nunley JA, Glisson RR. A new option for intramedullary fixation of Jones fractures: the Charlotte Carolina Jones fracture system. Foot Ankle Int. 2008;29(12):1216–21.
28. Glasgow MT, Naranja RJ Jr, Glasgow SG, et al. Analysis of failed surgical management of fractures of the base of the fifth metatarsal distal to the tuberosity: the Jones fracture. Foot Ankle Int. 1996;17(8):449–57.
29. Larson CM, Almekinders LC, Taft TN, et al. Intramedullary screw fixation of Jones fractures. Analysis of failure. Am J Sports Med. 2002;30(1):55–60.
30. Wright RW, Fischer DA, Shively RA, et al. Refracture of proximal fifth metatarsal (Jones) fracture after intramedullary screw fixation in athletes. Am J Sports Med. 2000;28(5):732–6.
31. Towne LC, Blazina ME, Cozen LN. Fatigue fracture of the tarsal navicular. J Bone Joint Surg Am. 1970;52:376–8.
32. Brukner P, Bradshaw C, Khan KM, White S, Crossley K. Stress fractures: a review of 180 cases. Clin J Sport Med. 1996;6(2):85–9.
33. Torg JS, Pavlov H, Cooley LH, et al. Stress fractures of the tarsal navicular. A retrospective review of twenty-one cases. J Bone Joint Surg Am. 1982;64:700–12.
34. Saxena A, Fullem B, Hannaford D. Results of treatment of 22 navicular stress fractures and a new proposed radiographic classification system. J Foot Ankle Surg. 2000;39:96–103.
35. Fitch KD, Blackwell JB, Gilmour WN. Operation for non-union of stress fracture of the tarsal navicular. J Bone Joint Surg Br. 1989;71:105–10.
36. Khan KM, Brukner PD, Kearney C, Fuller PJ, Bradshaw CJ, Kiss ZS. Tarsal navicular stress fracture in athletes. Sports Med. 1994;17:65–76.
37. Saxena A, Fullem B. Navicular stress fractures: a prospective study on athletes. Foot Ankle Int. 2006;27(11):917–21.
38. Mann J, Pedowitz D. Evaluation and treatment of navicular stress fractures, including non-unions, revision surgery and persistent pain after treatment. Foot Ankle Clin. 2009;14:187–204.
39. Potter NJ, Brukner PD, Makdissi M, Crossley K, Kiss ZS, Bradshaw C. Navicular stress fractures: outcomes of surgical and conservative management. Br J Sports Med. 2006;40(8):692–5.
40. Burne SG, Mahoney CM, Forster BB, Koehle MS, Taunton JE, Khan KM. Tarsal navicular stress injury: long-term outcome and clinicoradiological correlation using both computed tomography and magnetic resonance imaging. Am J Sports Med. 2005;33(12):1875–81.
41. Kaeding CC, Yu JR, Wright R, Amendola A, Spindler KP. Management and return to play of stress fractures. Clin J Sport Med. 2005;15(6):442–7.
42. Sherbondy PS, Sebastianelli WJ. Stress fractures of the medial malleolus and distal fibula. Clin Sports Med. 2006;25(1):129–37.
43. Kor A, Saltzman AT, Wempe PD. Medial malleolar stress fractures. Literature review, diagnosis, and treatment. J Am Podiatr Med Assoc. 2003;93(4):292–7.

Chapter 7
Plantar Fasciitis

Brian W. Fullem and Amol Saxena

7.1 Introduction

Plantar fasciitis is one of the more common injuries in the general population and can be debilitating for an athlete. In a retrospective study of 2002 running injuries, it was a found that 157 of the injuries were plantar fasciitis (7.8%) and another study found that there are more than one million patient visits per year to medical professionals.[1,2] The plantar fascia is the main supporting structure of the foot and arch; it is vulnerable to injury.

Plantar fascia injuries typically occur from overuse with an insidious onset, though they can happen acutely without prodromal symptoms. Patients may not seek treatment until the injury becomes more chronic in nature. It is commonly cited that the majority of the time fasciitis resolves with conservative treatment with studies showing relief of symptoms between 46% and almost 100%.[3-6]

Clinical examination is of utmost importance in the diagnosis and treatment of plantar fasciitis. Diagnostic testing may include plain radiographs, ultrasound and magnetic resonance imaging (MRI). Differential diagnoses may include stress fracture of the calcaneus; nerve-related injuries including tarsal tunnel syndrome, neuroma, and neuritis of the first branch of lateral calcaneal nerve; soft tissue mass; bursitis; fat pad atrophy; systemic arthritidies; tumors; and ruptures of the fascia.

B.W. Fullem, D.P.M. (✉)
508 S. Habana Ave., Ste. 230,
Tampa, FL 33609, USA
e-mail: bfullem1@aol.com

A. Saxena, D.P.M.
Department of Sports Medicine,
PAFMG-Palo Alto Division,
Palo Alto, CA, USA

A. Saxena (ed.), *Sports Medicine and Arthroscopic Surgery of the Foot and Ankle*,   83
DOI 10.1007/978-1-4471-4106-8_7, © Springer-Verlag London 2013

7.2   Anatomy

The plantar fascia attaches distally at the sulcus of the foot and runs along the plantar surface of the foot with three insertions in the plantar calcaneus: medially, centrally, and laterally. Bøjsen-Möller and Flagstad described the structure as being triangular with the base proximal.[7] Pontious et al. described the fascia as a dense band of fibers with the lateral and medial bands simply being coverings of the abductor hallucis and abductor digiti minimi muscles while the central portion is the most prominent and considered to be the true plantar aponeurosis.[8] The attachments of the medial and central portions are the most common locations of plantar fasciitis symptoms near the medial calcaneal tubercle (Fig. 7.1).

7.3   Clinical Findings

Plantar fasciitis has a classic presentation of pain with ambulation after rest, also known as post-static dyskinesia. Athletic patients may feel more discomfort in the "warm-up" phase of their activity; symptoms may subside after a few minutes of initiating their sport. In the early stages in the injury, the pain will subside after a few minutes or even steps, but in the chronic stages, the pain may not subside with ambulation at all. There is often a point of maximal pain at the plantar medial aspect of the calcaneus.

Patients may or may not be able to relate a causative factor for the onset of the pain. Literature review fails to identify an exact cause or foot type for this injury, but theories for the etiology of this injury include pes cavus, pes planus, overpronation, underpronation, excess weight, improper shoe gear, training errors, ankle equinus, lack of proper fat padding, and occupations that require standing for long periods of time.

Plain radiographs may show the presence of a calcaneal heel spur. The spur has little effect on the cause or treatment of plantar fasciitis. Radiographs may be of clinical importance in ruling out fracture, erosive changes associated with a systemic

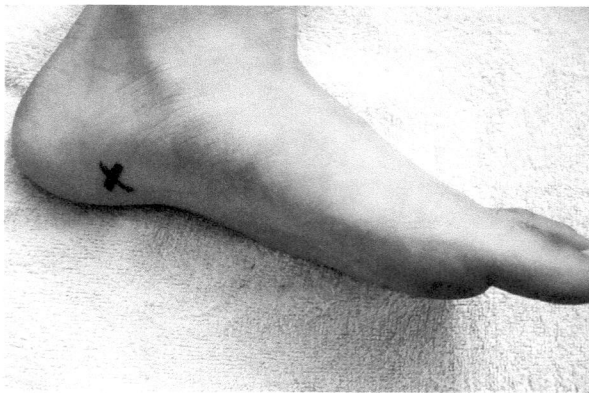

Fig. 7.1 Typical location of plantar fasciitis

arthritis or bone tumors. MRI and diagnostic ultrasound will show thickening of the fascia to at least twice the normal thickness[9,10] (Fig. 7.2).

7.4   Plantar Fascia Rupture

Rupture of the fascia may follow chronic long-term plantar fasciitis, occur acutely, or as a sequella of treatment such as after injection.[11-14] Most often the patient will relate feeling a pop or sudden sharp pain at the insertion of the medial or central band. Saxena and Fullem found an average return to activity of 9 weeks for athletes following this injury.[11] Patients often have bruising in the arch associated with the rupture (Fig. 7.3). Correlation of patients symptoms with the bruising is more than enough evidence of rupture but MRI provides more conclusive evidence (Fig. 7.4).

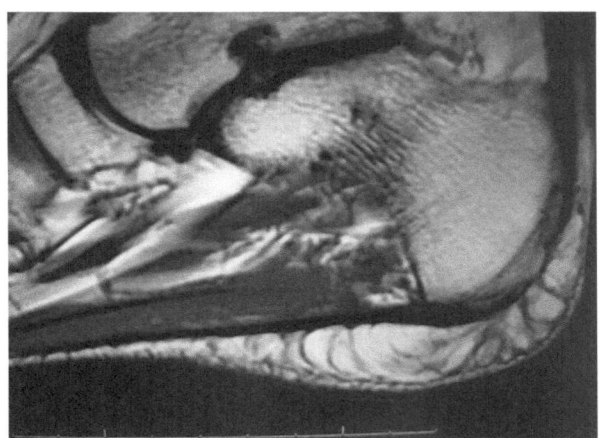

Fig. 7.2 MRI showing thickened plantar fascia

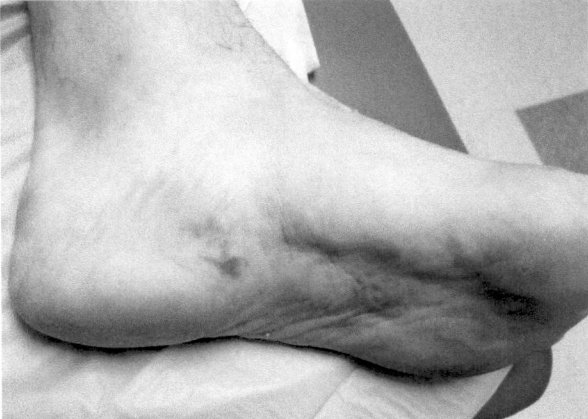

Fig. 7.3 Bruising associated with plantar fascia rupture

Fig. 7.4 (**a**) MRI sagittal
view showing plantar fascial
rupture. (**b**) MRI transverse
view showing medial plantar
fascia and abductor rupture

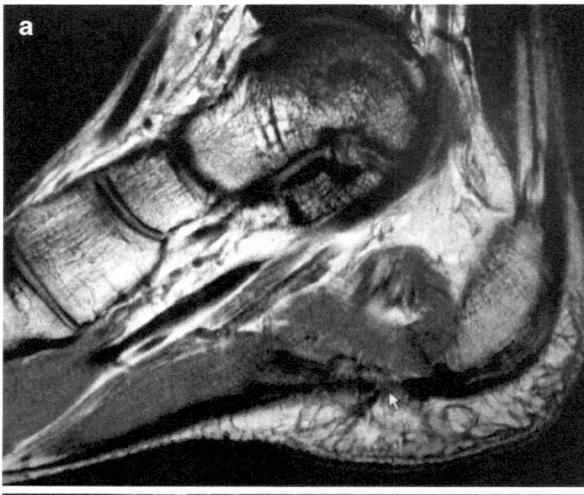

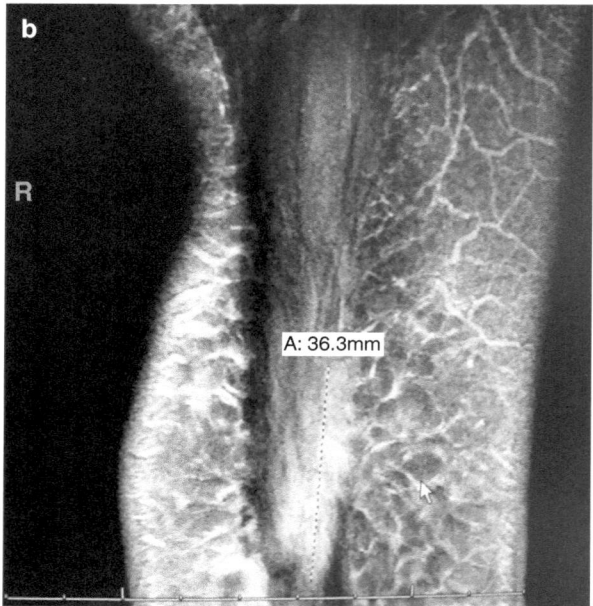

The treatment of a rupture differs greatly from the treatment of plantar fasciitis. Initial treatment should be aimed at reducing pain and inflammation through the use of non-weight-bearing, a below-knee walking boot, ice, and nonsteroidal anti-inflammatory drugs (NSAIDs) and/or narcotics if needed. Within 1–3 weeks, the patient should be able to progress to full weight-bearing in a boot and in another 1–3 weeks progress out of the boot to full weight-bearing. An arch support or foot orthosis placed inside the boot may be helpful. Physical therapy can be started very early in the process and should focus initially on helping to relieve symptoms through the use of electrical stimulation (for swelling and pain control), pulsed ultrasound, and soft tissue mobilization. It should then progress to strengthening the foot and leg to transition out of the boot and back to full activity.[11]

7.5   Nonsurgical Treatment of Plantar Fasciitis

Since a majority of patients with plantar fasciitis get better with nonsurgical (conservative) treatment, it is worthwhile for presentation. There are no universal protocols to eliminate all the symptoms. Initial treatment, particularly in athletic patients, is to focus on stretching, reduce activity, and add arch support. Patient should perform a simple wall stretch concentrating on improving the flexibility of the gastrocnemius–soleus complex. The fascia does not have any elastic fibers and attempting to stretch the fascia by hanging off a step or putting your toes up against the wall may actually prolong the injury. However, DiGiovanni et al. presented an alternative method of non-weight-bearing specific stretching of the fascia which in their study worked better than the wall stretching.[15]

Ice can help control symptoms and is best performed by freezing water in a round smooth plastic bottle and rolling the foot over the bottle for at least 10 min, twice a day. Oral anti-inflammatories, both steroidal and nonsteroidal, can be utilized, though recent research has shown, as is the case with Achilles tendonosis, acute inflammatory pathological findings do not exist. If NSAIDs relieve symptoms, it is likely they are providing an analgesic effect. It may also be likely an arthridity is involved.

Avoidance of barefoot and adherence to wearing shoes with good arch support is also important in the initial treatment phase. Taping can be very effective at reducing symptoms and also may help aid in the diagnosis. Plantar fasciitis pain can be relieved the majority of the time through taping consisting of a low-dye with a Campbell's rest strap over the top of the low-dye. Patient can be instructed to perform the taping themselves before activity. Alternative taping can be variations of the "plantar figure-of-eight" method (Fig. 7.5). Immobilization can be recommended for chronic cases, though ideally this should be reserved for calcaneal stress fractures and plantar fascia ruptures.

Corticosteroid injection can be very effective at reducing symptoms but is not without risks. Plantar fascia ruptures have been associated with injections, and multiple injections in the same area can lead to fat pad atrophy.[12-14] The associated ruptures could possibly be dose and type-of-steroid related. Higher doses of insoluble steroids may have a more deleterious effect. Acevedo and Beskin reported that 10% of their patients were injected for plantar fasciitis with 40 mg/mL of triamcinalone acetate.[12] One author (BF) prefers a mixture of 1.0 cc of 25% marcaine, 4 mg of Dexamethasone phosphate, and 5 mg of triamacinalone acetate with fewer than 10 post-injection fascial ruptures in 18 years of practice.

Over-the-counter arch supports should also be considered for the initial treatment phase. If symptoms persist, a custom orthotic device can be considered.

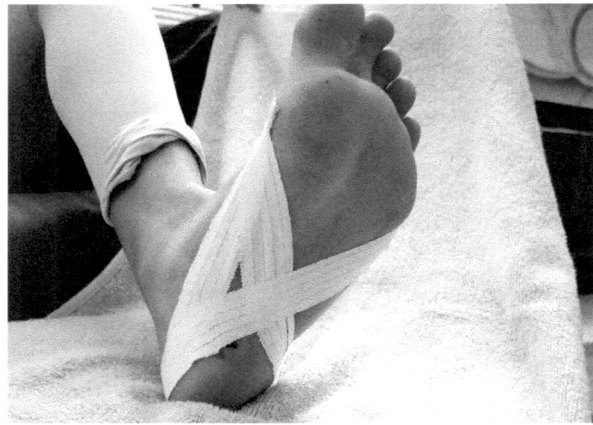

Fig. 7.5 Plantar "figure-of-8" taping. Additional reinforcement can be applied with traditional "low-Dye" taping

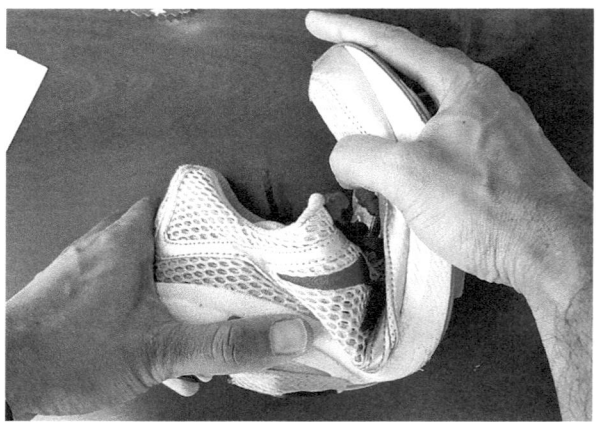

Fig. 7.6 Improper shoe flexibility predisposing plantar fascia or midfoot injury

A softer device should be used for the cavus/underpronated foot type while a more controlling device should typically be prescribed for the pes planus/overpronated foot type. Biomechanical examination and the patient's past experience should be combined with the physician's expertise to devise the best orthotic device. Examination of the athletic patient's shoe type is also paramount. Often sport shoes with arch cut-outs can instigate or aggravate plantar fascia conditions by allowing improper flexibility in the wrong region (Fig. 7.6).

Extracorporeal shock wave therapy (ESWT) is generally offered as a last resort in the United States before considering surgical management. Shock wave therapy is purported to ultimately work by improving the vascularization to the injured area. The treatment induces micro-trauma to the area, and during the repair process, new blood vessels develop to deliver nutrients to the area and heal the tissue. There are virtually no long-lasting negative effect from the treatment: cost and availability being the main deterrent in the United States. There are both high-energy and

Fig. 7.7 "Low-Energy"
D-Actor™ Soundwave
(Courtesy of Storz Medical
AG, Taegerwilen,
Switzerland. Used with
permission)

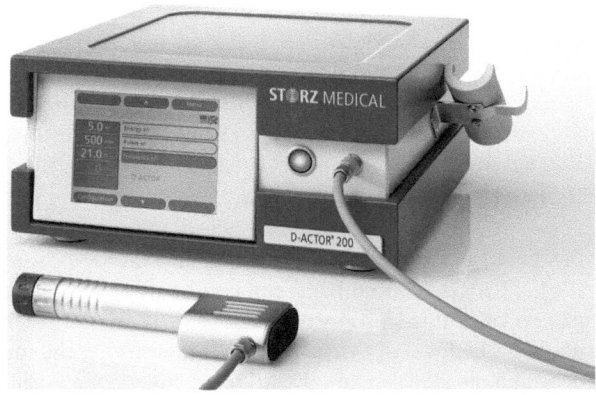

low-energy machines. High-energy machines use a protocol of one treatment but requires anesthesia. Critics of this method cite that the painful area, when under anesthesia, may actually not be treated. The low-energy machines (Storz AG, Taegerwilen, Switerzerland) do not require local anesthesia, thereby allowing for "patient-focused or -directed" treatment (Fig. 7.7). Low-energy protocol requires three treatments usually spaced 1 week apart. Athletic patients being treated with low-energy machines are often able to continue their sport. Evidenced-based medical literature mainly finds long-term success rates of over 70%.[16-20] Some studies show a high percentage of benefit from placebo (greater than 40%).[17,21]

7.6 Surgical Management of Plantar Fasciitis

Failed nonsurgical therapy for at least 6 months is generally acceptable for consideration of surgical intervention in athletic patients. Less than 5% of patients meet the authors' surgical criteria: rest, inserts, injections, sound wave as described above, along with at least 6 months or more of symptoms. Based on the authors' findings that plantar fascia rupture patients do well if they are immobilized and kept non-weight-bearing post-injury, we propose that surgical treatment in essence produces the same result: reduced tension and an acute inflammatory response at the plantar fascia attachment.

Surgical approaches may include endoscopic plantar fasciotomy (EPF), "instep" fasciotomy, and the traditional open approach over the medial aspect of calcaneus. There are advantages and disadvantages to each technique and surgeon preference should always be considered. The decision to perform surgery on an athletic patient is probably more critical than the actual technique. Based on the findings that patients with partial plantar fascia do well post-immobilization, the goal of surgery is to also create a "clean" partial rupture of the medial portion of the central plantar fascia band.[11] The concern of "weakening the arch" has not been clinically proven.[14,22]

In the absence of any nerve involvement, one author (BF) prefers the instep fasciotomy. This technique avoids the neurovascular bundle and has the advantage of being technically simple to perform. Woelffer and colleagues performed a retrospective analysis of 33 patients that underwent the instep fasciotomy and found at 5-year follow-up that 30 had good-to-excellent results.[23]

The instep fasciotomy procedure can be performed under local anesthesia. Boberg states "Proper placement of the incision is imperative to a satisfactory outcome".[24] The incision should be placed approximately 1 cm distal to the insertion at the heel, at the point where the arch begins to slope away from the calcaneus (Fig. 7.8). The central band can be identified in the arch and the incision should be placed over this portion of the fascia. A transverse incision is made and carried down to the level of the fascia. After identifying the medial and lateral border of the central band, the toes are dorsiflexed to place the fascia under tension and the fascia is severed. It is important to maintain the lateral band of the fascia to help avoid lateral column complications postoperatively. After irrigation, the wound is closed with a combination of simple and horizontal mattress sutures. The patient should be kept non-weight-bearing for a minimum of 2 weeks to facilitate proper healing of the skin incision and to allow the fascia to heal in an elongated state.

One can also perform a more traditional open approach which can incorporate a release of the first branch of the lateral calcaneal nerve, which is often implicated as a major cause of plantar heel pain. An oblique incision on the medial heel is placed from behind the medial malleolus near the junction of the medial skin and plantar fat pad, running into the plantar aspect of the foot. The fascia overlying the abductor hallucis muscle belly is incised and the septa in the porta pedis is also released allowing for a complete release of the first branch of the lateral calcaneal nerve. The fascia is then resected at the attachment and the plantar calcaneal spur is removed if present. It is advisable to keep deep closure to a minimum with emphasis on excellent skin closure technique with simple and interrupted mattress type sutures.[24]

Unfortunately, there is scant literature on performing plantar fascia surgery in athletes whether open, percutaneously, or endoscopically. Saxena reported on an

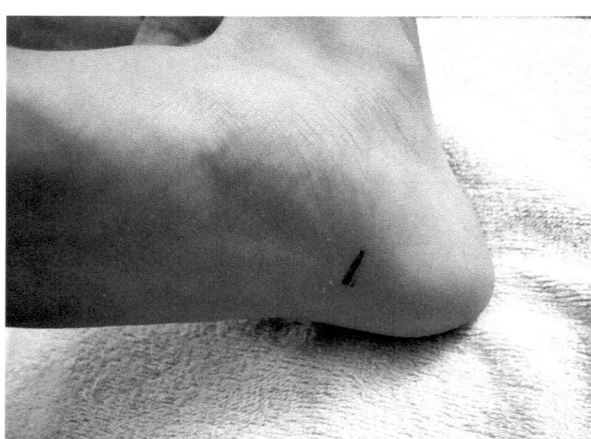

Fig. 7.8 Instep fasciotomy incision

Fig. 7.9 (**a**) Medial
endoscopic portal; (**b**) Lateral
endoscopic portal;
(**c**) Endoscopic view of
medial portion of plantar
fascia being cut

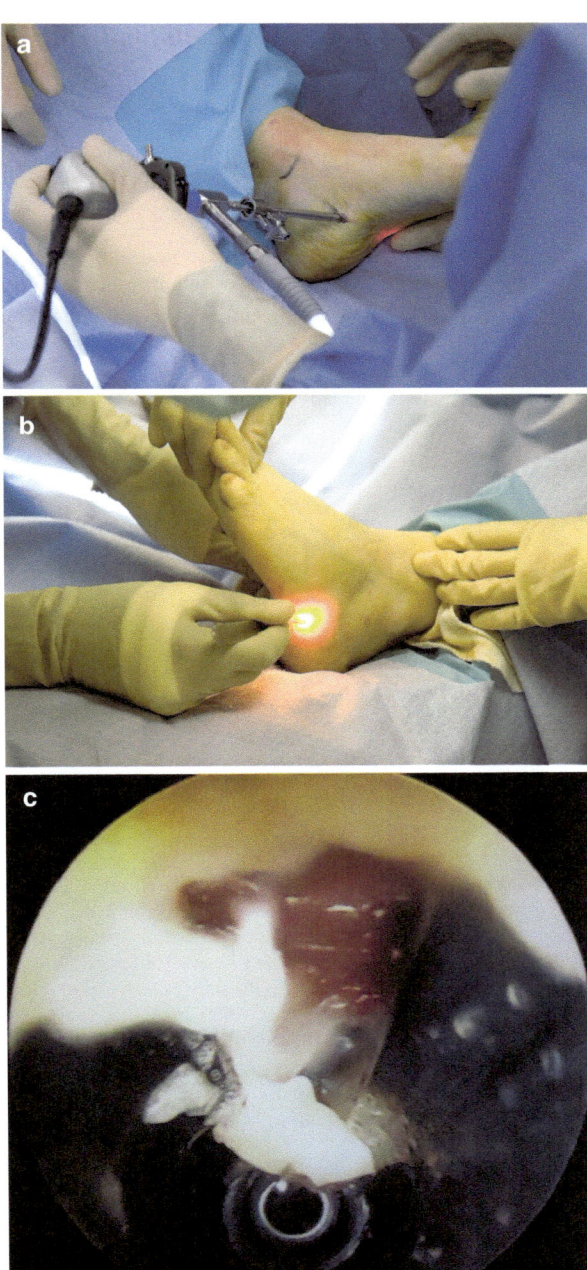

endoscopic approach on athletic patients in 2004. Overall, good and excellent results were obtained in over 90% of patients as long as their body-mass index (BMI) was <27.[22] The endoscopic approach had been criticized for inducing lateral column pain and nerve entrapment.[25] One author's (AS) preferred technique is the endoscopic approach. However, some critical differences are adhered to as compared to historical endoscopic approaches. With the two-portal approach using a 4.0-mm endoscope, only the medial one half of the central band is transected. A longitudinal lateral incision is made; so, the cannula is not placing undue tension on the lateral structures (Fig. 7.9). Postoperatively, patients are kept in a boot, non-weight-bearing for 2 weeks when skin sutures are removed, and then weight-bearing occurs for additional 2 weeks or until pain-free. This is critical as early weight-bearing may induce lateral compensation. Usually an arch support is used as well. Physical therapy is initiated at 5 or more weeks post-plantar fascia surgery. Return to sports with endoscopic technique can occur as soon as 7 weeks, but typically ranges around 12 weeks.[22]

References

1. Taunton JE, Ryan MB, Clement DB, McKenzie DC, Lloyd-Smith DR, Zumbo B. A retrospective case-control analysis of 2002 running injuries. *Br J Sports Med.* 2002;36(2):95–101.
2. Riddle DL, Schappert SM. Volume of ambulatory care visits and patterns of care for patients diagnosed with plantar fasciitis: a national study of medical doctors. *Foot Ankle Int.* 2004;25:303.
3. Wolgin M, Cook C, Graham C, et al. Conservative treatment of plantar heel pain: long-term follow-up. *Foot Ankle Int.* 1994;15:97.
4. O'Brien D, Martin WJ. A retrospective analysis of heel pain. *J Am Podiatr Med Assoc.* 1985;75:416.
5. Scherer PR. Biomechanics graduate research group for 1988: heel spur syndrome: pathomechanics and nonsurgical treatment. *J Am Podiatr Med Assoc.* 1991;81(2):68–72.
6. Lynch DM, Goforth WP, Martin JE, et al. Conservative treatment of plantar fasciitis: a prospective study. *J Am Podiatr Med Assoc.* 1998;88:375.
7. Bøjsen-Möller F, Flagstad KE. Plantar aponeurosis and internal architecture of the ball of the foot. *J Anat.* 1976;121:599.
8. Pontious J, Flanigan KP, Hillstrom HJ. Role of the plantar fascia in digital stabilization. A case report. *J Am Podiatr Med Assoc.* 1996;86:43–7.
9. Vohra PK, Kincaid BR, Japour CJ, Sobel E. Ultrasonographic evaluation of plantar fascia bands: a retrospective study of 211 symptomatic feet. *J Am Podiatr Med Assoc.* 2002;92:444–9.
10. Berkowitz JF, Kier R, Rudicel S. Plantar fasciitis: MR imaging. Radiology. 1991; 179(3):665–7.
11. Saxena A, Fullem B. Plantar fascia ruptures in athletes. Am J Sports Med. 2004;32(3):662–5.
12. Acevedo JI, Beskin JL. Complications of plantar fascia rupture associated with corticosteroid injection. Foot Ankle Int. 1998;19(2):91–7.
13. Sellman JR. Plantar fascia rupture associated with corticosteroid injection. Foot Ankle Int. 1994;15:376.
14. Leach R, Jones R, Silva T. Rupture of the plantar fascia in athletes. J Bone Joint Surg Am. 1978;60:537–9.

15. DiGiovanni BF, Nawoczenski DA, Lintal ME, et al. Tissue-specific plantar fascia-stretching exercise enhances outcomes in patients with chronic heel pain: a prospective, randomized study. J Bone Joint Surg Am. 2003;85:1270.
16. Chuckpaiwong B, Berkson EM, Theodore GH. Extracorporeal shock wave for chronic proximal plantar fasciitis: 225 patients with results and outcome predictors. J Foot Ankle Surg. 2009;48(2):148–55.
17. Marks W, Jackiewicz A, Witkowski Z, Kot J, Deja W, Lasek J. Extracorporeal shock-wave therapy (ESWT) with a new-generation pneumatic device in the treatment of heel pain. A double blind randomised controlled trial. Acta Orthop Belg. 2008;74(1):98–101.
18. Rompe JD, Meurer A, Nafe B, Hofmann A, Gerdesmeyer L. Repetitive low-energy shock wave application without local anesthesia is more efficient than repetitive low-energy shock wave application with local anesthesia in the treatment of chronic plantar fasciitis. J Orthop Res. 2005;23(4):931–41.
19. Gerdesmeyer L, Frey C, Vester J, et al. Radial extracorporeal shock wave therapy is safe and effective in the treatment of chronic recalcitrant plantar fasciitis: results of a confirmatory randomized placebo-controlled multicenter study. Am J Sports Med. 2008;36(11):2100–9. Epub 2008 Oct 1.
20. Gollwitzer H, Diehl P, von Korff A, Rahlfs VW, Gerdesmeyer L. Extracorporeal shock wave therapy for chronic painful heel syndrome: a prospective, double blind, randomized trial assessing the efficacy of a new electromagnetic shock wave device. J Foot Ankle Surg. 2007;46(5):348–57.
21. Ho C. Extracorporeal shock wave treatment for chronic plantar fasciitis (heel pain). Issues Emerg Health Technol. 2007;96(Part 1):1–4.
22. Saxena A. Uniportal endoscopic plantar fasciotomy: a prospective study on athletic patients. Foot Ankle Int. 2004;25(12):882–9.
23. Woelffer KE, Figura MA, Sandberg NS, Snyder NS. Five-year follow-up results of instep plantar fasciotomy for chronic heel pain. J Foot Ankle Surg. 2000;39(4):218–23.
24. Boberg J. Plantar fascia surgery. In: Chang T, editor. Master techniques in podiatric surgery: the foot and ankle. Philadelphia: Lippincott; 2005. p. 222–4.
25. Shapiro S. Endoscopic plantar fasciotomy. In: Scuderi G, Tria A, editor. Minimally invasive surgery in orthopedics. New York: Springer; 2009. p. 427–36.

Chapter 8
Osteochondral Lesions of the Talus

Amol Saxena

Talar lesions are extremely common with all types of ankle injuries including sprains and fractures. Some report that in up to 50% of ankle fractures and severe sprains, some type of talar lesion will occur. These are common sports injuries and are found with all types of ankle sprains and fracture/dislocations.[1-3] When talar lesions occur acutely, they are typically operated on immediately post-injury if there is a significantly displaced fragment. Most lesions are dealt with sub-acutely or chronically.

The term "osteochondral lesion" of the talus is often used for all lesions of the talus, whether they are transchondral or truly osteochondral. Further confusing the terminology is the use of the term "osteochondritis dissecans," which should be used for pediatric aseptic necrosis of the talus which is not usually traumatically induced. These erroneous terms are misleading and may be responsible for the variability in the results of treatments. In essence, one needs to compare "apples to apples."

Transchondral lesions are essentially "scuffs," de-laminations, or tears of talar articular cartilage that generally do not involve bone (Fig. 8.1).[3-5] Full-thickness tears can yield bare exposed subchondral bone. There are various classifications of these lesions. The main differentiation should be: If the lesion involves bone loss, it is a true osteochondral lesion. The classic Berndt and Hardy talar dome classification system is a hybrid of these two pathologies, as Type I lesions just involve cartilage, whereas Types II–IV involve cartilage and bone.[4] Other classification schemes involve describing progressive degradation of articular cartilage.[6]

Osteochondral lesions are also classified with other various systems. Often radiographic findings are used to assess lesions. Hepple et al described their magnetic resonance imaging (MRI) staging system of talar dome injury. Stages 1–4 consist of progressively worse injury to the chondral surface. Specifically Stage 1 is a lesion

A. Saxena, D.P.M.
Department of Sports Medicine, PAFMG-Palo Alto Division,
Clark Bldg., 3rd Flr, 795 El Camino Real, Palo Alto, CA 94301, USA
e-mail: heysax@aol.com

A. Saxena (ed.), *Sports Medicine and Arthroscopic Surgery of the Foot and Ankle*,
DOI 10.1007/978-1-4471-4106-8_8, © Springer-Verlag London 2013

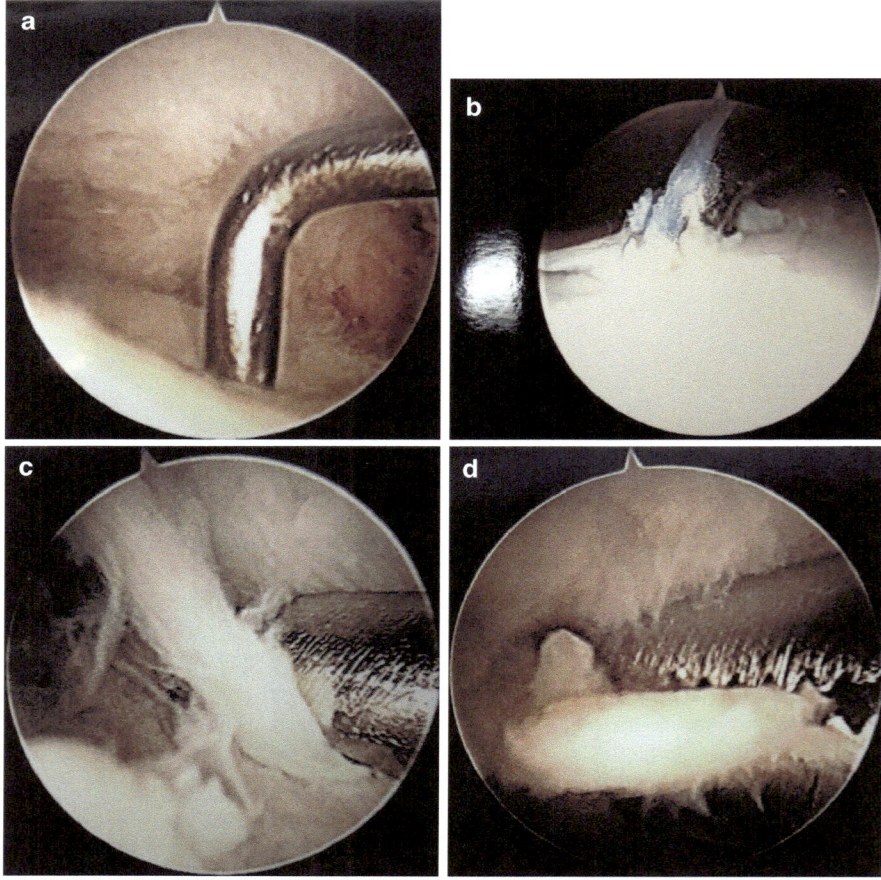

Fig. 8.1 Transchondral lesion "flap" softened cartilage being probed (**a**), separating flap (**b**), excising flap with shaver (**c**), and removing flap with grasper (**d**)

only within the articular cartilage. Stage 2 injuries represent bony trabecular compression with (2A) or without (2B) surrounding bony edema. Stages 3 and 4 describe increasing degrees of osteochondral fragment separation (Fig. 8.2). These injuries can be treated with microfracture. Stage 5 indicates subchondral cysts and avascular bone (Fig. 8.3). These type of lesions are often treated with bone grafting, either autogenous or allograft.[7]

Other classification systems have been described often to help base treatment. Scranton and McDermott added a fifth stage to Berndt and Hardy's system for lesions having an intact cartilage cap, but cystic underlying bone. "Bone bruises" occur with ankle injuries and are visible via MRI in up to 39% of cases. Asymptomatic lesions can occasionally be seen, but may not require treatment, though the incidence of this is not well studied. Chondral injuries are visible arthroscopically in 66% of acutely arthroscoped ankles.[8] Ferkel and Cheng created a specific arthroscopic classification system for chondral injuries having six grades (A-F) ranging from smooth cartilage (A), rough (B), fibrillated/fissured (C), flap or exposed bone (D), loose undisplaced fragment (E), or displaced fragment (F).[6]

The talo-tibial articulation is very critical. It has less room for derangement as 1 mm of displacement can create load imbalance due to toss of talar contact of 30–40%. This subsequent malalignment leads to premature wear, and is common with lateral ankle sprains. This can induce chondral and osteochondral injury.[9]

Recent literature has increased significantly in the past decade as to the results of treatment of talar lesions. Nonsurgical treatment can be attempted and may be successful for early chondral injuries and true "bone bruises" (i.e., micro-trabecular fractures), which generally consists of a period of non-weightbearing and immobilization. There is no uniform nonsurgical treatment regimen for talar injuries, partly due to variability in classification. Unfortunately, just as the preoperative classification and nomenclature vary, so does the postoperative assessment scoring systems. When dealing with athletic patients, one has to take into consideration "down-time" and return to activity (RTA) time frames. In general, treatment of osteochondral lesions has a longer RTA than chondral lesions.[3]

Surgical treatment is recommended for most talar articular lesions that are deep, large, involve bony defects, and/or are displaced. Osteotomy may be required in many cases to gain access to talar lesions. In fact, recent studies have shown accessibility of talar osteochondral lesions can be limited, and which osteotomies may be needed.[10-13] Lesion location traditionally has been classified as antero-lateral and poster-medial on the talar dome. This recently has been refuted by studies. Central lateral and medial locations are actually the most common, whereas the

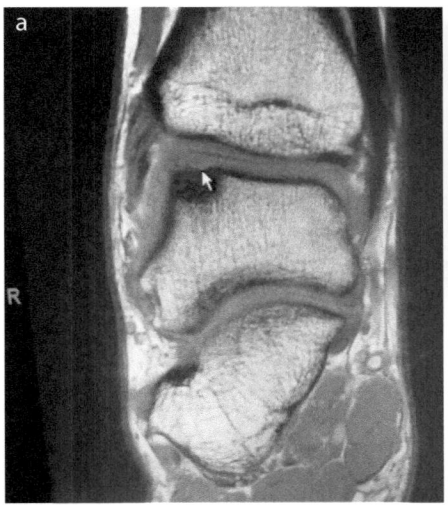
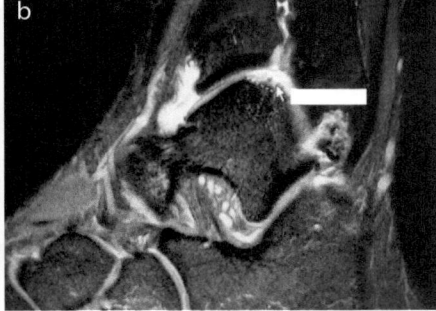

Fig. 8.2 AP T1 MRI (**a**) and lateral T2 (**b**) showing lateral transchondral lesion. Debridement of same lateral transchondral lesion (**c**), after debridement (**d**), introduction of microfracture pick (**e**), placement of microfracture pick (**f**), after performing microfracture: note bleeding (**g**)

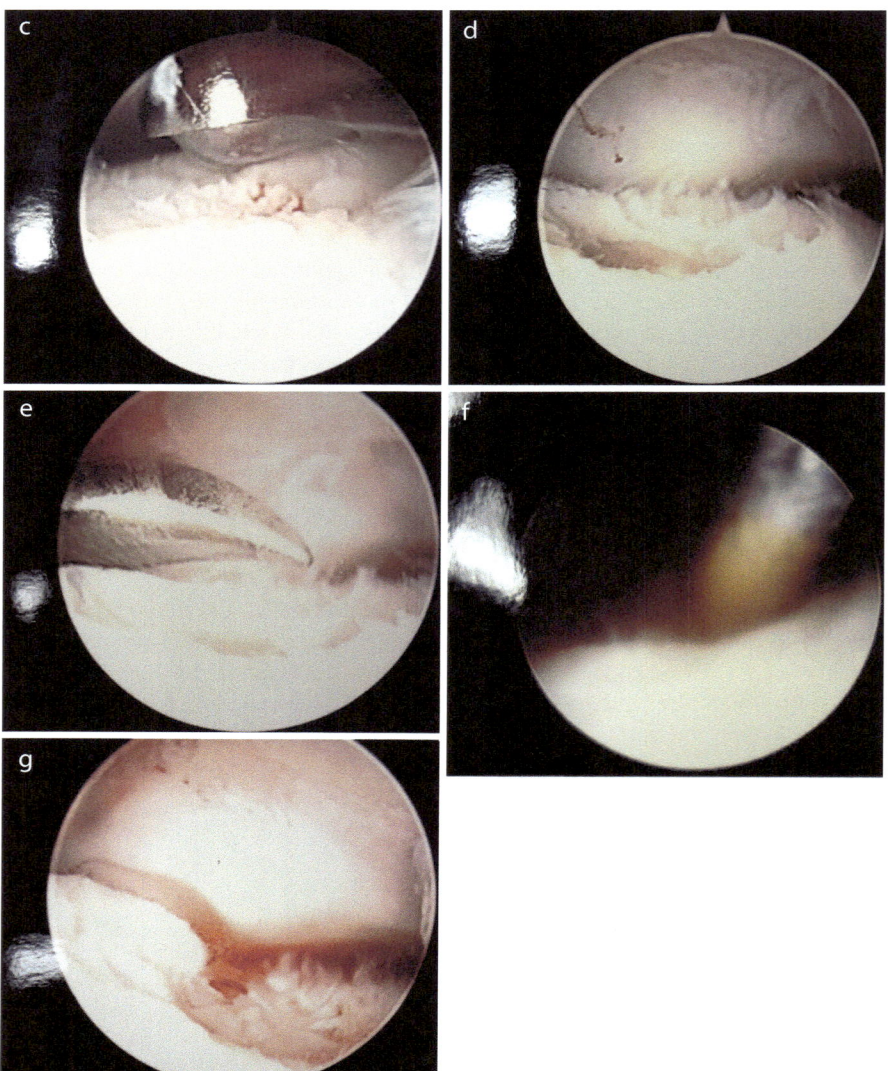

Fig. 8.2 (continued)

classic locations are actually less common. Elias et al reviewed 428 MRI studies
of ankle with talar dome injuries. Mid-medial lesions were the most common
occurring 227 times (53%) while true posterior medial lesions only occurred 58
times (14%). Central lateral defects were the second most common lesion, making
up 26% of the cohort.[14] Osteotomy may be needed to gain access to central lesions.
In addition to medial malleolar and fibular osteotomies to gain access to medial
and lateral lesions respectively, other oblique osteotomies may be preferred

Fig. 8.3 Osteochondral lesions with cystic and avascular bone. AP T1 (**a**) and lateral T1 (**b**)

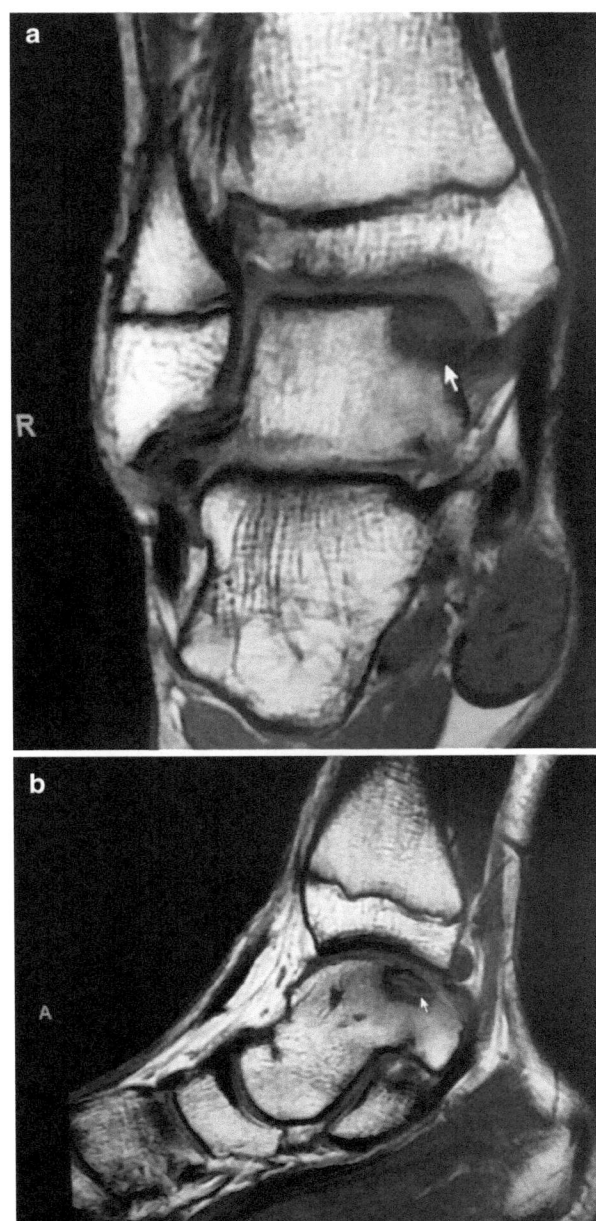

(Fig. 8.4).[10-15] Recent study of postero-lateral lesion access has shown fibular osteotomy gives significantly increased access.[10] Another study on accessibility showed a unique anterior tibial wedge osteotomy gives good access for central and medial lesions.[11]

Procedures for large osteochondral deficits could also require either fresh allograft or a second surgery for articular cartilage re-implantation, which has even longer RTA.[15-17] Microfracture and drilling are typical first-line treatment for chondral defects and smaller osteochondral lesions.[18-22] Furthermore, long-term evaluation of the traditional debridement and drilling of "osteochondral" lesions has shown that 35% of patients note deterioration over time.[23] This gives credence to bone grafting procedures for true osteochondral defects. Authors have shown favorable results from autogenous bone graft without cartilage transfer.[3,24] Retrograde drilling with insertion of bone graft for lesions with intact articular cartilage has shown favorable results as well.[20,25] Other treatment methods such as cartilage re-implantation and osteochondral allograft have been studied, but due to increased morbidity and cost are not recommended as first-line treatment.[15-18]

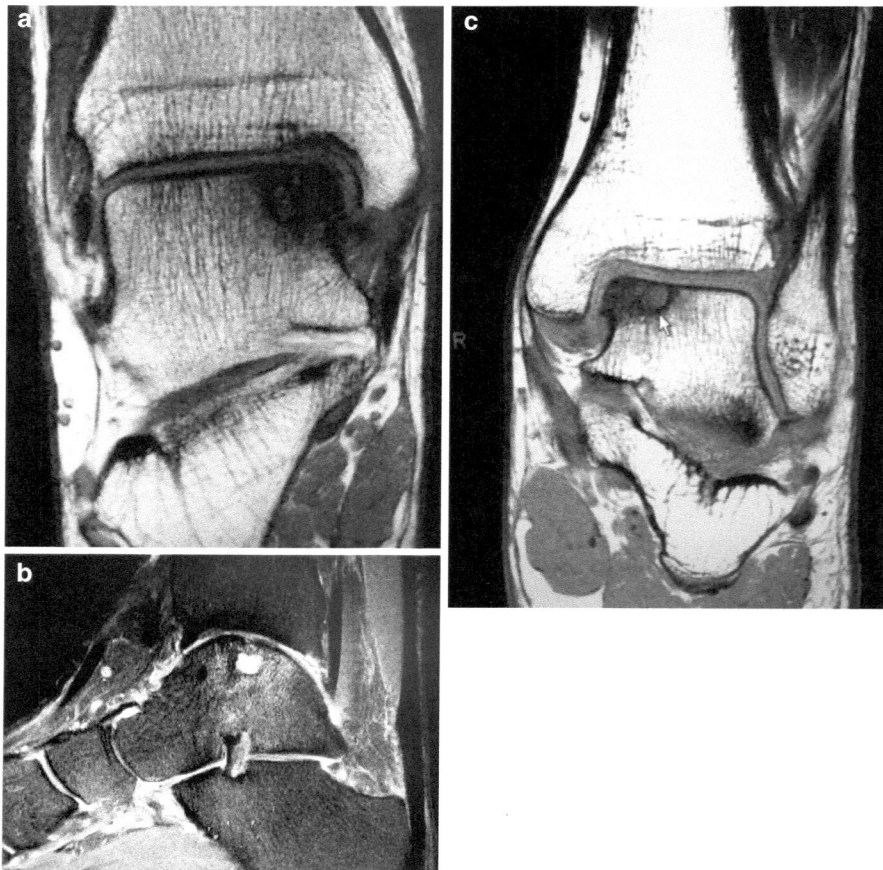

Fig. 8.4 OCDs requiring osteotomies. Medial malleolar (**a–c**), central pyramidal (**d**) and lateral malleolar (**e, f**)

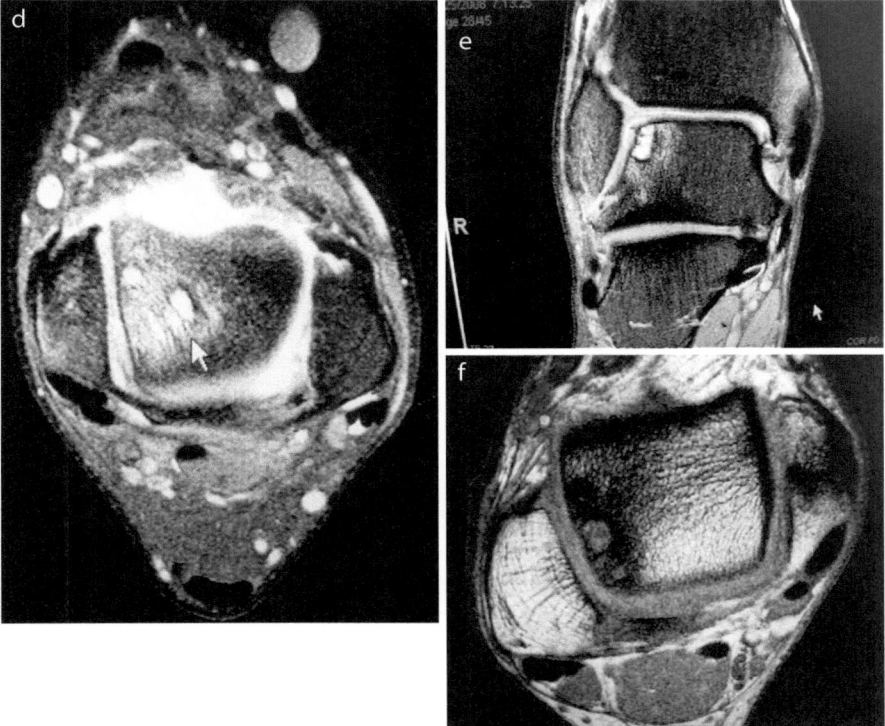

Fig. 8.4 (continued)

8.1   Treatment Protocols

Based on current research outcomes and RTA, the author recommends the following protocols.

8.1.1   *Transchondral Talar Lesions*

Typical treatment of transchondral talar lesions (TLTs) involves debridement and microfracture of the lesion when there is full-thickness cartilage loss (Fig. 8.5). Generally this is done arthroscopically visualizing with either a 2.7- or 4.0-mm 30° arthroscope. Standard antero-lateral and antero-media portals are created. Other accessory portals are used as needed. Transmalleolar drilling can be performed either with image-guidance or directly through visualization of an osteochondral trephine hole opposite the lesion for medial defects.[26] Details of this procedure are found elsewhere in this text. If the cartilage lesion is a large viable flap, fixation to

Fig. 8.5 Microfracture pick for a transchondral lesion

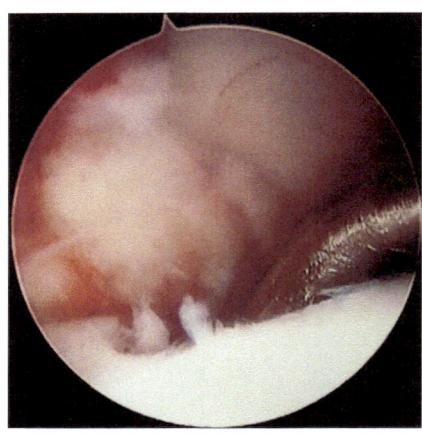

the talus can be performed. This is often performed with bio-fixatives. In cases where the cartilage appears to be grossly intact under direct inspection, retrograde drilling can be performed. This is done under image and arthroscopic control (Fig. 8.6). Newer arthroscopic equipment allows for easier performance of these techniques in the ankle (Fig. 8.7). Postoperatively, patients are kept non-weight-bearing for a minimum of three to six weeks, using a below-knee cast boot unless an osteotomy was performed. In those cases, patients are kept non-weightbearing for six weeks, with the first three weeks in a cast. After weightbearing is initiated, patients are maintained in the boot until 6–12 weeks post-surgery. (The longer time frame is for those undergoing osteotomy.) Physical therapy is initiated at 6–10 weeks post-surgery. Return to sports typically takes three or more months.

Difficult TLT cases are those lesions that involve a large portion of the talar surface area, bipolar lesions and corner lesions. Initial treatment can include above proposed methods. However, if lesions do not yield asymptomatic relief, other options described below may be needed.

8.1.2   *Osteochondral Lesions of the Talus*

True osteochondral lesions of the talus involve bone loss. The supporting surface of the talus is stressed more due to this loss of structure. Research supports the theory that replacing the bone both with (i.e., OATS or osteochondral autologous/allograft transfer) and without cartilage provides good relief.[3,25] Based on Ferkel et al's long-term study which showed drilling and currettement alone of osteochondral lesions yields favorable results only 72% of the time, supports the need for bone replacement.[24] The author prefers to perform autologous morselized bone graft to these defects. Osteotomy may be needed to gain access, along with metallic fixation for postoperative stabilization. (Ideally titanium screws and plates are used so as to

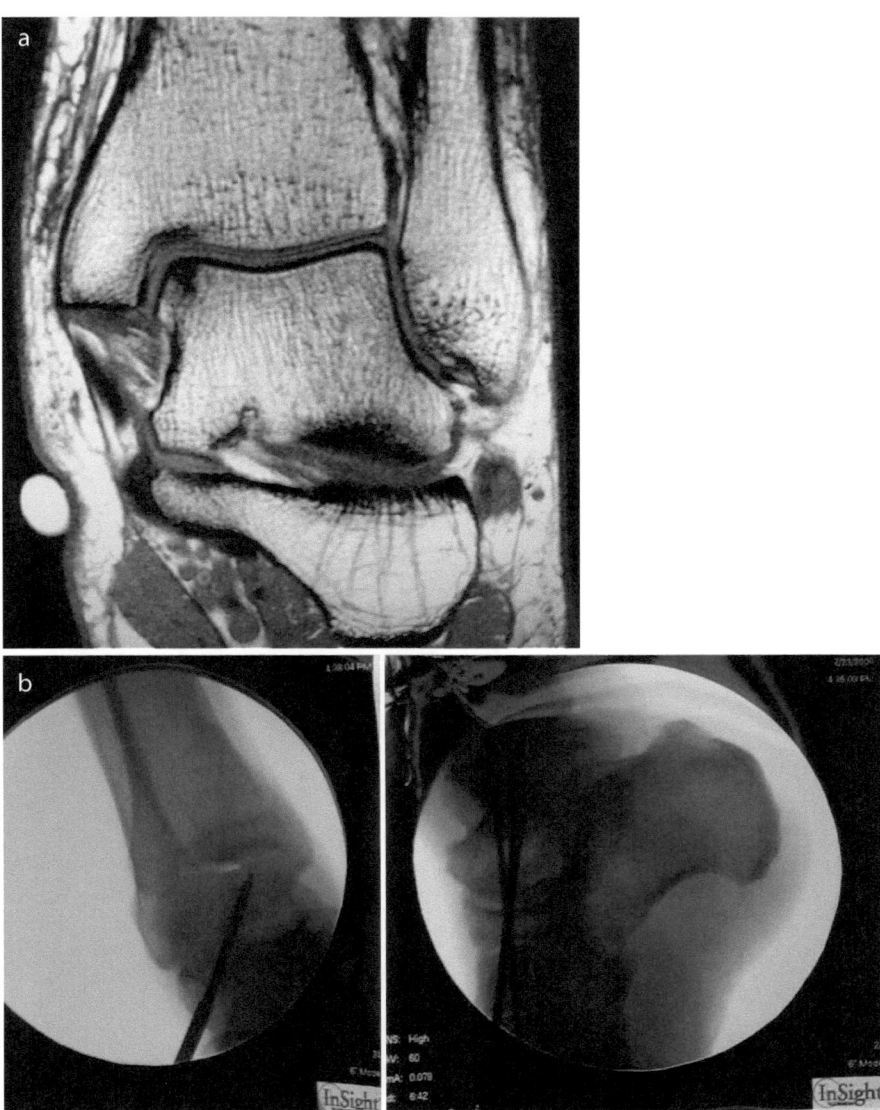

Fig. 8.6 MRI of a lesion (**a**) requiring retrograde drilling via image (**b**, **c**)

allow for additional MRI evaluation.) After curettage of the lesion, often via open arthrotomy, autogenous bone is harvested from the medial malleolus (for medial lesions), lateral calcaneus (lateral lesions), or ipsilateral iliac crest (large lesions), and tamped into the defect (Fig. 8.8). In some cases, retrograde drilling and bone grafting can be performed. Bone can be tamped into place when articular cartilage is intact but bone void exists (Fig. 8.6). Longer-term study is needed of these

Fig. 8.7 Radiolucent guide
(Arthrex, Inc., Naples, FL
USA) to assist with
retrograde drilling and bone
grafting (Courtesy Arthrex,
Inc., used with permission)

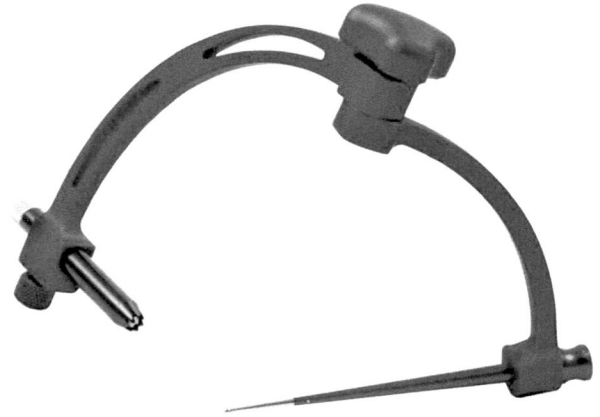

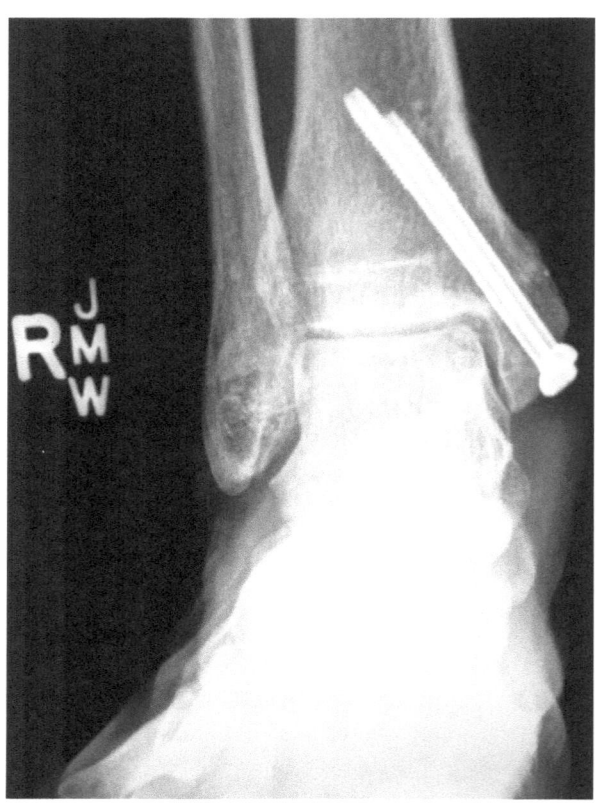

Fig. 8.8 Postoperative bone
graft (patient in Fig. 8.4a, b)

techniques but short-term results of retrograde drilling for talar osteochondral defects (OCDs) appear promising and have the benefit of preserving the cartilage surface.[27]

Though the autogenous OATS procedure shows reasonable results in the talus, donor site morbidity from the knee leaves patients with significant deficits; in some studies, more than 50% of patients complained of significant knee pain.[28-32] Allograft OATS adds to the cost of the procedure and given that 30% of the cartilage cells may not be viable 24 h after implantation, harvesting from the knee may be an unnecessary step. One study described autogenous bone graft from a non-weight-bearing portion of the talus with favorable results, which may be a better option in some situations since the cartilage thickness is similar.[31,33]

The author does utilize osteochondral allograft for corner or edge lesions, failed microfracture cases and sub-total ankle arthroplasty for large lesions (Figs. 8.9 and 8.10). Fresh talar allograft requires side matching and sizing. Recent studies show good results. The technique with fresh allografts involves matching the excised portion of the talus. Intraoperative imaging may show a "step-off" due to the difference in donor subchondral plate thickness. Therefore, clinical intraoperative inspection is mandatory on all sides of the donor placement. Fixation is generally with bio-screws or pins. Raikin recently reported on 15 cases with average defect size of over 6,000 mm^3 with good results.[16] He found graft stability and viability were maintained both structurally and functionally after mean follow-up 4.5 years post-implantation. He used metallic fixation and average patient age was 41.9 years. Metallic screws make subsequent re-imaging with MRI difficult. "Second-look" arthroscopies can show viable articular cartilage, but few studies relate this.[3,16,24,34]

8.2   Postoperative Management

Postoperative management of osteochondral lesion repair is typically six weeks non-weightbearing in a cast or boot, and then an additional 10–12 weeks in the boot until pain-free, or if an osteotomy was performed, bony healing has been achieved. Allograft incorporation could take several weeks longer (than 12 weeks). X-rays of bone graft incorporation and of the osteotomy if performed are obtained. Osteotomies that are fixed with resorbable screws may have persistent lucencies within the screw "tracks" (Fig. 8.11). Formal physical therapy starts at 10 weeks. Impact activities and sport resumption take approximately six months or even longer, especially for allograft patients. Most patients use an ankle brace or tape for sports postoperatively. One should note that similar treatments can be employed for chondral and osteochondral lesions of the tibial plafond and malleolar articular portions of the ankle as well. A treatment algorithm based on current literature and the author's experience is presented in Fig. 8.12. Treatment for failed OCDs can include ankle arthrodiastasis, realignment osteotomies, total ankle arthroplasty, and arthrodesis, discussed elsewhere in this text.

Fig. 8.9 X-ray (**a**) and MRI (**b**, **c**) of a patient undergoing fresh osteochondral allograft (**d**)

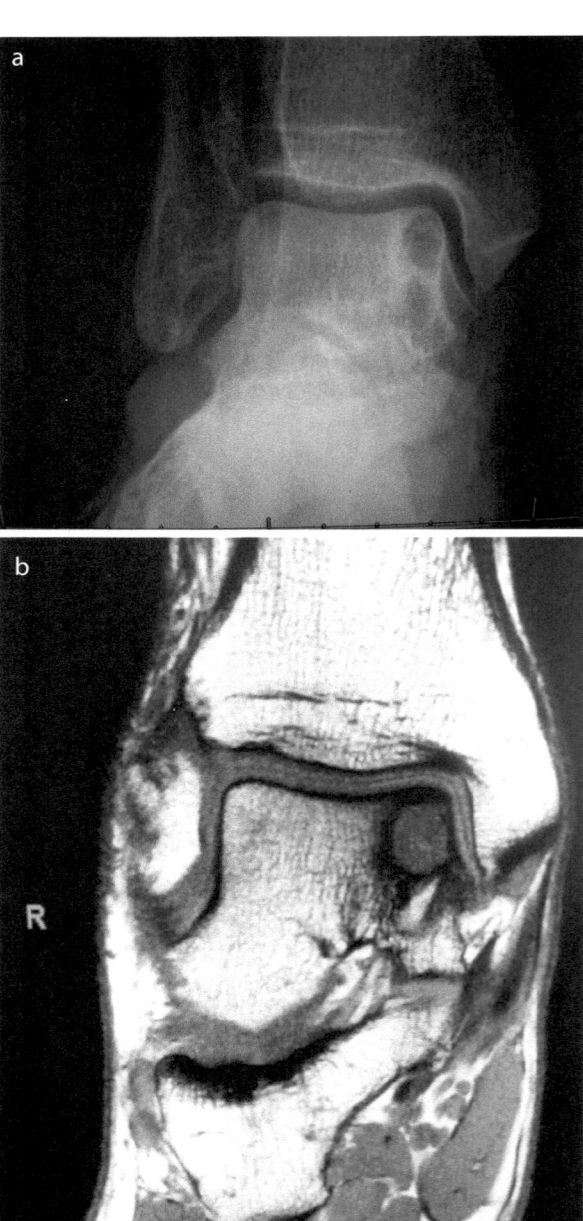

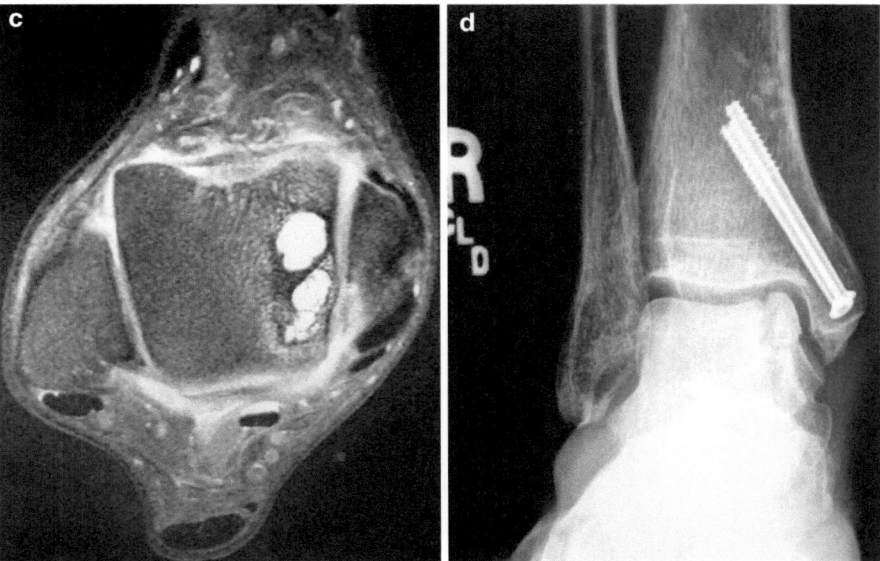

Fig. 8.9 (continued)

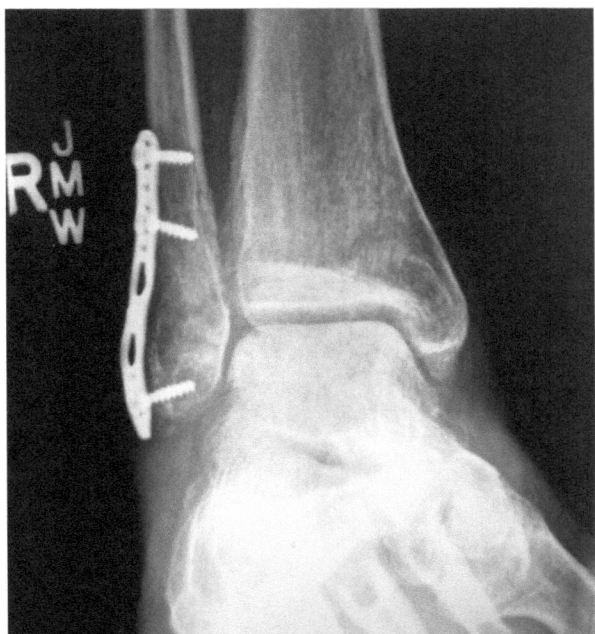

Fig. 8.10 Osteochondral allograft for lateral corner OCD (patient in Fig. 8.4e, f)

Fig. 8.11 Antero-pyramidal osteotomy for autogenous bone graft of a central-medial OCD (patient in Fig. 8.4c, d). Note lucency in distal tibia from bioresorbable screw used to fixate osteotomy immediate (**a**) and three month post-op X-rays (**b**)

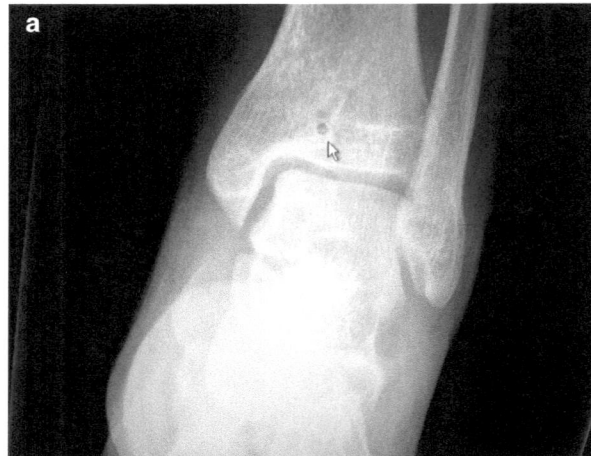

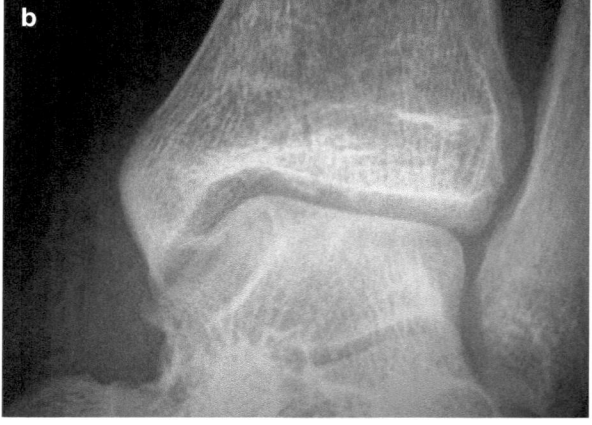

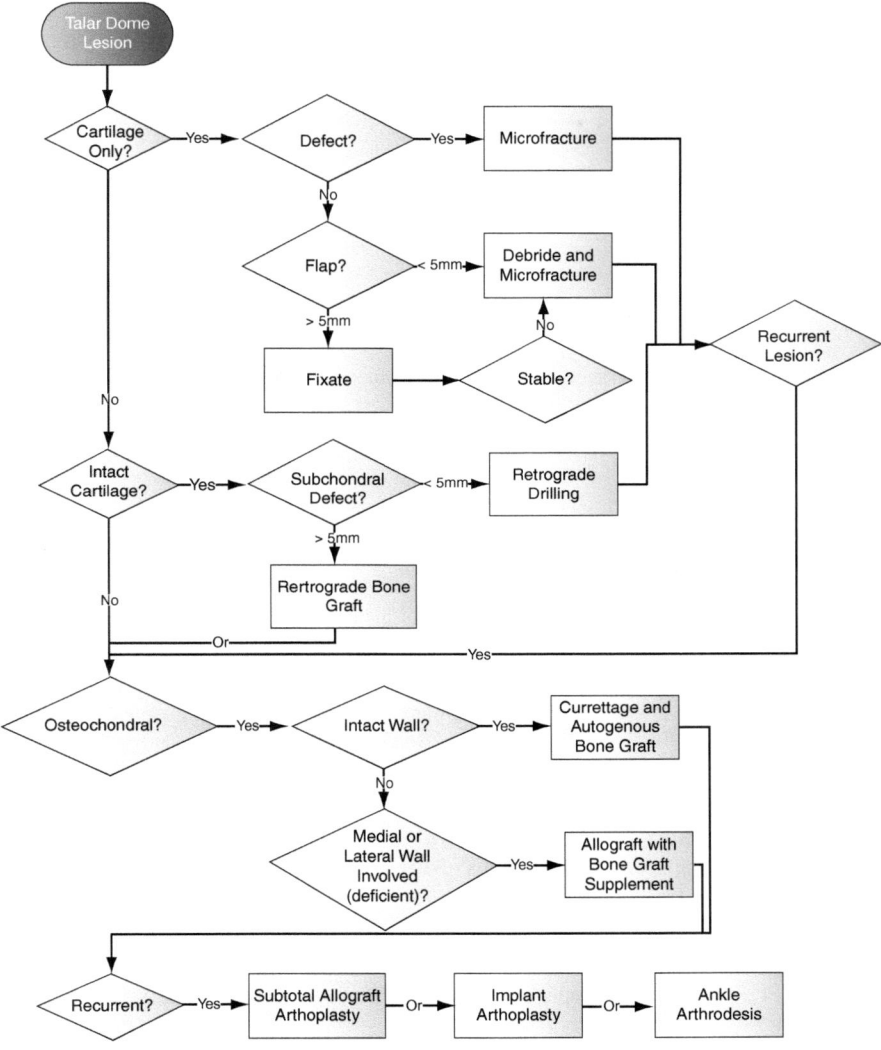

Fig. 8.12 Algorithm for Treatment of Talar Dome Lesions. Note: Most microfracture and retrograde drilling procedures are performed arthroscopically while autogenous bone grafting is performed via open arthrotomy. 5 mm refers to the diameter of the lesion measured intraoperatively. In addition, lesion location determines if an osteotomy is necessary with a lateral fibular, anterior tibial (pyramidal), or medial malleolar (inverted chevron) approach

References

1. DeLee JC. Fractures and dislocations of the foot. In: Mann RA, Coughlin MJ, editors. Surgery of the foot and ankle. 6th ed. St. Louis: Mosby; 1991. p.1465–518.

2. Ferkel RD. Arthoscopy of the ankle and foot. In: Mann RA, Coughlin MJ, editors. *Surgery of the foot and ankle*. St. Louis: Mosby; 1993. p. 1277–312.
3. Saxena A, Eakin C. Articular talar injuries in athletes: results of microfracture and autogenous bone graft. *Am J Sports Med*. 2007;35:1680–7.
4. Berndt AL, Harty M. Transchondral fractures (osteochondritis dissecans) of the talus. *J Bone Joint Surg Am*. 1959;4:988–1020.
5. Labovitz J, Scweitzer M. Osseous occult injuries after ankle sprains: incidence, location, pattern, and age. *Foot Ankle Int*. 1998;19:661–7.
6. Ferkel R, Cheng J. Ankle and subtalar arthroscopy. In: Kelikian A, editor. *Operative treatment of the foot and ankle*. New York: Appleton-Croft; 1999. p. 321.
7. Hepple S, Winson I, Glew D. Osteochondral lesions of the talus; a revised classification. *Foot Ankle Int*. 2000;21(12):789–93.
8. Scranton P, McDermott J. Treatment of type V osteochondral lesions of the talus with ipsilateral knee osteochondral autografts. *Foot Ankle Int*. 2001;22:380–4.
9. Caputo AM, Lee JY, Spritzer CE, et al. In vivo kinematics of the tibiotalar joint after lateral ankle instability. *Am J Sports Med*. 2009;37(11):2241–8.
10. Garras DN, Santangelo JA, Wang DW, Easley ME. A quantitative comparison of surgical approaches for posterolateral osteochondral lesions of the talus. Foot Ankle Int. 2008;29(4):415–20.
11. Kreuz P, Steinwachs M, Erggelet C, Lahm A, Henle P, Niemeyer P. Mosiacplasty with autogenous talar autograft for osteochondral lesions of the talus after failed primary arthroscopic management. Am J Sports Med. 2006;34(1):55–63.
12. Muir D, Saltzman C, Tochigi Y, Amendola N. Talar dome access for osteochondral lesions. Am J Sports Med. 2006;34:1457–63.
13. Navid DO, Myerson MS. Approach alternatives for treatment of osteochondral lesions of the talus. Foot Ankle Clin. 2002;7(3):635–50.
14. Elias I, Zoga AC, Morrison WB, Besser MP, Schweitzer ME, Raikin SM. Osteochondral lesions of the talus: localization and morphologic data from 424 patients using a novel anatomical grid scheme. Foot Ankle Int. 2007;28(2):154–61.
15. Zengerink M, Szerb I, Hangody L, Dopirak RM, Ferkel RD, van Dijk CN. Current concepts: treatment of osteochondral ankle defects. Foot Ankle Clin. 2006;11(2):331–59.
16. Raikin S. Fresh osteochondral allografts for large volume cystic osteochondral defects of the talus. J Bone Joint Surg. 2009;91-A(12):2818–26.
17. Whittaker JP, Smith G, Makwana N, et al. Early results of autologous chondrocyte implantation in the talus. J Bone Joint Surg Br. 2005;87(2):179–83.
18. Giannini S, Buda R, Vannini F, DiCaprio F, Grigolo B. Arthroscopic autologous chondrocyte implantation in osteochondral lesions of the talus: surgical technique and results. Am J Sports Med. 2008;36:873–80.
19. Becher C, Thermann H. Results of microfracture in the treatment of articular defects of the talus. Foot Ankle Int. 2005;26(8):583–9.
20. Kono M, Takao M, Naito K, Uchio Y, Ochi M. Retrograde drilling for osteochondral lesions of the talar dome. Am J Sports Med. 2006;34:1450–6.
21. Tol J, Struijs P, Bossuiyt P, Verhagen R, van Dijk C. Treatment strategies in osteochondral defects of the talar dome: a systematic review. Foot Ankle Int. 2000;21:119–26.
22. Van Dijk C, Verhagen R, Struijs P. Systematic review of treatment strategies for osteochondral defects of the talar dome. Foot Ankle Clin. 2003;2:233–42.
23. Ferkel RD, Zanotti RM, Komenda GA, et al. Arthroscopic treatment of chronic osteochondral lesions of the talus: long-term results. Am J Sports Med. 2008;36(9):1750–62.
24. Draper S, Fallet L. Autogenous bone grafting for the treatment of talar dome lesions. J Foot Ankle Surg. 2000;39(1):15–23.
25. Taranow W, Bisignani G, Towers J. Retrograde drilling of osteochondral lesions of the medial talar dome. Foot Ankle Int. 1999;20(8):474–80.

26. Grady J, Hughes D. Arthroscopic management of talar dome lesions using a transmalleolar approach. J Am Podiatr Med Assoc. 2006;96(3):260–3.
27. Gobbi A, Francisco R, Lubowitz J, Allegra F, Canata G. Osteochondral lesions of the talus: randomized controlled trial comparing chondroplasty, microfracture and osteochondral autograft transplantation. J Arthos Rel Surg. 2006;2210:1085–92.
28. Baltzer AW, Arnold JP. Bone-cartilage transplantation from the ipsilateral knee for chondral lesions of the talus. Arthroscopy. 2005;21(2):159–66.
29. Hangody L, Fules P. Autologous osteochondral mosaicplasty for the treatment of full-thickness defects of weight-bearing joints: ten years of experimental and clinical experience. J Bone Joint Surg Am. 2003;85:25–32.
30. Kreuz PC, Steinwachs M, Edlich M, et al. The anterior approach for the treatment of posterior osteochondral lesions of the talus: comparison of different surgical techniques. Arch Orthop Trauma Surg. 2005;5:1–6.
31. Reddy S, Pedowitz D, Parekh S, Sennett B, Okereke E. The morbidity associated with osteochondral harvest from asymptomatic knees for the treatment of osteochondral lesions of the talus. Am J Sports Med. 2007;35:80–5.
32. Valderabano V, Leumann A, Rasch H, Egelhof T, Hintermann B, Pagenstert G. Knee-to-ankle mosaicolasty for the treatment of osteochondral lesions of the ankle joint. Am J Sports Med. 2009;37(Supp 1):105S–11.
33. Kreuz PC, Steinwachs M, Erggelet C, Lahm A, Henle P, Niemeyer P. Mosaicplasty with autogenous talar autograft for osteochondral lesions of the talus after failed primary arthroscopic management: a prospective study with a 4-year follow-up. Am J Sports Med. 2006;34(1):55–63.
34. Lee B, Bai L, Yoon T, Jung S, Seon J. Second-look arthroscopic findings and clinical outcomes after microfracture for osteochondral lesions of the talus. Am J Sports Med. 2009;37(Supp 1):63S–70.

Chapter 9
Os Trigonum Injuries

Amol Saxena

Os trigonum and posterior talar process injuries are common in sports, especially soccer, football,and basketball, along with dancers, particularly those who go "en pointe."[1-3] Symptoms can be precipitated by an ankle sprain, with hyper-plantarflexion often causing a "nutcracker" effect displacing the os trigonum or creating a posterior talar fracture. The os trigonum occurs in up to 30% of the population as a normal variant.[2] It lies intra-articularly adjacent to the posterior talar process. Both the posterior ankle and subtalar joint capsules adhere to this bone. The flexor hallucis longus (FHL) tendon generally courses medial to it and can be aggravated by injury to this ossicle or the posterior talus itself. The injury should be differentiated from stenosing tenosynovitis of the FHL tendon. Because of the proximity of these anatomical structures, patients may confuse their symptoms to emanate from the Achilles tendon; however with careful inspection, symptoms and swelling will be located in the deep posterior ankle recess. Symptoms will increase with hyper-plantarflexion of the ankle and range of motion of the FHL. X-rays should reveal the os trigonum or enlarged posterior talar process (Fig. 9.1). Computed tomography (CT) or magnetic resonance imaging (MRI) maybe needed to show fracture or displacement of the ossicle (Fig. 9.2). Nonsurgical treatment is often recommended for non-displaced injuries (that do not involve a large portion of the ankle or subtalar joint surface) and usually for first-time "events." Immobilization in a below-knee cast or boot for 4–6 weeks is recommended. If patients still have symptoms from the posterior ankle after 3 months of rehabilitation, one soluble steroid injection can be administered.

In recalcitrant cases of symptomatic os trigonum injuries, surgical excision can result in good relief. Open surgical approach is typically posterolateral, unless preoperative imaging reveals that the ossicle or fracture is displaced medially.[2] Arthroscopic excision is described elsewhere in this text but has recently been

A. Saxena, D.P.M.
Department of Sports Medicine, PAFMG-Palo Alto Division,
Clark Bldg., 3rd Flr, 795 El Camino Real, Palo Alto, CA 94301, USA
e-mail: heysax@aol.com

A. Saxena (ed.), *Sports Medicine and Arthroscopic Surgery of the Foot and Ankle*,
DOI 10.1007/978-1-4471-4106-8_9, © Springer-Verlag London 2013

Fig. 9.1 X-ray showing an os trigonum

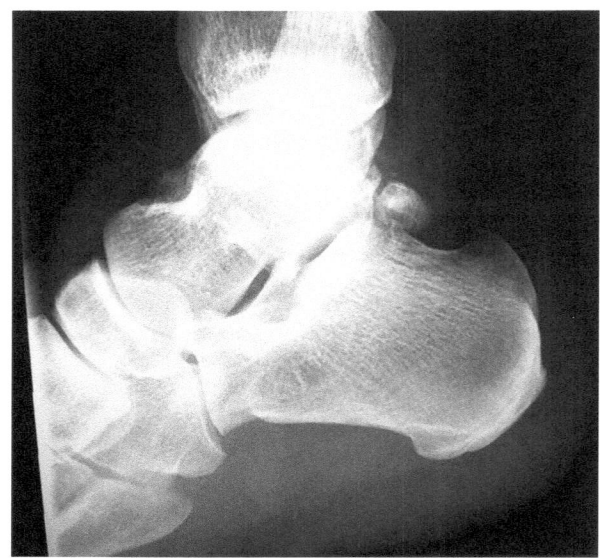

Fig. 9.2 MRI of os trigonum

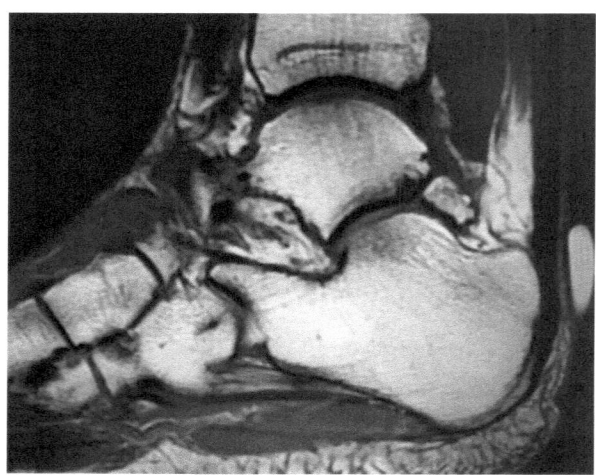

proven to have good results in athletes.[3] The patients can be placed prone to get better visualization with both open and arthroscopic excision, and in case another incision can be made, otherwise, lateral position is preferred. Some authors describe surgical extirpation of the bone arthroscopically as well, which is explained elsewhere in this text. The typical lateral open approach gains access to the posterior ankle and subtalar joint, when making the incision just behind the peronei (Fig. 9.3). This avoids the posterolateral neurovascular structures. The peronei are retracted anteriorly and a posterior capsulotomy is performed. A rongeur is often needed to remove the associated posterior synovitis. Care is taken to protect the FHL medially.

Fig. 9.3 (**a**, **b**) Posterolateral incision for recurrent posterior impingement of os trigonum in a dancer who had a previous medial approach

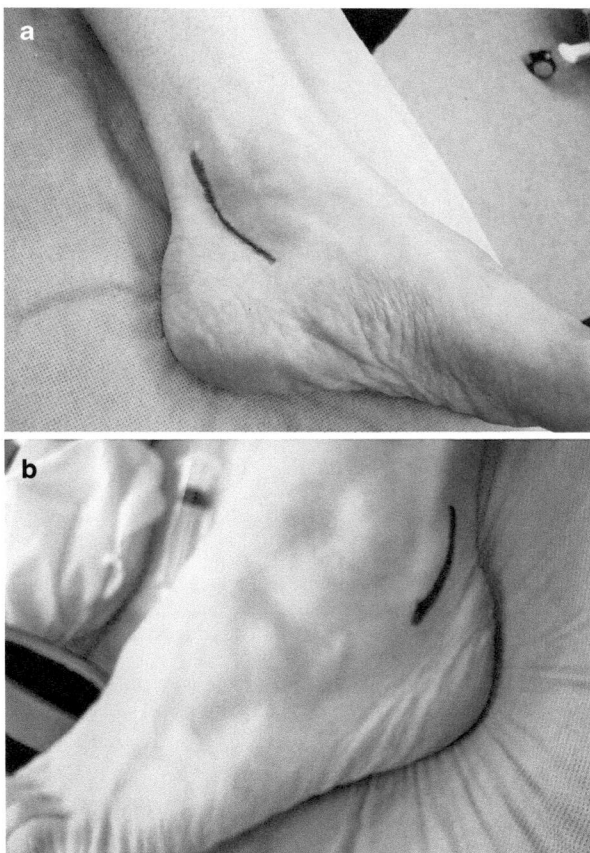

A small osteotome can be used to free up the posterior ossicle or fracture talar process. Dorsiflexion and plantarflexion of the foot can help identify the posterior joints and the offending ossicle. It should be removed in toto (Fig. 9.4). The posterior talus is smoothed with a rasp, particularly the portion which comes in contact with the FHL. The tendon itself is inspected for any tears or stenosing tenosynovitis, which can be repaired or debrided as needed. Potential complications are excessive scarring and fibrosis of the FHL tendon and neurovascular injury. The area of resected bone can be covered with bone wax. The posterior articular surfaces are inspected for chondral defects and smaller loose bodies. Also, 1 cc of dexamethasone phosphate can be injected to decrease any adhesions. The capsule and peroneal retinaculum is re-approximated with absorbable suture. If additional lateral ankle procedures are needed, the incision can be extended anteriorly. Skin is closed with nonabsorbable suture. Patients can weight-bear post-surgery with a cast boot, generally for 4 weeks unless other procedures dictate otherwise. Formal physical therapy is initiated at 4 weeks. Patients can return to sports and dance between 6 and 12 weeks.

Fig. 9.4 Postoperative X-ray after os trigonum excision

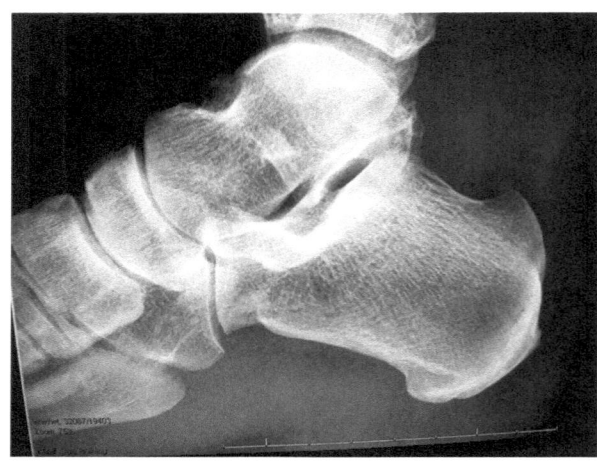

References

1. Horibe S, Kita K, Natsu-ume T, Hamada M, Mae T, Shino K. A novel technique of arthroscopic excision of a symptomatic os trigonum. *Arthroscopy*. 2008;24(1):121–4.
2. Blake R, Lallas P, Ferguson H. The os trigonum syndrome: a literature review. *J Am Podiatr Med Assoc*. 1992;82(3):154–61.
3. Calder JD, Sexton SA, Pearce CJ. Return to training and playing after posterior ankle arthroscopy for posterior impingement in elite professional soccer. *Am J Sports Med*. 2010;38(1):120–4.

Chapter 10
Syndesmosis Injuries

George Tye Liu and Marque A. Allen

10.1 Epidemiology

Injuries of the distal tibiofibular syndesmosis comprise approximately 1–18% of all ankle sprains and are involved in 10% of all ankle fractures.[1] A low reported incidence may be due to poor sensitivity in identifying subtle widening of the syndesmosis on radiograph, as these injuries are often unnoticed in the absence of frank diastasis. Though they represent a low percentage of ankle injuries, syndesmotic injury is the single most predictive factor for long-term disability and chronic ankle pain regardless of grade.[2] In athletes, syndesmosis injuries significantly increase the time to return to activity compared to lateral ankle sprains and can be a source of significant disability.[3]

10.2 Anatomy and Function

The distal tibiofibular syndesmotic complex consists of four ligaments which tighten as the ankle dorsiflexes, locking the talus into a "closed and packed" position for the propulsive phase of gait. The anterior inferior tibiofibular ligament originates from the anterior tubercle of the tibia and descends obliquely to the anterior border of the lateral malleolus. This ligament is often multi-fasicular and occasionally will have a branch of the perforating peroneal artery penetrating the ligament. In cadaveric studies, isolated sectioning of this ligament allows 2.3 mm of diastasis and 2.7° of external rotation.[4]

G.T. Liu, D.P.M. (✉)
Department of Orthopaedic Surgery, University of Texas Southwestern Medical Center,
1801 Inwood Rd., Dallas, TX 75390-8883, USA
e-mail: liugt401@aol.com

M.A. Allen, D.P.M.
Texas Center for Athletes,
San Antonio, TX, USA

A. Saxena (ed.), *Sports Medicine and Arthroscopic Surgery of the Foot and Ankle*,
DOI 10.1007/978-1-4471-4106-8_10, © Springer-Verlag London 2013

The posterior tibiofibular ligament is composed of the superficial and deep components. The superficial portion descends posterolaterally from the posterior tubercle of the tibia and attaches to the digital fossa of the lateral malleolus. The deep component, also known as the transverse tibiofibular ligament, is located more inferior to its superficial counterpart, is more fibrocartilage in composition, and serves as the primary restraint against syndesmotic widening.[5]

The interosseous tibiofibular ligament is formed by dense short elastic fibers originating from the medial aspect of the fibular shaft inserting along the lateral tibia. This ligament continues superiorly forming the aponeurotic fibers of the interosseous ligament which ascends the remaining interval between the tibia and fibula. The vertical and concave groove along the distal lateral tibia formed between the anterior and posterior tibial tubercles, known as the fibular notch or the tibial incisura, allows a structural fit of the medial distal fibula.

10.3   Biomechanics

The fibula at the level of the tibiofibular joint is dynamic throughout the gait cycle in both translational and rotational movements. The tibiofibular syndesmosis tightens as the ankle dorsiflexes to accommodate the wider anterior portion of the talar dome. Concomitant tension of the deltoid and lateral collateral ligaments with ankle dorsiflexion creates a tightly restrained position of the talus within the ankle mortise for stable forward translation of body weight. Additionally, as the ankle dorsiflexes, there is intermalleolar widening approximately 1.25 mm and 2.5° of external rotation to accommodate anterior widening of the talar dome.[6,7]

10.4   Mechanism of Injury

Most syndesmotic injuries are commonly reported in athletic sports such as skiing, ice hockey, football, and basketball.[3,8,9] Sporting activities have been considered a risk factor for these injuries compared to the non-sporting population. Injury to the syndesmosis commonly occurs with a forced external rotation of the foot on the ankle and may be completely ligamentous, but is commonly associated with fractures of the malleoli.

10.5   Clinical Diagnosis

Patients with syndesmotic injuries will often report more difficulty bearing weight compared to patients with isolated lateral ankle sprains. In contrast to lateral ankle sprains, pain is located along the syndesmosis and is often accompanied by supramalleolar swelling with or without ecchymosis. Several clinical maneuvers have been described

Fig. 10.1 Temporarily restoration of ankle function with standing, walking, or heel rises after circumferential taping of syndesmosis is considered diagnostic of syndesmosis injury

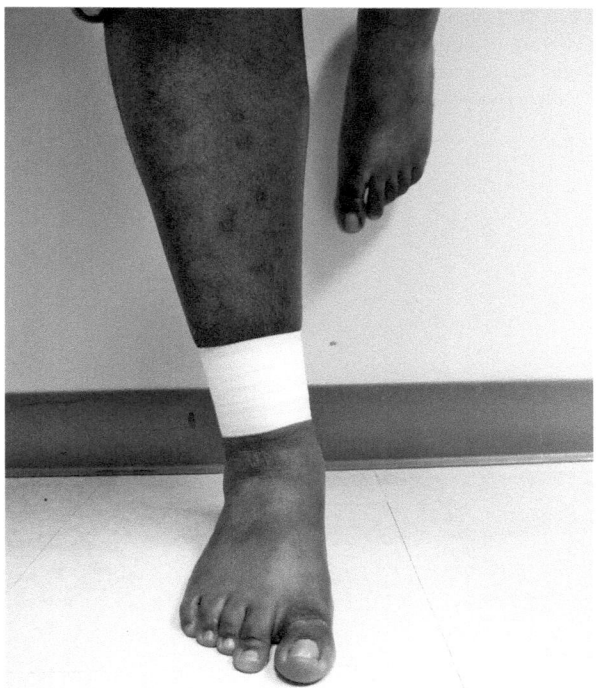

to identify injury at the ankle syndesmosis including the fibular squeeze, fibular translation, Cotton, and external rotation test.[10] Fibular squeeze test is performed by squeezing the fibula against the tibia at the proximal leg attempting to widen and elicit pain at the distal syndesmosis. A variation of this maneuver is the "cross-legged test" which is performed by having the patient rest the injured leg on the thigh of the contralateral limb to reproduce pain along the syndesmosis.[11] Another diagnostic test is the "stabilization test" which involves circumferential taping to stabilize the ankle syndesmosis (see Fig. 10.1). The test is considered positive for syndesmosis injury if the patient is able to perform standing, walking, and heel rises after taping.[12] The external rotation test or the Kleiger's test involves externally rotating the foot on the leg attempting to elicit pain by widening the syndesmosis (see Fig. 10.2). In cadaveric studies, the external rotation test achieved the most widening of the syndesmosis and therefore is considered the most clinically provocative test for syndesmosis injury.[10] The interosseous tenderness length, which measures the distance of palpated pain from the syndesmosis, has been shown to correlate well with time to return to activity.[13]

10.6 Radiographs

Medial clear space, tibiofibular clear space, and tibiofibular overlap are com mon radiographic parameters used to measure anatomic joint alignment and syndesmosis integrity. Though commonly used, these radiographic parameters have

Fig. 10.2 External rotation of the foot on the leg can elicit acute pain to an injured ankle syndesmosis

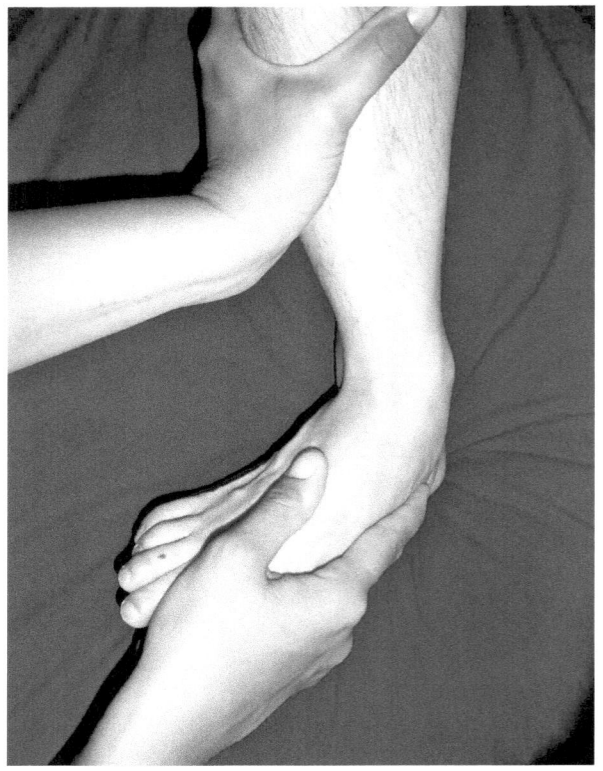

sensitivity for identifying occult syndesmosis injuries. In a study correlating radiographic and magnetic resonance imaging (MRI) for syndesmotic injuries, only medial clear space widening greater than 4 mm correlated with syndesmotic and deltoid ligament rupture (Fig. 10.3).[14]

10.7   Computed Tomography and Magnetic Resonance Imaging

Occult syndesmosis injuries are often subtle and difficult to identify with conventional radiographic studies in the absence of frank diastasis. Axial views of the syndesmosis from computed tomography (CT) can improve detection of syndesmotic widening by quantitatively comparing tibial fibular distance to the contralateral limb. A difference of 2 mm or greater is considered abnormal.[15] Magnetic resonance imaging (MRI) can identify specific syndesmotic ligament

Fig. 10.3 Radiographic
findings of an increased
medial clear space and
tibiofibular clear space
widening are both indicators
of both deltoid and
syndesmotic disruption,
respectively

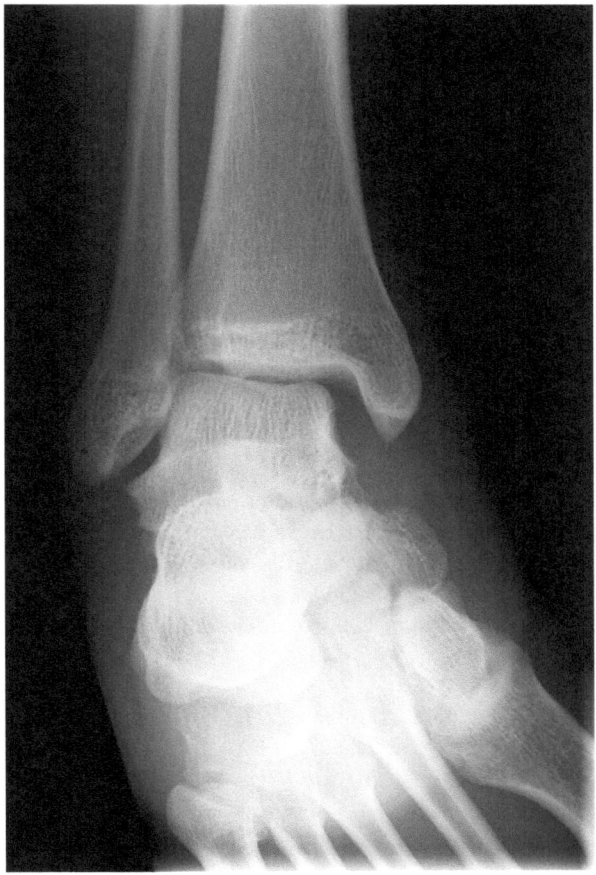

Fig. 10.3 Radiographic findings of an increased medial clear space and tibiofibular clear space widening are both indicators of both deltoid and syndesmotic disruption, respectively

tears with high sensitivity and specificity and can be used in conjunction with biomechanical criteria to predict degree of syndesmosis injury and level of instability.[16]

10.8 Stress Imaging

Stress imaging of ankle injuries can improve identification of syndesmosis injuries previously undetected by plain radiograph.[17] Ligamentous insufficiency can be detected with stress testing demonstrating increased medial clear space or tibiofibular clear space widening under radiograph or fluoroscopic imaging. The lateral stress test reproduces the greatest increase in tibiofibular clear space in experimentally induced syndesmotic ligaments injuries.[36] Results of stress testing may vary due to inconsistency of projection beam angle and stabilizing the proximal limb from motion during stress maneuver.

10.9   Nonsurgical Treatment

There is no consensus regarding the duration and method of treatment for nondisplaced syndesmotic injuries; however, most agree that these injuries recover well with a short course of immobilization followed by progressive stages of non-weight-bearing mobilization, resistance training, and functional rehabilitation.[13,18] A period of non-weight-bearing with the foot kept in slight plantarflexion, protected in a below-knee cast or brace should be rendered. Early institution of physical and manipulative therapy has been proposed in the rehabilitation of syndesmotic injuries; however, its role remains controversial and undocumented.

10.10   Surgical Treatment

Surgical intervention for tibiofibular syndesmotic injuries is indicated if greater than 2 mm of syndesmotic widening or greater than 4 mm of medial clear space widening of the ankle mortise is identified on radiograph or stress imaging. The authors also recommend stabilization when two or more syndesmotic ligaments are compromised with concomitant deltoid ligament injury, regardless of fibular position.

10.10.1   Surgical Technique

10.10.1.1   Positioning

Patient is placed in the supine position on the radiolucent operating room table. A bump may be placed beneath the hip of the surgical limb to internally rotate the ankle allowing surgical access to the lateral ankle and proper positioning of fluoroscopic C-arm imaging. Folded blankets are used to elevate the surgical limb to avoid obstruction of contralateral limb during lateral imaging.

10.10.1.2   Reduction of the Syndesmosis

The tips of the medial and lateral malleoli of the ankle are identified. The syndesmosis is reduced by placing a reduction clamp across the medial and lateral malleoli matching the biomechanical axis of the ankle. This axis is approximately 25° from posterolateral to anteromedial direction (Fig. 10.4). Once clamp is tightened, reduction is verified with mortise and anterior-posterior views under fluoroscopy (Fig. 10.5).

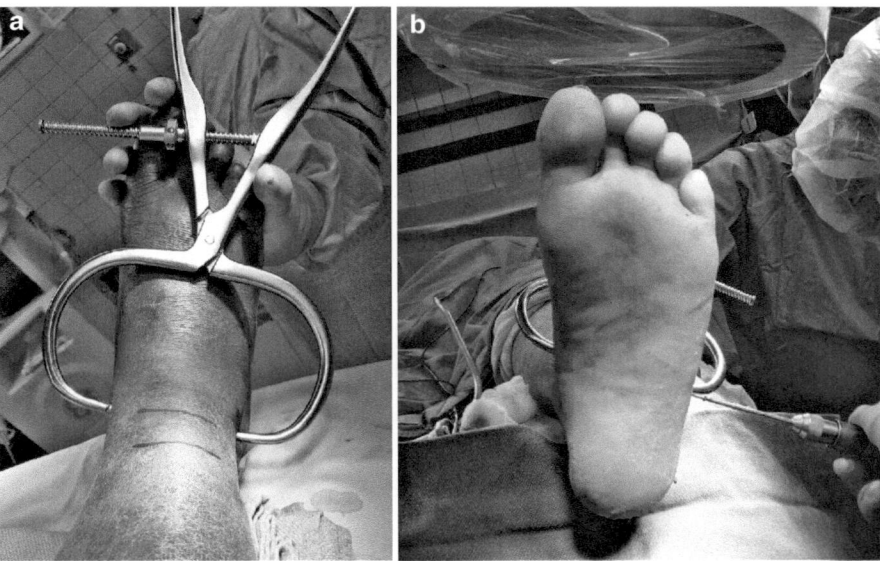

Fig. 10.4 (**a**) Periarticular reduction clamp traverses the bi-malleolar axis of the ankle. (**b**) The tips of the reduction clamp are positioned approximately 20–25° posterolateral to anteromedial matching the bi-malleolar axis

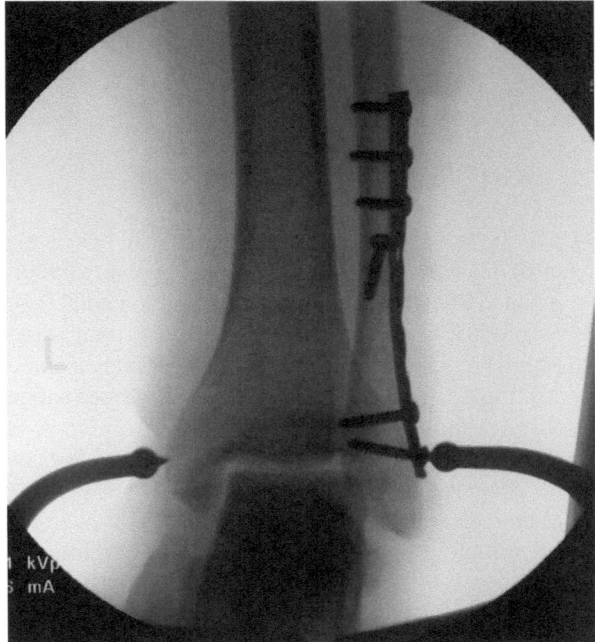

Fig. 10.5 Once the periarticular clamp is tightened, fluoroscopic imaging is used to verify syndesmotic reduction

Fig. 10.6 Two 3.5 fully threaded cortical screws are placed through a one-third tubular plate to increase torsional stability and purchase of the screws

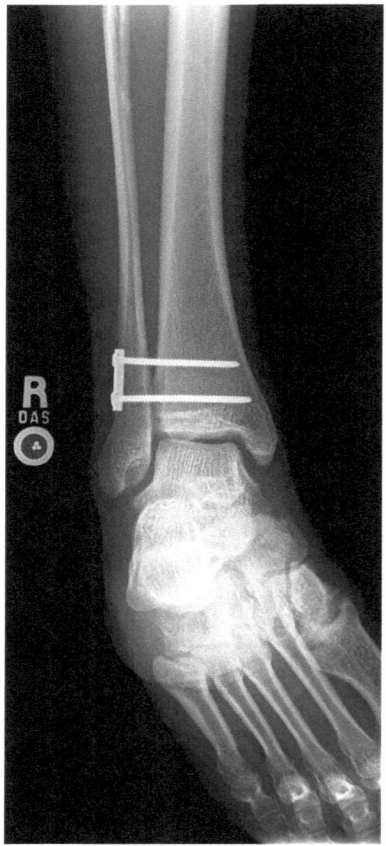

10.10.1.3   Screw Fixation

Under fluoroscopic imaging, a 2.5-mm drill hole is made from the fibula to the tibia approximately 1.5–2.0 cm superior as well as parallel to the tibiotalar joint line and angulated 25° from posterolateral to anteromedial trajectory. The cortices are tapped to avoid distraction of the fibula from the tibia when engaging the 3.5-mm screw through the third cortex and to achieve non-lag technique. The hole is measured and a 3.5-mm fully threaded cortical screw is placed tricortically maintaining the reduction of the tibiofibular syndesmosis. Two 3.5-mm fully threaded cortical screws with tricortical purchase or one 4.5-mm fully threaded cortical screw tetracortical have equivocal purchase strength.[19]

Screw fixation through a one-third tubular plate can increase stability of fixation by distributing the stress of screw head purchase to the fibula.[20] For an isolated syndesmotic disruption without distal fibula fracture or syndesmotic disruptions with a Maisonneuve fracture, a 2-hole one-third tubular plate may be incorporated with transsyndesmotic fixation (Fig. 10.6).

10.10.1.4 Suture Button

A proposed advantage of tensioned suture button fixation of the syndesmosis was that it did not require removal. Though mechanical studies comparing the stability of suture versus screw fixation reveal that screw fixation better resists syndesmotic widening and external rotation compared to suture, there are no significance differences with clinical outcomes of either technique.[21–23]

Using the same drill hole orientation as described for transsyndesmotic screw fixation and with the reduction clamp in place, all four cortices are drilled. The straight needle attached to the suture-button fixation is passed from lateral to medial through the drill hole and out of the intact medial skin while avoiding injury of the saphenous nerve and vein. The oblong button is advanced through the drill hole of the medial tibial cortex. The two medial lead sutures are pulled in opposite directions to seat the oblong button flush to the medial tibial cortex. Both lead sutures are cut and removed. The suture attached to the trailing lateral button is tensioned by pulling on either free end of the suture tightening the syndesmosis. Once the lateral button is flush to the fibula, the suture ends are secured with 4–5 ties and cut 1 cm long to allow the knot to lay flush, reducing suture prominence. Position of the buttons is confirmed with fluoroscopy. A second tightrope may be placed 1 cm proximal using the same method but divergent angle to improve rotational stability (Fig. 10.7).

10.10.2 Postoperative Course

Though there is little consensus regarding postoperative weight-bearing status surgeons generally instruct patients to be non-weight-bearing for 6 weeks, then transition into a weight-bearing walking boot for 2 weeks, followed by a soft lace-up ankle brace thereafter. Despite studies reporting similar clinical outcomes whether syndesmosis screws were retained, removed, or eventually failed, the convention of practice is to remove the screws at 6–12 weeks.[24–27]

10.11 Rehabilitation

Early return to function is often the goal of either conservative or surgical treatment; however, timing of return may vary with the degree of injury and type of activity. Most rehabilitation programs involve three progressive phases of therapy. In the acute phase, protection of the limb by immobilization is needed to reduce the inflammatory response and pain of the acute injury or the immediate postoperative period. Goals of the second phase are to restore strength, mobility, and normal gait.

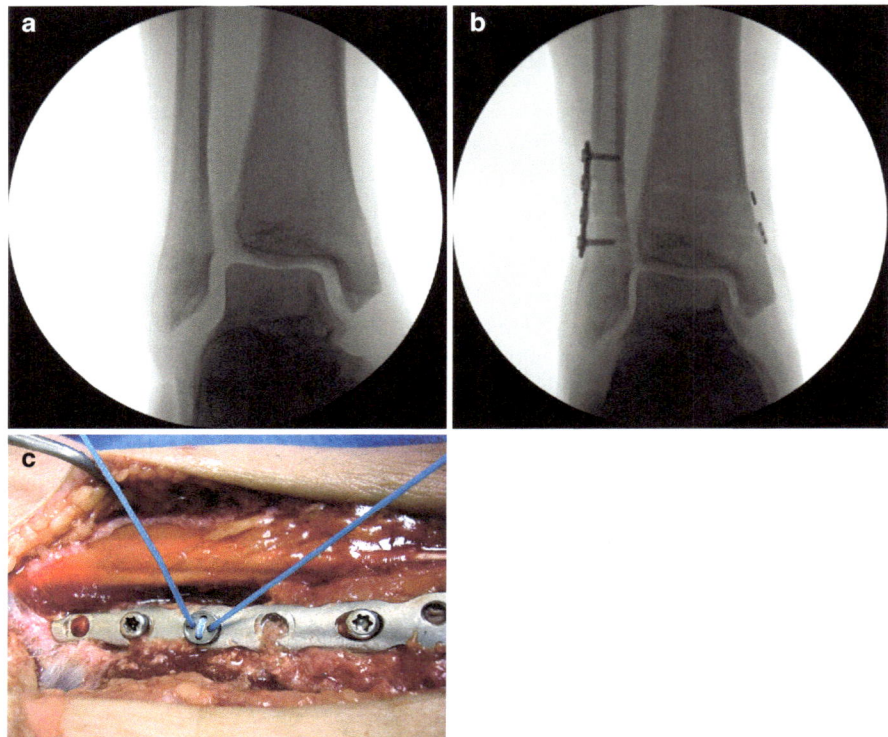

Fig. 10.7 (**a**) Widening of the syndesmosis with decreased tibiofibular overlap is identified. (**b**) Suture button is shown maintaining syndesmotic reduction. (**c**) Suture-button fixation provides adequate stability and more physiologic rehabilitation of the syndesmosis

Patients who are able to perform repetitive hopping without pain proceed to the final phase of rehabilitation which involves increasing strength, proprioception, neuro-muscular control, and sport-specific training.[2,13]

10.12 Outcomes

Anatomic reduction of the syndesmosis is the most important factor prognostic of outcomes regardless of method of stabilization. Nonanatomic reduction of the syn-desmosis correlates with fair-to-poor functional outcomes.[28,29] Mechanical studies simulating physiologic cyclic loading of both syndesmosis disruptions repaired with one tricortical 3.5-mm screw or Tightrope™ suture button (Arthrex Inc., Naples FL USA) demonstrate no significant changes in syndesmotic gapping between the two groups.[30] Though transsyndesmotic screw fixation exhibits improved stiffness and higher load to failure, clinical observational studies demonstrate no significant differences in outcomes between screw fixation and suture-button methods.[21,22,30]

10.13   Chronic Syndesmosis Injuries

Delayed diagnosis of syndesmosis injuries may lead to chronic ankle pain, instability, and eventually posttraumatic arthritis.[29,31–34] Symptoms of chronic syndesmosis injuries may include continued low-to-moderate grade pain, sensation of instability, and inability to return to pre-injury activities. Clinical findings are often less specific; therefore, diagnostic studies including bilateral weight-bearing radiographs and stress radiographs are often useful in identifying diastasis. CT is the diagnostic study of choice to quantitatively detect widening of the syndesmosis. MRI can identify chronic ligament tears of the syndesmosis, incongruencies of the tibiofibular joint, and syndesmotic widening.[35]

Open or arthroscopic debridement of the syndesmotic ligaments, without addressing the functional insufficiency of the syndesmotic ligaments, may lead to continued instability. Conventional treatment of chronic syndesmosis injuries entails debridement of the disorganized scarred ligamentous tissues, anatomic reduction of the fibula into the tibial incisura, and stable transsyndesmotic fixation in hopes to achieve stable fibrosis of the syndesmosis. Ligamentoplasty or ligament reconstruction of the tibiofibular syndesmosis can be performed in chronically unstable syndesmosis injuries in young, high demand patients without manifestations of degenerative arthritis or if little viable ligaments remain for adequate healing of the ankle syndesmosis. Ligamentoplasty with split peroneus longus tendon autograft weaved through distal tibial and fibular canals reproducing anatomic locations of the anterior, posterior tibiofibular, and interosseous ligaments has been reported to be effective in reduction of ankle pain and eliminating instability associated with chronic syndesmotic ankle injuries[31] (Fig. 10.8).

Fig. 10.8 Peroneus longus tendon allograft is routed circumferentially about the distal tibiofibular syndesmosis through anterior-posterior drill holes in both tibia and fibula. The allograft is tightened and secured with an interference screw within the tibia and depending on the fibula's width, either an interference screw or an anchor laterally

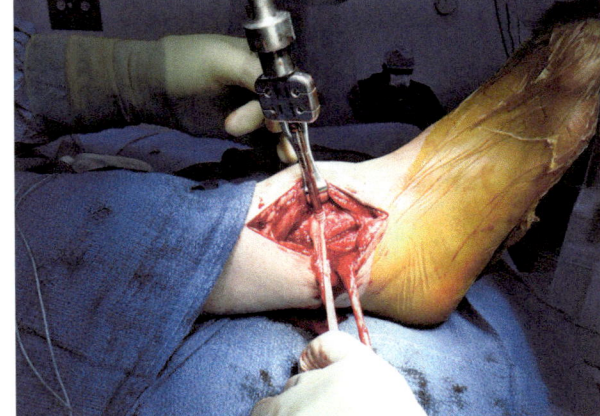

References

1. Jensen SL, Andresen BK, Mencke S, et al. Epidemiology of ankle fractures. A prospective population-based study of 212 cases in Aalborg, Denmark. Acta Orthop Scand. 1998;69(1):48–50.
2. Gerber JP, Williams GN, Scoville CR, et al. Persistent disability associated with ankle sprains: a prospective examination of an athletic population. Foot Ankle Int. 1998;19(10):653–60.
3. Hopkinson WJ, St Pierre P, Ryan JB, et al. Syndesmosis sprains of the ankle. Foot Ankle. 1990;10(6):325–30.
4. Xenos JS, Hopkinson WJ, Mulligan ME, et al. The tibiofibular syndesmosis. Evaluation of the ligamentous structures, methods of fixation, and radiographic assessment. J Bone Joint Surg Am. 1995;77(6):847–56.
5. Ogilvie-Harris DJ, Reed SC, Hedman TP. Disruption of the ankle syndesmosis: biomechanical study of the ligamentous restraints. Arthroscopy. 1994;10(5):558–60.
6. Close JR. Some applications of the functional anatomy of the ankle joint. J Bone Joint Surg Am. 1956;38-A(4):761–81.
7. Peter RE, Harrington RM, Henley MB, et al. Biomechanical effects of internal fixation of the distal tibiofibular syndesmotic joint: comparison of two fixation techniques. J Orthop Trauma. 1994;8(3):215–9.
8. Boytim MJ, Fischer DA, Neumann L. Syndesmotic ankle sprains. Am J Sports Med. 1991;19(3):294–8.
9. Stuart MJ, Smith A. Injuries in Junior A ice hockey. A three-year prospective study. Am J Sports Med. 1995;23(4):458–61.
10. Beumer A, van Hemert WL, Swierstra BA, et al. A biomechanical evaluation of clinical stress tests for syndesmotic ankle instability. Foot Ankle Int. 2003;24(4):358–63.
11. Kiter E, Bozkurt M. The crossed-leg test for examination of ankle syndesmosis injuries. Foot Ankle Int. 2005;26(2):187–8.
12. Williams GN, Jones MH, Amendola A. Syndesmotic ankle sprains in athletes. Am J Sports Med. 2007;35(7):1197–207.
13. Nussbaum ED, Hosea TM, Sieler SD, et al. Prospective evaluation of syndesmotic ankle sprains without diastasis. Am J Sports Med. 2001;29(1):31–5.
14. Nielson JH, Gardner MJ, Peterson MG, et al. Radiographic measurements do not predict syndesmotic injury in ankle fractures: an MRI study. Clin Orthop Relat Res. 2005;436:216–21.
15. Ebraheim NA, Lu J, Yang H, et al. Radiographic and CT evaluation of tibiofibular syndesmotic diastasis: a cadaver study. Foot Ankle Int. 1997;18(11):693–8.
16. Oae K, Takao M, Naito K, et al. Injury of the tibiofibular syndesmosis: value of MR imaging for diagnosis. Radiology. 2003;227(1):155–61.
17. Jenkinson RJ, Sanders DW, Macleod MD, et al. Intraoperative diagnosis of syndesmosis injuries in external rotation ankle fractures. J Orthop Trauma. 2005;19(9):604–9.
18. Brosky T, Nyland J, Nitz A, et al. The ankle ligaments: consideration of syndesmotic injury and implications for rehabilitation. J Orthop Sports Phys Ther. 1995;21(4):197–205.
19. Hoiness P, Stromsoe K. Tricortical versus quadricortical syndesmosis fixation in ankle fractures: a prospective, randomized study comparing two methods of syndesmosis fixation. J Orthop Trauma. 2004;18(6):331–7.
20. Ho JY, Ren Y, Kelikian A, et al. Mid-diaphyseal fibular fractures with syndesmotic disruption: should we plate the fibula? Foot Ankle Int. 2008;29(6):587–92.
21. Forsythe K, Freedman KB, Stover MD, et al. Comparison of a novel fiberwire-button construct versus metallic screw fixation in a syndesmotic injury model. Foot Ankle Int. 2008;29(1):49–54.
22. Cottom JM, Hyer CF, Philbin TM, et al. Transosseous fixation of the distal tibiofibular syndesmosis: comparison of an interosseous suture and endobutton to traditional screw fixation in 50 cases. J Foot Ankle Surg. 2009;48(6):620–30.
23. Thornes B, Shannon F, Guiney AM, et al. Suture-button syndesmosis fixation: accelerated rehabilitation and improved outcomes. Clin Orthop Relat Res. 2005;431:207–12.

24. Miller AN, Paul O, Boraiah S, et al. Functional outcomes after syndesmotic screw fixation and removal. J Orthop Trauma. 2010;24(1):12–6.
25. Manjoo A, Sanders DW, Tieszer C, et al. Functional and radiographic results of patients with syndesmotic screw fixation: implications for screw removal. J Orthop Trauma. 2010;24(1):2–6.
26. Bell DP, Wong MK. Syndesmotic screw fixation in Weber C ankle injuries – should the screw be removed before weight bearing? Injury. 2006;37(9):891–8.
27. Moore JA Jr, Shank JR, Morgan SJ, et al. Syndesmosis fixation: a comparison of three and four cortices of screw fixation without hardware removal. Foot Ankle Int. 2006;27(8):567–72.
28. Weening B, Bhandari M. Predictors of functional outcome following transsyndesmotic screw fixation of ankle fractures. J Orthop Trauma. 2005;19(2):102–8.
29. Chissell HR, Jones J. The influence of a diastasis screw on the outcome of Weber type-C ankle fractures. J Bone Joint Surg Br. 1995;77(3):435–8.
30. Klitzman R, Zhao H, Zhang LQ, et al. Suture-button versus screw fixation of the syndesmosis: a biomechanical analysis. Foot Ankle Int. 2010;31(1):69–75.
31. Grass R, Rammelt S, Biewener A, et al. Peroneus longus ligamentoplasty for chronic instability of the distal tibiofibular syndesmosis. Foot Ankle Int. 2003;24(5):392–7.
32. Edwards GS Jr, DeLee JC. Ankle diastasis without fracture. Foot Ankle. 1984;4(6):305–12.
33. Endean T, King W, Martin R. Syndesmotic rupture without ankle fracture: a report of two cases in professional football players. J Am Podiatr Med Assoc. 2003;93(4):336–9.
34. Kennedy JG, Soffe KE, Dalla Vedova P, et al. Evaluation of the syndesmotic screw in low Weber C ankle fractures. J Orthop Trauma. 2000;14(5):359–66.
35. Brown KW, Morrison WB, Schweitzer ME, et al. MRI findings associated with distal tibiofibular syndesmosis injury. AJR Am J Roentgenol. 2004;182(1):131–6.
36. Stoffe K, Wysocki D, Baddour E, et al. Comparison of two Intraoperative assessment methods for injuries to the ankle syndesmosis: a cadaveric study. J Bone Joint Surg Am. 2009;91:2646–52.

Chapter 11
Acute Repair of Ruptured Foot and Ankle Tendons in Athletic Patients

Amol Saxena

Acute tendon ruptures in the sports medicine population occur most commonly in the Achilles tendon. Literature supports surgical treatment of acute complete Achilles tendon tears, particularly in athletic and hi-demand individuals.[1-4] Partial tears in high-level athletes may also warrant surgical treatment. Achilles ruptures occur in many sports and patients often recount feeling and even hearing a "pop." A palpable dell or soft spot is noted. Diagnosis is often confirmed via the calf squeeze ("Thompson" test) or "Matles" sign which are positive for rupture if the foot does not plantarflex (Fig. 11.1). Inability to heel-raise on the injured limb is also noted (though this may be present with other ankle tendon ruptures). Other diagnostic tests such as ultrasound and magnetic resonance imaging (MRI) are often not needed. It should be noted that medications such as quinolones and steroids, along with medical conditions such as gout and inflammatory arthropathies, can induce tendon rupture.

11.1 Surgical Treatment of Acute Achilles Tendon Ruptures

The acutely ruptured Achilles can be repaired by open, "mini-open," and percutaneous techniques. Research has shown that open repair has lower incidence of re-rupture but greater wound complications. Predominantly, a medial longitudinal approach for an open procedure is utilized. The surgery is performed with the patient in the prone position and can be performed without a tourniquet and with local anesthesia or regional block. The frayed tendons' ends are debrided (Fig. 11.2). Krackow suture technique on both ruptured ends is used to re-approximate the

A. Saxena, D.P.M.
Department of Sports Medicine, PAFMG-Palo Alto Division,
Clark Bldg., 3rd Flr, 795 El Camino Real, Palo Alto, CA 94301, USA
e-mail: heysax@aol.com

A. Saxena (ed.), *Sports Medicine and Arthroscopic Surgery of the Foot and Ankle*,   131
DOI 10.1007/978-1-4471-4106-8_11, © Springer-Verlag London 2013

Fig. 11.1 Positive Matles' sign of the near Achilles tendon confirming rupture as represented by the inability of the foot to stay passively plantarflexed

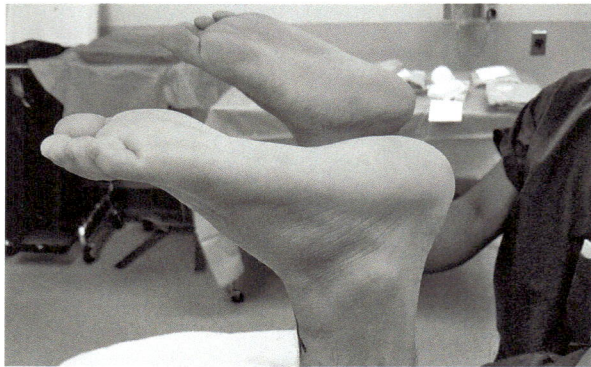

Fig. 11.2 Achilles tendon rupture

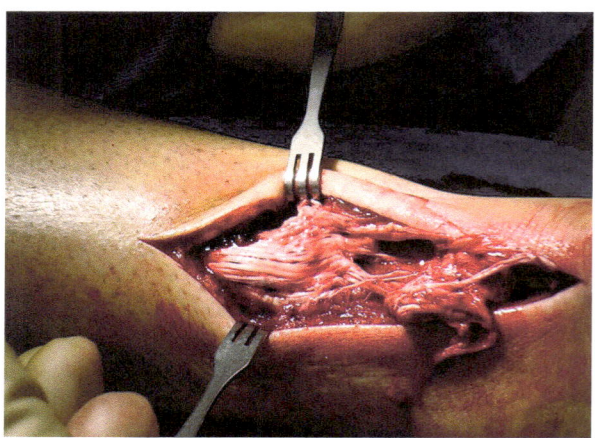

ruptured Achilles tendon with the foot maintained in a plantarflexed position generally with #2 suture (Fig. 11.3).[1] Additional reinforcement can be performed with smaller gauge suture such as 2–0, and subcutaneous tissues are closed in layers, avoiding tension over the tendon and skin (Fig. 11.4). Both open and percutaneous techniques can be performed with absorbable or nonabsorbable sutures, with the former more prevalent in Europe and the latter more common in North America. Granuloma and suture reaction can occur regardless of suture material.[5] Percutaneous and "mini-open" techniques may be beneficial in females and those with history of keloid formation.[3,4] The re-rupture incidence and nerve entrapment occurrence are higher with these techniques as compared to open repair. Maffulli et al. modified the traditional percutaneous technique to avoid sural nerve entrapment. They biased the proximal percutaneous incisions more medially (Fig. 11.5).[4] Gaps larger than 5 cm that cannot be bridged by turn-down flaps or gastrocnemius recession may need to be addressed by flexor tendon (usually FHL) or peroneus brevis transfer, the latter

Fig. 11.3 Krackow suture technique

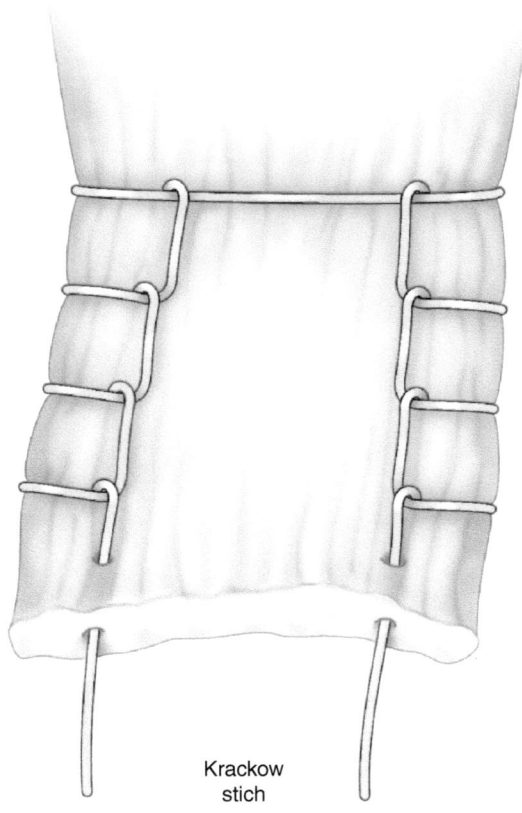

Krackow
stich

of which may be better in athletic patients though not yet critically studied.[4,5] Postoperatively, the ruptured Achilles tendon is protected by a below-knee cast/ boot, or an anterior splint to prevent dorsiflexion, with the foot in equinus, and kept non-weight-bearing for approximately 2 weeks. Randomized study comparing non-weight-bearing of 1 week versus 3 weeks showed no difference.[2] Progression to weight-bearing occurs with gradual reduction of equinus over the next several weeks, often in a boot with heel wedges that can be gradually decreased. Physical therapy consists of progressive strengthening (initially with surgical tubing and/or a towel at 3 weeks) including single-legged heel raises. A heel cushion (6-mm heel lift) may be maintained (bilaterally) for 6 or more months post-op. Return to daily activities takes at least 8–12 weeks with return to sports occurring at 12–26 weeks. A detailed physical therapy regimen is found in Chap. 18 [Rehabilitation].

Fig. 11.4 (**a**) Repaired
tendon. (**b**) Skin suture

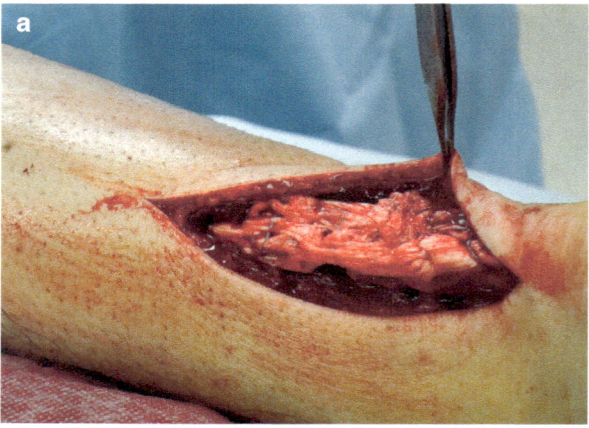

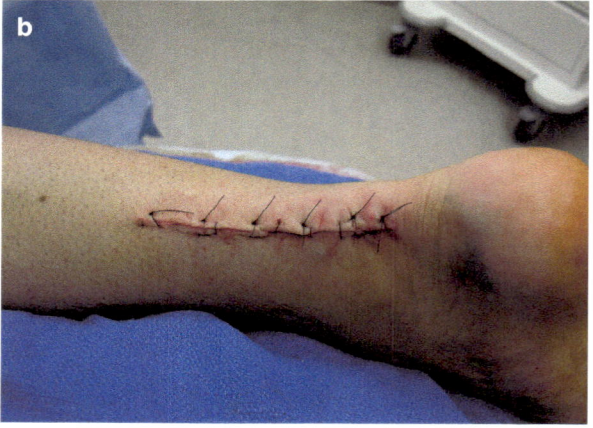

Fig. 11.5 Modified
percutaneous Achilles tendon
repair incisions as described
by Carmont and Maffulli[4]

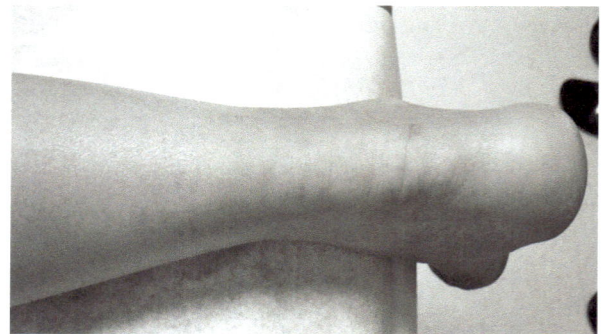

11.2 Miscellaneous Foot and Ankle Tendon Ruptures

Other ankle tendon ruptures such as with peroneal tendons can occur acutely particularly with inversion ankle injuries in sports.[6-12] These are discussed in detail, elsewhere in this text, as well as surgical treatment of chronic Achilles tendinopathy. Acute tendon ruptures of the anterior and posterior tibial tendons, though somewhat rare in sports, are often dealt with surgically. This usually involves primary repair, generally using suture anchors for avulsion type injuries. Though tibialis anterior ruptures with significant gapping, it can be repaired with transfer of extensor hallucis longus (EHL) (and tenodesis of the distal stump to the extensor hallucis brevis [EHB]); loss of dorsiflexion strength may be an issue in athletes. A free graft of "doubled" EHB (first extensor tendon of extensor digitorum brevis) can be used to bridge the defect (Figs. 11.6 and 11.7). Similarly, transfer of flexor digitorum longus (FDL) for posterior tibial tendon tears may not be ideal in athletic patients, and direct repair should be attempted when possible.

Acute posterior tibial ruptures and accessory navicular/os tibiale externum injuries occur in athletes as well. Excision of the displaced ossicle, (particularly if it results in functional loss of strength of the posterior tibial tendon and is a re-injury or significantly gapped), débridement of the degenerated tendon, and reattachment of the insertion to a more plantar location are recommended. Manipulating the foot in a supinated position while inserting the anchor to the inferior navicular (instead of medial) is helpful when reattaching the posterior tibial tendon (Fig. 11.8).[7-9] Assessment as to the patient's foot structure and potential need for concomitant procedures is paramount. Some recent studies show re-fixation of a displaced accessory navicular may be worth considering as an alternative to excision (i.e., "Kidner" procedure).[10,11]

Less common are acute flexor and extensor tendon injuries in the region of the ankle, though these can be associated with prior corticosteroid injection in the vicinity of the rupture. Traumatic laceration of ankle tendons can occur in athletes, often as open injuries in martial arts, cycling, and occasionally in contact sports. The standard principles of wound débridement and primary tendon repair are performed. Elsewhere in this text are descriptions of secondary tendon repair and transfer techniques that can be utilized as the situation deems.

Generally, athletic patients with tendon tears are protected with non-weight-bearing immobilization for 3 weeks. They are able to utilize a stationary bike with a boot or cast during this time. After 3 weeks, progressive weight-bearing and strengthening occurs. Active range-of-motion exercises can occur at this time, though tendons that tend to get adhered, such as the extensor hallucis longus at the level of the first metatarsal phalangeal joint (MPJ), can be mobilized sooner. Hallux dorsiflexion is important particularly for athletes, and extensor injuries to the great toe should not be trivialized, even in children. If rehabilitated properly, most athletic patients with acute foot and ankle tendon ruptures can return to sports, though full return can take 1 year. Details on rehabilitation techniques are found in Chap. 18.

136

A. Saxena

Fig. 11.6 (**a**) Lateral. (**b**) Axial MRI of complete tibialis anterior rupture

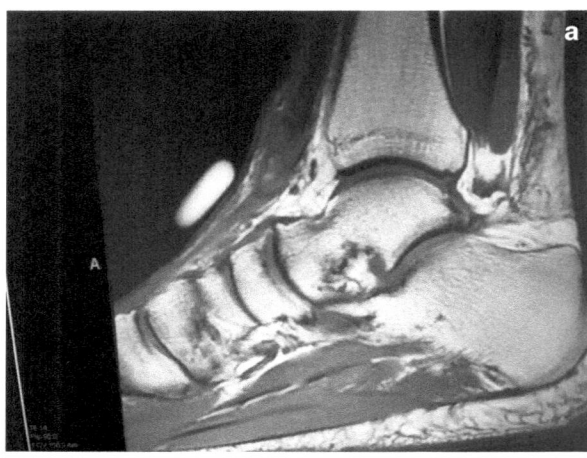
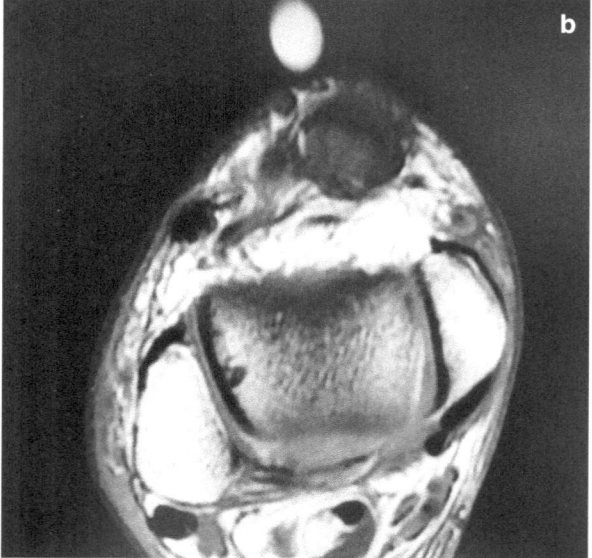

Fig. 11.7 (**a**) and (**b**) Tibialis anterior rupture repaired with free graft of doubled extensor hallucis brevis (first tendon of extensor digitorum brevis)

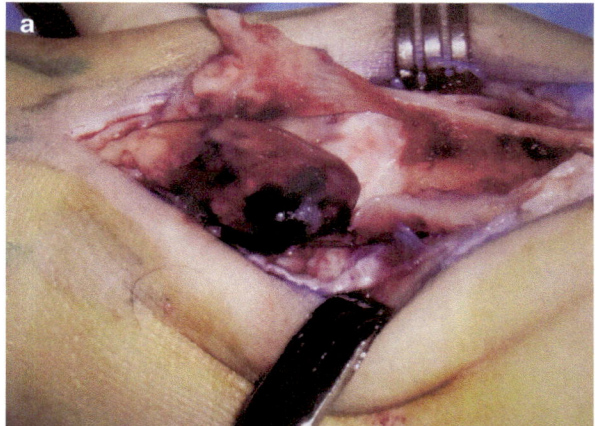

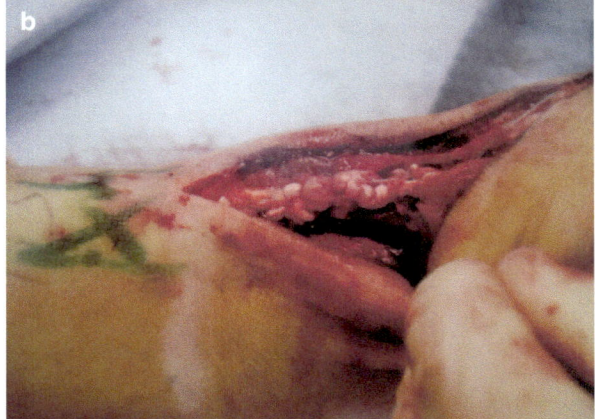

Fig. 11.8 (**a**) and (**b**) Avulsed posterior tibial tendon reattachment with anchor in an athletic patient. Foot is supinated to allow for more plantar reattachment of the tendon. Note placement of subtalar arthroereisis due to his flexible but significantly pronated foot structure. He is still playing tennis with the implant intact 4 years post-op

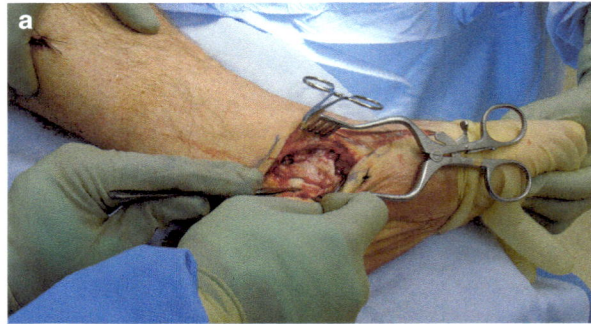

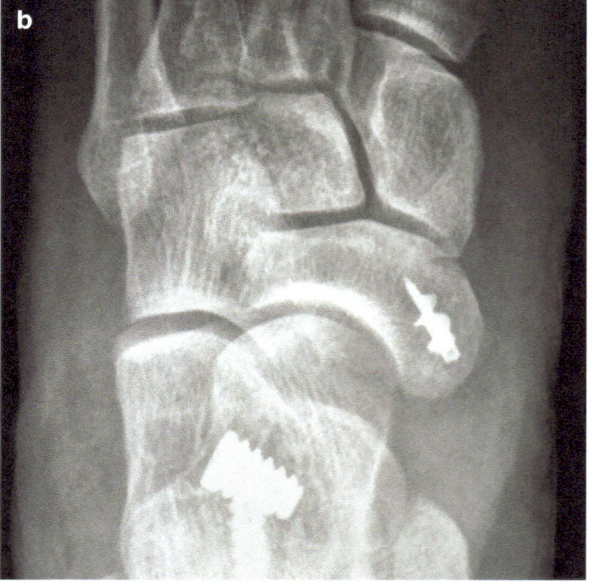

References

1. Mandelbaum BR, Myerson MS, Forster R. Achilles tendon ruptures: a new method of repair, early range of motion, and functional rehabilitation. Am J Sports Med. 1995;23:392–5.
2. Maffulli N, Tallon C, Wong J, Lim K, Bleakney R. Early weightbearing and ankle mobilization after open repair of acute midsubstance tears of the Achilles tendon. Am J Sports Med. 2003;31:692–700.
3. Bradley J, Tibone J. Percutaneous and open surgical repairs of Achilles tendon ruptures. a comparative study. Am J Sports Med. 1990;18(2):188–95.
4. Carmont M, Maffulli N. Modified percutaneous repair of ruptured Achilles tendon. Knee Surg Sports Traumatol Arthrosc. 2008;16:199–203.
5. Saxena A, Maffulli N, Nguyen A, Li A. Wound complications from surgeries pertaining to the Achilles tendon: an analysis of 219 surgeries. J Am Podiatr Med Assoc. 2008;98:95–101.
6. Saxena A, Cassidy A. Peroneal tendon injuries: an evaluation of 49 tears in 41 patients. J Foot Ankle Surg. 2003;42(4):215–20.
7. Porter DA, Baxter DE, Clanton TO, Klootwyk TE. Posterior tibial tendon tears in young competitive athletes: two case reports. Foot Ankle Int. 1998;19(9):627–30.
8. Subotnick S. Ankle tendons in sports medicine of the lower extremity. New York: Churchill Livingstone; 2004. p. 261–76.
9. Title CI, Schon LC. Achilles tendon disorders including tendinosis and tears. In: Porter DA, Schon LC, editors. Baxter's the foot and ankle in sports. 2nd ed. Philadelphia: Elsevier; 2008. p. 147–81.
10. Chung JW, Chu IT. Outcome of fusion of a painful accessory navicular to the primary navicular. Foot Ankle Int. 2009;30(2):106–9.
11. Scott AT, Sabesan VJ, Saluta JR, Wilson MA, Easley ME. Fusion versus excision of the symptomatic Type II accessory navicular: a prospective study. Foot Ankle Int. 2009;30(1):10–5.
12. Coughlin MJ, Schon LC. Disorders of tendons. In: Coughlin MJ, Mann RA, Saltzman CL, editors. Surgery of the foot and ankle. 8th ed. Philadelphia: Mosby; 2007. p. 1149–277.

Chapter 12
Chronic Compartment Syndrome of Leg and Foot

Richard T. Bouché

12.1 Introduction

As endurance sports and training continue to be popular, exercise-induced leg and foot pathologies have mandated increased attention from sports physicians – common and uncommon causes should be considered.[1,2] One uncommon entity that has gained popularity and is being recognized earlier in the clinical course is chronic compartment syndrome (CCS).[3] CCS has been reported in various lower extremity locations with the leg far and away being the most common location.[4] This section will review basic though important concepts about CCS as it applies to the leg and foot. Emphasis will be on clinical presentation and management.

12.2 Definition

Generically speaking, compartment syndrome (CS) is a condition in which increased pressure within a closed anatomical space (compartments of foot and/or leg) compromises the circulation (resulting in ischemia) which in turn compromises the function of muscle and nerve tissues within that space.[5] This compromise in circulation can result in temporary or permanent damage to the involved nerve and muscle tissues depending on the type of CS involved.[6]

R.T. Bouché, D.P.M.
The Sports Medicine Clinic, Northwest Hospital,
10330 Meridian Ave. N., Suite 300, Seattle, WA 98133, USA
e-mail: rbouche@nwhsea.org

A. Saxena (ed.), *Sports Medicine and Arthroscopic Surgery of the Foot and Ankle*, 141
DOI 10.1007/978-1-4471-4106-8_12, © Springer-Verlag London 2013

12.3   Classification

CS can be classified as acute or chronic. Acute compartment syndrome (ACS) is commonly due to trauma and rarely to exercise.[6] ACS is a medical emergency requiring prompt recognition and treatment. Absolute pressure measurement, symptom duration, and careful clinical assessment and monitoring are key factors in determining need for fasciotomy. In contrast, CCS is a chronic, exercise-induced condition characterized by recurrent pain and disability and is commonly encountered in military and sports populations. A transient (temporary) form of CCS has also been encountered by the author in the leg and foot. Onset of the problem coincides with initiation of a new activity (usually running) with no previous history of CCS symptoms being related.

12.4   Etiology/Pathophysiology

Though speculative, all previous theories concerning the pathophysiology of CS propose that an increase in intra-compartment pressure to a critical level results in a compromise in tissue perfusion[5,7-10] though this concept has been challenged.[11] Increased tissue pressure may result from various situations including limited or decreased compartment volume (i.e., tight, noncompliant fascia), increased compartment content (i.e., muscle swelling and hypertrophy), and externally applied pressure (i.e., constricting hosiery, shoes, casts, etc.).[12] CCS is likely caused by a congenitally tight, thickened, and noncompliant fascia affecting the leg and foot which does not allow an increase in compartment volume during exercise. Transient CCS is probably the result of excessively swollen muscles due to lack of conditioning resulting in decreased compartment content. To explain the compromise in tissue perfusion, the author (RTB) favors Matsen's arteriovenous-gradient theory as this theory correlates well with the clinical findings of CCS and emphasizes the interrelationships of tissue pressure, local venous pressure, local blood flow, and metabolic tissue demands.[5] According to this theory, increase in tissue pressure increases local venous pressure, reducing the local arteriovenous gradient. This results in reduced blood flow and oxygenation, compromising tissue function and viability. Because compartment pressure is usually less than arterial blood pressure, distal arterial blood flow and peripheral pulses remain intact. The digital capillary bed drains into extra-compartmental veins, and the digital arteriovenous gradient and blood flow remain intact. Thus, peripheral pulses and digital circulation are poor indicators of blood flow within the compartment as they are typically intact.

12.5   Clinical Presentation

Being consistent with the definition,[13] there are four criteria that need to be met to make a clinical diagnosis of CCS[8]:

- Specific anatomic location (signs and symptoms localized to one or more of the four-leg compartments or ten-foot compartments)
- Evidence of increased tissue pressure (patient relates severe tightness and pain and exam will reveal induration to touch of involved compartment)
- Compromised circulation (patient relates pain out of proportion with pain elicited on passive stretch of involved compartment)
- Neuromuscular dysfunction (patient relates numbness and weakness, exam reveals weakness of muscles, and hyperesthesia of involved intra-compartmental nerves)

12.5.1   History

Patients with CCS all relate similar complaints of long-standing exercise-induced leg or arch pain (with the exception of transient CCS which is short lived) aggravated by sports activity and relieved by rest. In the leg, anterior and lateral compartments are more involved than deep and superficial posterior compartments. In the foot, involvement of the medial, superficial, and calcaneal compartments predominates with the medial compartment being most commonly implicated.[14-17] Activities of daily living are usually well tolerated. Consistent, reproducible, localized symptoms include an onset of tightness, intense pain (cramping), numbness, and weakness after a specific amount of exercise as measured by time or distance. Patients cannot exercise through the pain because it is so severe and they must stop to rest. Complete relief is obtained after a short period of rest (minutes to hours) before exercise can be resumed. Symptoms can be induced in less time if the leg or foot is constricted externally by tight shoes, hosiery, taping, etc.

12.5.2   Physical Examination

Examination for CCS mandates a static and especially a dynamic exam after exercise. Exam at rest (before exercise) is typically unremarkable. A prominent muscle or a muscle herniation may be apparent. Pulses and capillary refill time are normal.

Symptoms are reproduced after an exercise challenge involving the offending sports specific activity. Again circulation is checked with pulses and capillary refill typically being normal. If pulses are abnormal or digital pallor is observed, then a vascular etiology should be sought. Exam after activity reveals induration (firmness) of the involved compartment with pain on passive stretch of the involved intra-compartment muscles of leg or foot. Nerve exam reveals hyperesthesia of the involved nerves, and muscle exam statically and dynamically reveals weakness with probable gait abnormality (i.e., foot slap with steppage gait for anterior CCS of leg).

12.6   Differential Diagnosis

CCS of the leg and foot should be considered under the broad category of claudication syndromes. Problems in this category all present classically with no pain at rest and pain induced by exercise relieved by rest. Claudication syndromes can be divided into vascular and nonvascular problems.[18] Vascular problems would include arterial disorders (i.e., arterial occlusive disease, popliteal artery entrapment, adductor outlet, external ilio-femoral endofibrosis, etc.), venous claudication (secondary to previous ilio-femoral deep venous thrombosis), and CCS (leg and foot). Nonvascular problems would include neurogenic disorders (i.e., spinal stenosis [pseudoclaudication], common peroneal nerve entrapment, etc.), systemic problems (i.e., anemias, congestive heart failure), vitamin deficiencies (i.e., vitamin B1), and muscle enzyme disorders (muscle phosphorylase deficiency).

Other common musculoskeletal problems are commonly confused with CCS. A careful evaluation will differentiate these problems as the problems listed below all present with signs and symptoms at rest. Tibialis anterior muscle soreness/strain and tibial stress syndrome (shin-splints) are commonly mistaken for CCS of the leg. Plantar fascial strain, and abductor hallucis muscle soreness/strain are commonly mistaken for CCS of the foot.

12.7   Diagnostic Testing

The role of diagnostic testing is to objectively confirm the suspicion of CCS surmised from the history and physical examination. Though magnetic resonance imaging (MRI) has been explored recently,[11,19] the gold standard remains compartment pressure measurement (CPM). A noninvasive technique called near-infrared radiofrequency has shown promise on initial studies and correlates well with CPM.[20,21] Based on previous publications[22,23] and the author's experience with CCS of the leg and foot, the following criteria are recommended for confirming the diagnosis of CCS:

• Resting pressures greater than 10 mmHg (normal resting measurements before exercise should be 10 mmHg or less)

Fig. 12.1 Compartment
pressure measuring device

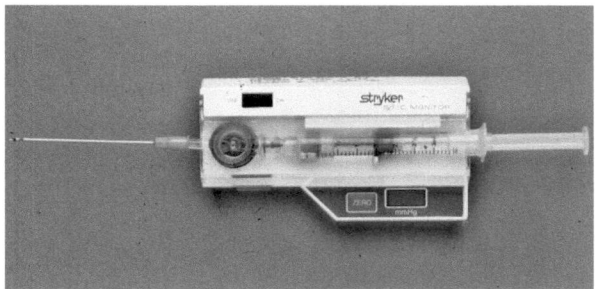

- Immediate static pressure measurements greater than 35 mmHg (obtained within 30 s after provocative exercise and with reproduction of symptoms)
- 5 minute reading greater than 20 mmHg
- Prolonged return to resting measurement greater than 6 min

These are all consistent with a diagnosis of CCS. CPM is typically performed with commercially available instrumentation that allows accurate and reproducible measurements (Fig. 12.1). The four compartments of the leg and the multiple compartments of the foot can all be measured though care must be taken to appreciate local anatomy and location of vital neurovascular structures. Special care needs to be taken when measuring the deep posterior compartment of the leg and the superficial and calcaneal compartments of the foot. The posterior tibial neurovascular bundle in the deep posterior leg compartment and the medial and lateral plantar neurovascular bundle in the superficial and calcaneal foot compartments, respectively, need to be protected.

12.8   Treatment

Treatment options for CCS include living with the problem, conservative treatment, and definitive surgical fasciotomy of the involved leg and foot compartments. If the patient opts to live with their problem, they must be made aware that they will be at increased risk of ACS due to the patient being less tolerant to increases in compartment pressure.[24] Education about both forms of ACS is mandatory so that the patient knows what to expect if this medical emergency occurs.

12.8.1   Conservative Treatment

Conservative care is symptomatic and mainly consists of avoidance of offending activities and participating in other activities "to tolerance." Anecdotal reports of deep massage have been shown to be beneficial for CCS of the leg.[25] Foot orthoses

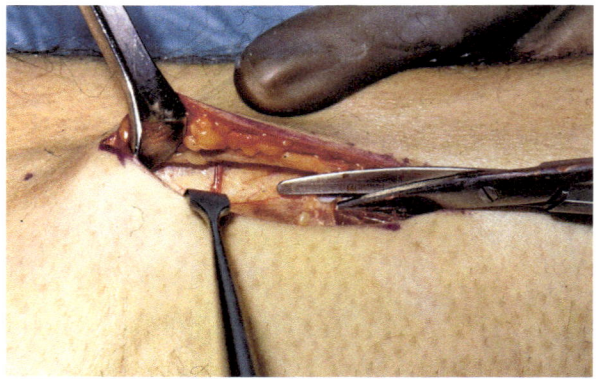

should be avoided as they have been shown to aggravate the symptoms of CCS of the leg by increasing intra-compartment pressure during exercise.[26] If foot orthoses are attempted for CCS of the foot, then at least a half-size larger shoe is recommended to avoid further shoe constriction. Elimination of external factors causing constriction is paramount. Transient CCS typically responds to conservative treatment and surgery should not be needed. An initial period of rest is followed by a graduated exercise program designed for the desired activity.

12.8.2 Surgical Treatment

Based on the author's clinical experience with CCS of the leg and foot and supported by results reported in the literature,[4,14-17,27-33] surgical open fasciotomy of the involved compartments (confirmed with CPM) is curative and should be considered the treatment of choice.

Surgery for CCS of the leg requires a fasciotomy through a distal anterolateral approach to decompress the anterior and/or lateral compartments and a distal posteromedial approach to decompress the deep and superficial posterior compartment. The fasciotomy is extended proximally and distally over each involved compartment to encompass the entire length of the leg. A proximal accessory incision can be made to supplement the distal incisions if proximal exposure is needed. Care needs to be taken to protect the superficial peroneal nerve anteriorly and the saphenous nerve and greater saphenous vein posteriorly (Fig. 12.2). Once the vital structures are protected, fasciotomy with Metzenbaum scissors is performed (Fig. 12.3).

Surgery for CCS of the foot requires a medial approach using a longitudinal linear incision centered over the abductor hallucis muscle belly extending distally to

Fig. 12.3 Fasciotomy of
deep posterior compartment

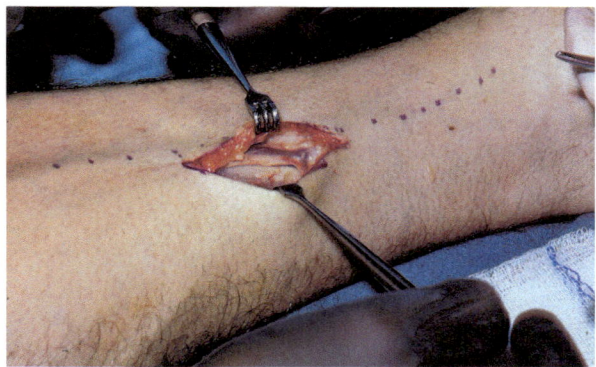

the myotendinous junction (Fig. 12.4). If a hypertrophic or accessory muscle is encountered, then a muscle debulking or accessory muscle excision can be performed respectively. By mobilizing the abductor hallucis muscle, the superficial and calcaneal compartments can be decompressed as well if indicated. Care needs to be taken to avoid injury to the medial and lateral neurovascular bundles during this procedure.

Postoperatively, a Jones compression dressing is applied for 1 week, followed by use of a removable splint for up to 3 additional weeks. The patient is kept non-weight-bearing during this time followed by 2 additional weeks in a short leg walking boot. Physical therapy is usually initiated at 3 weeks with emphasis on gentle stretching, early range of motion exercises, soft tissue mobilization, and general conditioning. Though considered on a case-by-case basis, return to running sports can usually be considered at 8–12 weeks post surgery.

12.9   Summary

CCS of the leg and foot is an uncommon though important cause of lower extremity pain. CCS is classified as a claudication syndrome characterized by no symptoms at rest though symptoms occur with exercise. A broad differential diagnosis of various entities that comprise claudication syndrome should be considered and appropriately ruled out in a systematic fashion. The four criteria for diagnosis of CCS should be apparent, and if these criteria are met, then CPM should be obtained to validate the diagnosis. If a course of conservative care is not successful, then compartment decompression via fasciotomy is indicated and should be curative. Expected result from surgery should be excellent with few complications.

Fig. 12.4 (**a**) Medial incision
for foot fasciotomy in a
patient with CCS of medial
and central compartments.
(**b**) After dissecting below
abductor hallucis, vessels are
evident. (**c**) Fasciotomy
exposing central
compartment musculature
(Photos courtesy of Amol
Saxena, DPM)

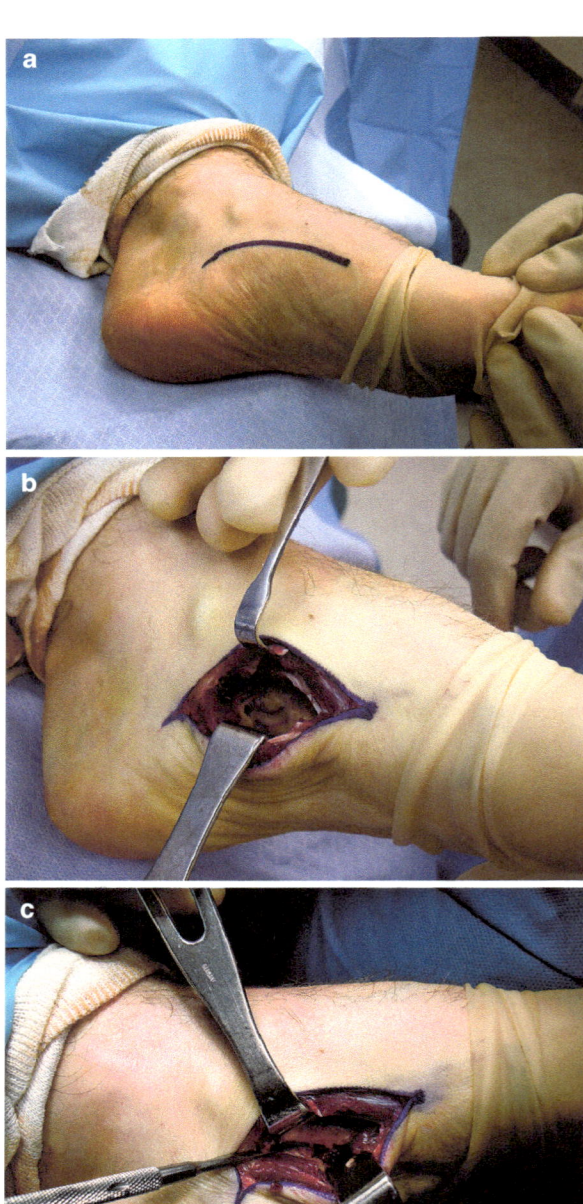

References

1. Bouché RT. Exercise-induced leg pain- common etiologies (Feature Article). Foot Ankle Q. 1995;5:1–9.
2. Bouché RT, Reeves M, Smith LJ. Exercise-induced leg pain: uncommon etiologies (Feature Article). Podiatry Tracts. 1992;5:289–300.
3. Styf J. Diagnosis of exercise-induced leg pain in the anterior aspect of the lower leg. Am J Sports Med. 1988;16:165–9.
4. Detmar DE, Sharpe K, Sufit RL, et al. Chronic compartment syndrome: diagnosis, management and outcomes. Am J Sports Med. 1988;13:162–70.
5. Matsen FA III. Compartmental syndrome: a unified concept. Clin Orthop. 1975;113:8–14.
6. Mubarak SJ, Hargens AR. Compartment syndromes and Volkmann's contracture. Philadelphia: WB Saunders; 1981.
7. Eaton RG, Green WT. Epimysiotomy and fasciotomy in the treatment of Volkmann's ischemic contracture. Orthop Clin North Am. 1972;3:175–86.
8. Ashton H. The effect of increased tissue pressure on blood flow. Clin Orthop. 1975;113: 15–26.
9. Burton AC. On the physical equilibrium of small blood vessels. Am J Physiol. 1951;1674:319–29.
10. Hargens AR, Akeson WH, Mubarak SJ, et al. Fluid balance within the canine anterolateral compartment and its relationship to compartment syndromes. J Bone Joint Surg. 1978; 60A:499.
11. Amendola A, Rorbeck CH, Vellett D, et al. The use of magnetic resonance imaging in exertional compartment syndromes. Am J Sports Med. 1990;18(1):29–34.
12. Matsen FA. Etiologies of compartmental syndrome. In: Matsen FA, editor. Compartmental syndromes. New York: Grune & Stratton; 1980.
13. Matsen FA. Definition of the compartmental syndrome. In: Matsen FA, editor. Compartmental syndromes. New York: Grune & Stratton; 1980.
14. Lokiec F, Siev-Ner I, Pritsch M. Chronic compartment syndrome of both feet. J Bone Joint Surg. 1991;73B:178–9.
15. Seiler R, Guziec G. Chronic compartment syndrome of the foot – a case report. J Am Podiatr Med Assoc. 1994;84:91–4.
16. Muller GP, Masquelet AC. Chronic compartment syndrome of the foot. A case report. Revue de Chirurgie Orthopedique. 1995;81:549–52.
17. Mollica M. Chronic exertional compartment syndrome of the foot- a case report. J Am Podiatr Med Assoc. 1998;88:21–4.
18. Bouché RT. Exercise-induced leg pain. In: Subotnick S, editor. Fundamentals of lower extremity sports medicine. New York: 2nd Ed. Churchill-Livingstone; 1999:Chap 16.
19. Eskelin MK, Lotjonen JM, Mantysaari MJ. Chronic exetional compartment syndrome: MR imaging at 0.1 T compared with tissue pressure measurement. Radiology. 1998;206:333–7.
20. van den Brand JG, Nelson T, Verleisdonk JM, et al. The diagnostic value of intracomparmental pressure measurement, magnetic resonance imaging, and near-infrared spectroscopy in chronic exertional compartment syndrome – a prospective study in 50 patients. Am J Sports Med. 2005;33(5):699–704.
21. van den Brand JG, Verleisdonk EJ, Van der Werken C. Near infrared spectroscopy in the diagnosis of chronic exertional compartment syndrome. Am J Sports Med. 2004;32(2):452–6.
22. Dayton P, Goldman FD, Barton E. Compartment pressure in the foot – analysis of normal values and measurement technique. J Am Podiatr Med Assoc. 1990;80(10):521–5.
23. Pedowitz RA, Hargens AR, Mubarek SJ, et al. Modified criteria for the objective diagnosis of chronic compartment syndrome of the leg. Am J Sports Med. 1990;18(1):35–40.
24. Bouché RT. Chronic compartment syndrome of the leg. J Podiatr Med Assoc. 1990;80(12): 633–48.

25. Blackman P, Bradshaw C, Crossley K. Chronic exertional compartment syndrome in the lower leg: a comparison of treatment options and outcomes. In: 1994 international conference of science and medicine in Sport. Brisbane : Sports Medicine Australia; 1994. p. 56–7.

26. Padhiar N, King JB. Foot orthoses can change compartmental pressures in the leg. Br J Sports Med. 1998;32(1):89.

27. Veith RG, Matsen FA, Newell SG. Recurrent anterior compartmental syndromes. Phys Sports Med. 1980;8:80–8.

28. Reneman RS. The anterior and the lateral compartmental syndrome of the leg due to intensive use of muscles. Clin Othop. 1975;113:69–80.

29. Martens MA, Backaert M, Vermaut G, et al. Chronic leg pain in athletes due to a recurrent compartment syndrome. Am J Sports Med. 1984;12:148–51.

30. Rorabeck CH, Fowler PJ, Nott L. The results of fasciotomy in the management of chronic exertional compartment syndrome. Am J Sports Med. 1988;16:224–7.

31. Allen MJ, Barnes MR. Exercise pain in the lower leg. Chronic compartment syndrome and medial tibial stress syndrome. J Bone Joint Surg. 1986;68B:818–23.

32. Fronek J, Mubarak SJ, Hargens AR, et al. Management of chronic exertional anterior compartment syndrome of the lower extremity. Clin Orthop. 1987;220:217–27.

33. Styf JR, Korner LM. Chronic anterior-compartment syndrome of the leg. Results of treatment by fasciotomy. J Bone J Surg. 1986;68A:1338–47.

Chapter 13
Ankle Instability

Daniel R. Stephenson, Timothy P. Charlton, and David B. Thordarson

Ankle injuries are among the most commonly treated musculoskeletal injuries. In the United States, there are 23,000 ankle injuries each day, and the United Kingdom sees nearly 5,000.[1,2] Within orthopedics, estimates place the incidence of ankle sprains between 10% and 25% of all musculoskeletal injuries.[3,4] Of these, nearly 85% involve the lateral ankle complex.[5] The sequelae of these injuries can be variable. Conservative management with functional rehabilitation can lead to good-to-excellent results in 70–85% of these injuries,[6] but 20–40% will have persistent pain and instability.[7,8]

Ankle instability can be either mechanical or functional. Mechanical instability is a physical sign and is defined as abnormal ligamentous laxity, whereas functional instability is a symptom and refers to the sensation of the ankle giving way. As such, the terms "laxity" and "instability" should not be used interchangeably.

13.1 Anatomy of the Lateral Ligamentous Complex

The lateral ligamentous complex of the ankle comprises three major ligaments: the anterior talofibular ligament (ATFL), the calcaneofibular ligament (CFL), and the posterior talofibular ligament (PTFL).

The ATFL courses from the anterior edge of the fibula just lateral to the articular cartilage and inserts distal to the articular cartilage of the talar dome.[9] It is a

D.R. Stephenson, M.D. • D. B. Thordarson, M.D.
Department of Orthopaedic Surgery,
University of Southern California, Los Angeles, CA, USA

T.P. Charlton, M.D. (✉)
Department of Orthopaedic Surgery,
USC Keck School of Medicine Surgery of the Foot and Ankle,
1520 San Pablo Street, Suite 2000,
Los Angeles, CA 90033, USA
e-mail: timothy.charlton@usc.edu

A. Saxena (ed.), *Sports Medicine and Arthroscopic Surgery of the Foot and Ankle*,
DOI 10.1007/978-1-4471-4106-8_13, © Springer-Verlag London 2013

confluence of tissues of the anterior capsule of the ankle. The ATFL is the primary restraint to inversion throughout the complete arc of ankle motion, despite being the weakest of the three. It experiences increased strain as the ankle is placed in increased plantar flexion. The ATFL is generally injured with planter flexion, inversion, and internal rotation, and is injured in nearly all ankle sprains.

The CFL originates on the anterior edge of the fibula just distal to the ATFL.[10] It courses posteromedially deep to the peroneal tendons and inserts on the calcaneus distal to the subtalar joint. When the ankle is dorsiflexed, the fibers become more vertical; thus, it effectively functions as the primary lateral collateral ligament. It is most commonly injured with inversion and dorsiflexion[11] and is involved in 50–75% of ankle sprains.[5]

The PTFL runs from the posteromedial aspect of the lateral malleolus to the lateral talar tubercle, and is the strongest of the three ligaments. The strain on the PTFL is greatest in dorsiflexion, but it is involved in fewer than 10% of all ankle sprains.[12]

13.2   History and Physical

As with all orthopedic injuries, a thorough history and physical is essential to making the diagnosis of ankle instability. Most patients are able to give a clear history of one or more ankle injuries. There is a small subset, however, that has a foot deformity (varus or cavovarus) that lack a history of injury. The most common complaint is repeated giving way or recurrent sprains of the ankle. Often this is coupled with difficulty walking on uneven ground. Assessment of whether symptoms occur only on uneven ground or with all walking activity aids in the evaluation of its severity. It is also crucial to assess any pain the patient is having, particularly its location and its cause. Pain does not generally accompany ankle instability.

The physical examination should begin with observation. Examine the shape and alignment of the entire leg, ankle, and foot. Note any malalignment of the hind foot, particularly varus. Range of motion should be noted and any evidence of anterior or posterior impingement. One should perform the anterior drawer test for ATFL laxity. The anterior drawer test should compare the amount of anterior displacement between the injured and uninjured ankles. CFL ligament laxity should be assessed with the talar tilt maneuver by inverting the hindfoot while maintaining maximum talocrural dorsiflexion; however both of these are best seen with stress radiographs, particularly the tilt.

13.3   Radiographic Evaluation

One should obtain plain standing radiographs, and possibly stress radiographs to help discern instability. The two commonly used stress evaluations are the anterior drawer and the talar tilt. The former is considered abnormal if displacement is greater than 3 mm, and is grossly pathologic when greater than 6 mm. The CFL is assessed by looking at the talar tilt with a side-to-side difference of less than 9° considered as not significantly lax.[13] Often these radiographic evaluations help to rule out other injuries, rather than assist in the diagnosis.

The use of CT or MRI is not generally needed, but may be of use in patients with multiple potential etiologies present (i.e., osteochondral lesions, anterior capsular impingement).

13.4 Treatment Options

Most patients undergo nonoperative management in the initial stages/presentation of ankle instability. These efforts should focus on both proprioceptive training and ankle strengthening, particularly eversion strengthening. One may also consider bracing; however, this may risk deconditioning the musculature. If the patient fails to be relieved by these measures, then one may consider operative intervention. When one plans to address grade III ankle injuries, options include cast immobilization, functional management, and surgical repair. Cast immobilization usually entails up to 3 weeks in a short leg walking cast, followed by 12 weeks of therapy. This is generally avoided in high demand athletes. Functional management generally adheres to the principles of RICE (Rest, Ice, Compress, Elevate), followed by rehabilitation. A meta-analysis comparing casting to functional rehabilitation found that the symptoms, ability to return to play, and range of motion were better among those undergoing functional rehabilitation versus those that were initially treated with cast immobilization.[14] Unfortunately, there is no high-quality meta-analysis that compares nonsurgical to surgical management. However, in a prospective randomized trial where patients were assigned to operative versus nonoperative treatment, slightly superior results were found in the operative group.[15] The costs and complications unfortunately seemed to outweigh the benefits of recommending early operative intervention.

There are multiple options to treating these injuries surgically. The selection of the definitive surgery is largely dependent on the experience and training of the surgeon. There are also patient factors that may contribute to the decision of the surgeon, such as the demands and lifestyle of the patient. Basic issues that need to be addressed are: open versus less invasive methods, anatomic versus nonanatomic reconstruction, and what concomitant procedures to perform. The primary indication for operative intervention is the failure of nonsurgical management. Further, operative techniques are generally divided into anatomic repair and tenodesis stabilization.

There are several anatomic reconstructions to choose from including the Broström–Gould or a hamstring allograft reconstruction. Nonanatomic procedures include the Watson-Jones, Chrisman–Snook, modified Evans, and Elmsie. When selecting what type of reconstruction, high level athletes and professional dancers present unique demands. Sacrifice of the hamstrings or peroneal tendons can be extremely detrimental to their performance. The preservation of strong eversion is crucial, but each procedure has its limitations.

Fig. 13.1 Mark out anatomy

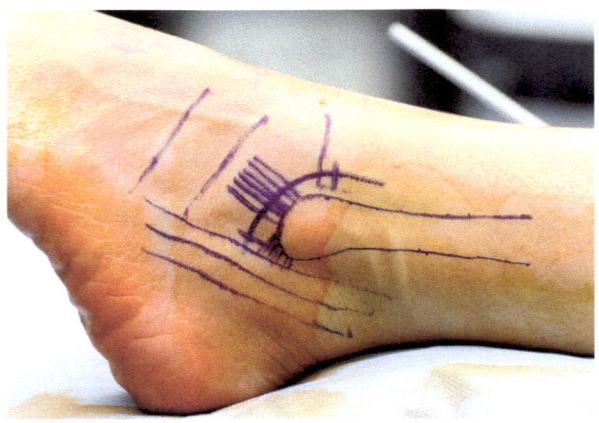

The Broström–Gould procedure is an anatomic reconstruction that yields consistently good to excellent outcomes, even with long-term follow-up. It is frequently considered the gold standard to which other treatments are compared. Broström initially described this procedure in 1966 as a direct repair of the lateral ankle ligaments,[16] and this was subsequently modified by Gould[17] to include subtalar stabilization by the advancement of the inferior extensor retinaculum to the fibula. It is relatively simple and appropriate for most patients. Relative contraindications include generalized ligamentous hyperlaxity, failed prior surgery, and some feel worker's compensation patients. These tend to be better managed by nonanatomic procedures.

The Chrisman–Snook procedure is generally indicated in those with chronic insufficiency of the ATFL and/or CFL. Candidates include those who are obese, large sportsmen such as football linemen and rugby players, as well as those with a correctable hindfoot deformity. Potential concerns include the inability to restore ankle flexibility and loss of subtalar motion.[18] Alternatives include the Elmsie or modified Evans procedure.

Further, currently era, several graft alternatives have been suggested for reconstructive procedures.[3,13,19-21] Possible grafts include: allograft, plantaris graft, and gracilis. These avoid the complications of weakening the peroneal tendons, but at the risk of donor site morbidity or, in the case of allograft, uncertain tissue composition and infectious disease transmission. Some authors have even recommended arthroscopic thermal shrinkage.[22]

13.4.1 Anatomic Reconstruction

The Broström–Gould incision can be either the traditional hockey stick shape, a longitudinal, or a J type incision. All of these incisions allow for an anterior tibiotalar cheilectomy, if indicated. Generally, a 4-cm incision is made out over the anterior border of the distal fibula (Fig. 13.1). Dissection should be carried out meticulously as the sural nerve and superficial peroneal nerve can be found near either end of the

Fig. 13.2 Extensor
retinaculum in blue

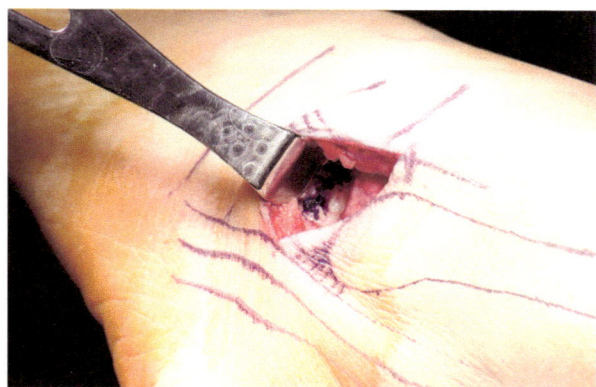

Fig. 13.3 ATFL cut

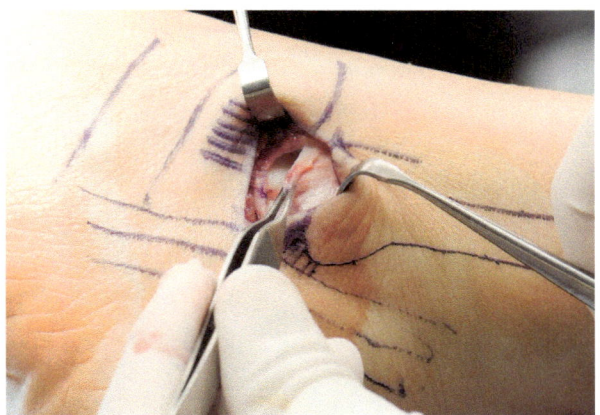

incision. Once the extensor retinaculum is exposed, it should be detached from its inferior insertion on the talar neck, and preserved for later in the procedure (Fig. 13.2). The peroneal sheath is opened inferiorly to allow for retraction of the peroneal tendons and exposure of the CFL. The ATFL should then be exposed by dissecting anteriorly within the incision. The ligaments and the capsule are incised leaving 2-mm cuff of tissue distal to the fibula (Fig. 13.3). Tensioning of the tissues should occur with the foot in an everted and dorsiflexed position. The anterior portion of the Broström is then coupled with the reinforcement with the inferior extensor retinaculum as it is advanced proximally (Gould procedure). The CFL can be tensioned using suture anchors or drill holes to provide fixation[23] (Fig. 13.4). Careful attention should be made not to place fixation too far laterally and potentially encroach on the peroneal groove. One author (TPC) will also reconstruct the lateral talocalcaneal ligament (Fig. 13.5), in an effort to reduce subtalar laxity, but imbrication with 2.0 nonabsorbable braided suture. The anterolateral capsule along with the ATFL and then extensor retinaculum are then imbricated. (Figs. 13.6–13.10). The subcutaneous tissues and skin are then closed in layers (Figs. 13.11 and 13.12).

Fig. 13.4 Lateral talocalcaneal

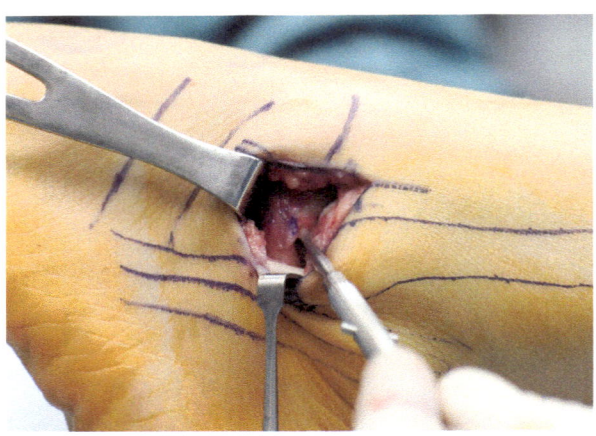

Fig. 13.5 Drill holes in the fibula for CFL tunnel

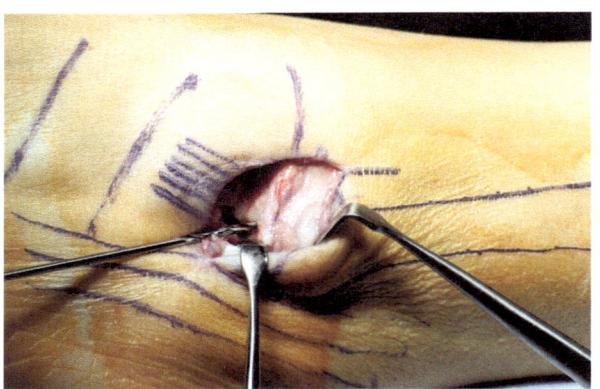

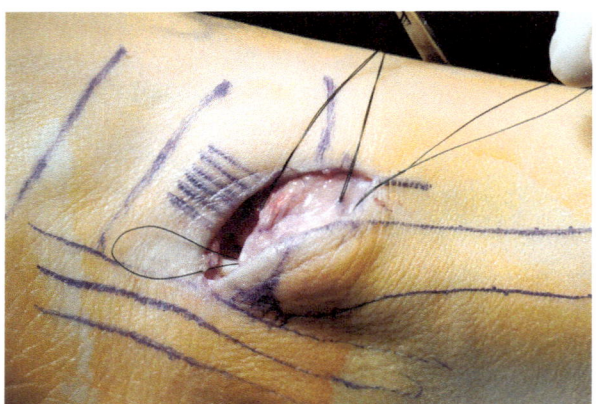

Fig. 13.6 Reinforcement of extensor retinaculum

Fig. 13.7 Reconstruction of the LTCL

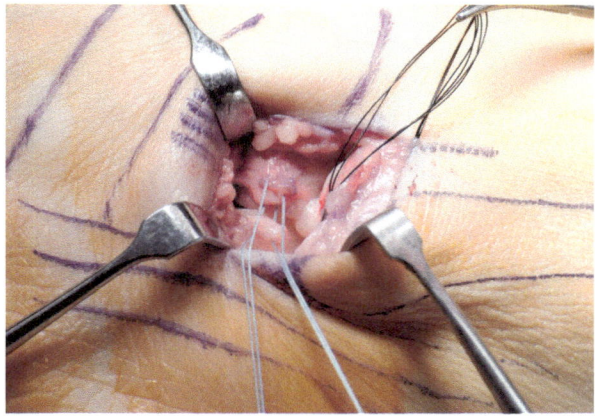

Fig. 13.8 Passage of CFL through drill holes

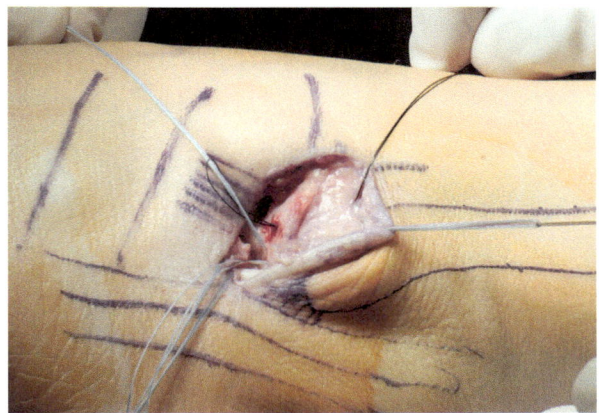

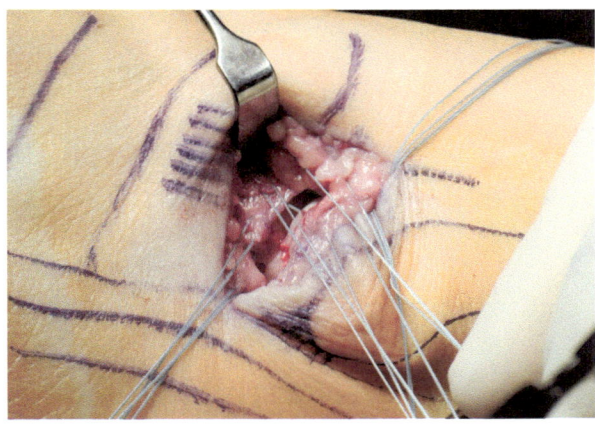

Fig. 13.9 LTCL at 8 o'clock; ATFL, CFL suture at 2 o'clock

Fig. 13.10 Extensor retinaculum with 2.0 Vicryl

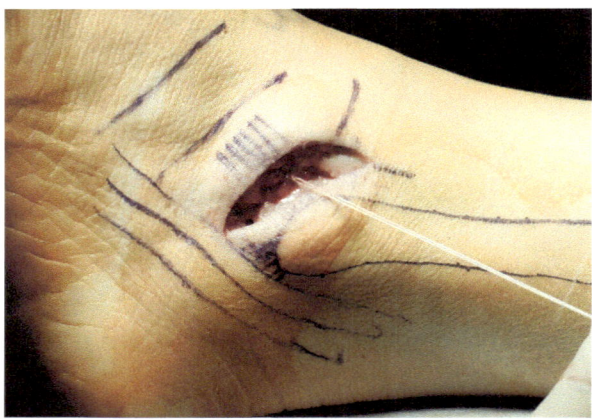

Fig. 13.11 The anterior lateral incision can have a very cosmetic closure

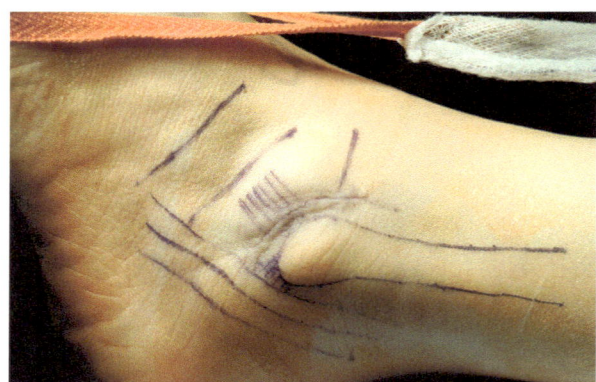

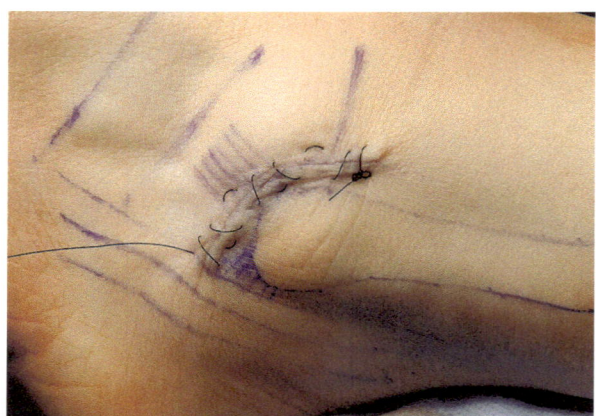

Fig. 13.12 Tulane two step

Fig. 13.13 Curette the
bottom of the fibula for CFL
attachment

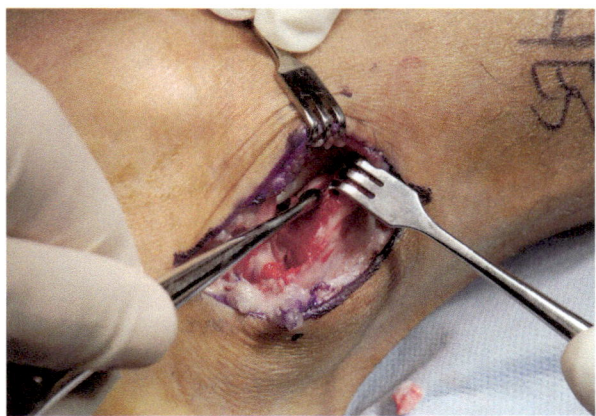

Fig. 13.14 Suture anchors
can be used for CFL
attachment

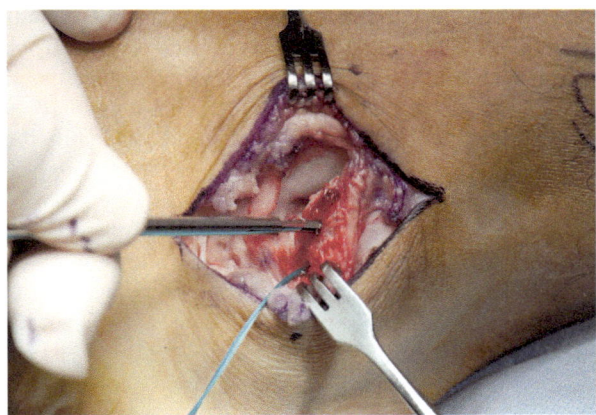

Tendon augmented ligament reconstruction can be done using gracilis or semi-tendinosis autograft or allograft. This is generally reserved for failed initial Broström reconstruction or primary reconstruction in patients with generalized ligamentous laxity. Tunnels are created in the fibula to allow for passage of a tubularized graft, with a typical graft measuring between 5 and 6 mm in diameter. Careful attention must be made to create tunnels that do not break the most distal portion of the fibula, as subsequent fixation can be quite difficult. Tunnels are placed at the insertion of the ATFL on the talus and CFL on the calcaneus (Figs. 13.13 and 13.14). Fixation is maintained with interference screws with the foot held in slight valgus position (Fig. 13.15).

13.4.2 Nonanatomic Tenodesis

Watson-Jones described the first of these procedures in 1952. He described a procedure where the peroneus brevis was woven through the calcaneus and fibula. Evans

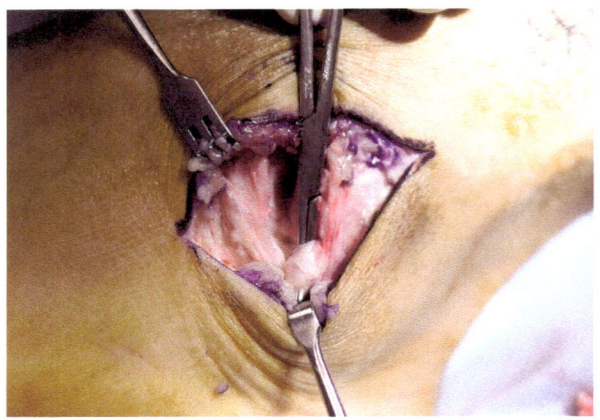

later simplified this procedure by placing the distally attached brevis through an oblique drill hole in the distal fibula and tenodesed this to the brevis stump.

The Chrisman–Snook procedure[24] performed through a curved incision over the course of the peroneal tendons from the myotendinous junction to the base of the fifth metatarsal. The sural nerve should be identified prior to dividing the ligament maintaining the peroneal tendons in their groove. Next the peroneus longus is retracted to expose the peroneus brevis in the groove. The brevis is split longitudinally from its insertion, leaving the attachment to the base of the fifth metatarsal intact. Then the half with the longest tendon component is divided at the myotendinous junction. At this point, an appropriately sized drill hole is made in the antero-posterior direction at or just proximal to the level of the tibiotalar joint, with the graft placed from anterior to posterior. With the foot in neutral with mild eversion, the graft is tensioned and sutured to the periosteal/ligamentous tissues adjacent to the anterior drill hole, reconstructing the ATFL. At this point, the peroneus longus and the remaining brevis are returned to their groove. The split tendon passes over their superficial border to help prevent dislocation. The surface of the calcaneus is then exposed and two drill holes are made 1.5 cm apart at the same diameter as the distal fibular holes. These are connected using curettes. The tendon is passed from posterior to anterior, with sutures at both ends of the tunnel. The remaining tendon is then attached to the anterior portion of the graft either near the base of the fifth metatarsal or at the anterior fibular drill hole.

13.5   Postoperative Protocols and Results

Generally, after any of these procedures, the patient is placed in a short leg splint or cast and made non-weight bearing for a period of 2 weeks. Following this, weight bearing is allowed in a cast. At 6 weeks after surgery, the patient is allowed to begin proprioceptive and strength training.

The results of the Broström–Gould procedure have been repeatedly good to excellent. Several studies examining the results find 91% excellent results at 2.6-year follow-up,[25] or 87% good-to-excellent results.[26] However, these authors note that failure of previous surgeries, generalized ligamentous laxity, and instability of greater than 10 years were relative contraindications. The Watson-Jones procedure yields good to excellent results at 10–18-year follow-up, despite the 18% complication rate (which excludes wound complications).[27]

Long-term results of the modified Evans procedure are not as favorable with one study showing that only 52% of patients had returned to pre-injury level of activity at 4.6 years after surgery.[28] Karlsson found that 50% of patients had unsatisfactory results with 14-year follow-up after the Evans procedure.[1]

13.6 Syndesmotic Instability

Syndesmotic injuries or "high ankle sprains" most commonly result from rotational injuries or forced abduction. They are seen with lesser frequency with inversion. The incidence of syndesmotic injuries is estimated 1–18% of all ankle injuries.[29,30] These injuries are not common, but misdiagnosed or undiagnosed injuries can lead to a chronic pain and disability. The syndesmosis is defined as the anterior inferior tibiofibular ligament (AITFL), the posterior inferior tibiofibular ligament (PITFL), the transverse tibiofibular ligament, and the interosseous membrane and ligament. The AITFL spans from Chaput's tubercle on the anterior tibia to the anterior distal fibula, with an average width of 20 mm. The interosseous ligament lies 0.5–2 mm above the tibiotalar joint and blends with the interosseous membrane. The PITFL lies on the posterior aspect of the tibia, Volkmann's tubercle, and inserts on the posterior portion of the distal fibula. The transverse tibiofibular ligament lies just superior and anterior to the PITFL and functions as a labrum. Together these ligaments function to provide stability to the ankle joint. The ankle allows a small degree of excursion of the fibula with normal ankle function. However, if two of these ligamentous structures are injured, there may be significant mechanical laxity.[31]

13.6.1 Clinical and Radiographic Evaluation

A detailed history, including the interval from injury to presentation, is taken. Common complaints include a sensation of giving way and difficulty walking on uneven ground. A focused clinical examination begins with inspection and palpation for tenderness. They also commonly have stiffness, particularly in dorsiflexion. The "squeeze test" is performed by squeezing the fibula at the level of the mid-calf.[32] While suggestive of injury, this test is not sensitive or specific enough to make a diagnosis. A more reliable examination is to have the patient sit with the hips and knees flexed at 90°. The examiner then places a gentle external rotation force, and pain is suggestive of a syndesmotic injury.

Radiographs include an AP, lateral and mortise view of the ankle, as well as a stress external rotation mortise view. Special attention should be paid to the following parameters: increased tibiofibular clear space, decreased tibiofibular overlap, and increased medial clear space.

Tibiofibular clear space is defined as the distance between the medial border of the fibula and the lateral border of the posterior tibia as it extends into the incisura fibularis. The measurement is made 1 cm proximal to the plafond and should be less than 6 mm in both the mortise and AP views. Increased tibiofibular clear space is considered the most reliable indicator of instability.[33]

The tibiofibular overlap is defined as the portion of the lateral malleolus that overlies the anterior tibial tubercle, measured 1 cm proximal to the plafond. In the AP view, this should be greater than 6 mm or 42% of the fibula width. In the mortise view, it should be greater than 1 mm.

The medial clear space, or the distance between the lateral border of the medial malleolus and medial border of the talus, is measured at the level of the talar dome. In the mortise view, this should be less than or equal to the superior clear space. An increase is more indicative of a deltoid injury than of a syndesmotic injury. Other modalities may be useful, such as computed tomography (CT) or magnetic resonance imaging (MRI). CT is able to assess minor syndesmotic diastasis but MRI is more sensitive and specific, especially since it visualizes the ligamentous structures.

13.6.2 Indications and Treatment

Patients that have persistent symptoms after conservative treatment for a syndesmotic sprain, have instability on stress radiographs, or present more than 3 months after injury should be treated with surgery. Standard syndesmotic treatment should be performed with screw or endobutton suture fixation in acute cases of instability. However, for chronic syndesmotic instability, the medial ankle joint should be opened with a medial arthrotomy. Any interposed tissue, which can be as fibrotic as cartilage, should be debrided from the medial gutter to allow reduction of the talus.

Following the reduction of the talus, a large reduction clamp should be used to maintain the reduction of the syndesmosis. The syndesmosis in then stabilized with two syndesmotic screws, with most advocating use of 3.5 cortical screws through four cortices. Another option is to hold the syndesmotic reduction with fiberwire-button constructs (Tightrope® Arthrex, Naples, Fl). The use of a fiberwire-button construct has been seen to be biomechanically equal to screw fixation.[34] Postoperatively, the patient is kept in a splint for 2 weeks and non-weight bearing for a total of 6 weeks. If screws were used, they are routinely removed after 12–16 weeks. Some patients may experience some postoperative complaints that are usually related to impingement of the AITFL in the joint. This can be treated arthroscopically, if necessary.

13.7 Chronic Medial (Deltoid) Instability

Injuries to the medial ligaments of the ankle are seen more often than originally believed according to Hintermann and colleagues.[35] These injuries can be caused by an array of activities, particularly with rotational injuries. While these types of injuries can be seen in association with lateral malleolar fractures, there is an element of deltoid insufficiency seen in some patients with advanced posterior tibial tendon disorder, traumatic and athletic injuries. Occasionally, there is also a valgus tilt seen in patients with a history of triple arthrodesis or total ankle arthroplasty.

Medial ankle instability can be acute or chronic, and its degree of severity can be variable. There are also various conditions that can lead to chronic medial ankle instability. An ankle sprain can contribute to chronic medial instability in addition to chronic overload from a fixed valgus hindfoot deformity and/or flatfoot deformity. Hintermann divides these types of lesions into three types: Type I is a proximal tear or avulsion of the deltoid, type II has an intermediate tear of the deltoid, and type III is a distal tear or avulsion of the spring ligament.[35]

The medial ligamentous complex of the ankle is extremely variable. The superficial components cross both the ankle and subtalar joints, whereas the deep deltoid ligament only crosses the ankle joint. The deltoid ligament functions as a strong restraint to valgus tilt of the talus.[36] The deltoid ligament only allows 2 mm of diastasis of the talus from the medial malleolus when all other medial structures are removed. Functionally, the superficial layers of the deltoid limit talar tilt. The deep fibers limit external rotation.

13.7.1 Clinical and Radiographic Evaluation

The history of deltoid injury generally includes an eversion and/or pronation mechanism with the foot planted. Chronic injuries will present with medial ankle instability and pain. A feeling of "giving way," particularly when walking downhill or stairs or when walking on even ground is frequently present. Medial tenderness over the gutter and visible valgus of the hindfoot that disappears with firing of the posterior tibial tendon (single heel rise) will usually be evident. Another clinical test is to have the patient in a seated position with the feet hanging freely.[35] The heel is then grasped in one hand, and the tibia in the other. Varus and valgus stress are compared to the contralateral side with increased medial laxity evident on the involved side. A subsequent comparison of the anterior drawer test is made.

Plain weightbearing radiographs are made to exclude other pathology. Stress radiographs are generally more useful for evaluating acute injuries as they are less informative in chronic cases. Similarly, CT scans may help in diagnosing an associated talocalcaneal coalition and other bony lesions but are less helpful to diagnose ligamentous incompetence. MRI can demonstrate the injury of the deltoid ligament in addition to associated pathology.

13.7.2   Treatment

Arthroscopy can be a useful tool in the evaluation of medial instability. The instability is graded as: (1) Stable when there is less than 2-mm translocation of the talus (2) Moderately unstable where the talus subluxes 5 mm (3) Grossly unstable where the talus easily subluxes out of the mortise, allowing for easy access to the posterior ankle joint. Seventy-five percent of patients with chronic medial instability also have an avulsion of the ATFL. Medial exploration is indicated following arthroscopic evaluation if there is visible medial ankle instability.

Hintermann recommends treatment based on the type of pathology. The most common type of acute rupture of the deltoid ligament is an avulsion of the proximal end ligament. This injury can be reinserted or repaired using suture anchors into the medial malleolus.

Chronic instability has a variety of treatment options. Chronic type I ruptures can be treated with a suture anchor placed about 6 mm above the tip of the medial malleolus and then retensioning the tibionavicular and tibiospring ligaments. Chronic Type II lesions generally have insufficient ligaments in two ligamentous ends, with the deep still attached distally and the superficial still attached proximally. One anchor is placed 6 mm proximal to the medial malleolus and one on the superior edge of the navicular tuberosity. This creates a strong, well-tensioned reconstruction. Chronic type III lesions require debridement, nonabsorbable suture repair of the spring ligament, and an anchor is placed in the navicular tuberosity. After tensioning, heavy absorbable sutures can be used to stabilize the reconstructed ligaments.

Chronic rupture of the deep deltoid ligament often involves the superficial deltoid as well. A posterior tendon autograft can be placed through drill holes, or a bone-tendon-bone allograft can be used to reconstruct the tendon with two distal limbs – one placed in the medial talus and the other in the sustentaculum tali. Proximally, it is fixed to the distal tibia (medially or laterally).[37] Other authors have described tunneling the peroneus brevis through the talus with its distal insertion left intact. It is passed through the medial malleolus and then tunneled back to the lateral tibia.[38]

Postoperatively, all of these procedures (with the exception of type I lesions) are placed in a short leg weight bearing cast for a period of 6 weeks. Rehabilitation with passive and active range of motion at the ankle joint is then begun. Type I lesions are treated with functional mobilization. In Hintermann's study, they had good to excellent results in 89% of their patients (48 total), 7% fair, and 2% poor. Clearly this is an evolving area of foot and ankle instability and further study will be necessary.

13.8   Conclusion

Ankle instability is a frequently seen problem to foot and ankle surgeons as well as the general orthopedic or trauma surgeon. Key aspects of the physical exam are understanding the pathologic anatomy, as well as anatomic considerations that may predispose the patient to injury, such as a varus heel alignment. Surgical strategies should be focused on anatomic reconstruction of the lateral ligament complex. Rehabilitation should be focused on proprioception and returning the patient to the pre-injury level, with a return to stability and minimal recurrence of ankle sprains.

References

1. Karlsson J, Eriksson BI, Bergsten T, Rudholm O, Swärd L. Comparison of two anatomic reconstructions for chronic lateral instability of the ankle joint. Am J Sports Med. 1997;25(1): 48–53.
2. van Rijn RM, van Os AG, Bernsen RM, Luijsterburg PA, Koes BW, Bierma-Zeinstra SM. What is the clinical course of acute ankle sprains? A systematic literature review. Am J Med. 2008;121(4):324–31.
3. Caprio A, Oliva F, Treia F, Maffulli N. Reconstruction of the lateral ankle ligaments with allograft in patients with chronic ankle instability. Foot Ankle Clin. 2006;11(3):597–605.
4. Kerkhoffs GMMJ, Handoll HHG, de Bie R, Rowe BH, Struijs PAA. Surgical versus conservative treatment for acute injuries of the lateral ligament complex of the ankle in adults. Cochrane Database Syst Rev. 2008;2:1–66.
5. Ferran NA, Maffulli N. Epidemiology of sprains of the lateral ankle ligamentous complex. Foot Ankle Clin North Am. 2006;11:659–62.
6. Kannus P, Renstrom P. Treatment for acute tears of the lateral ligaments of the ankle. Operation, cast or early controlled mobilization. J Bone Joint Surg Am. 1991;73(2):305–12.
7. Ajis A, Maffulli N. Conservative management of chronic ankle instability. Foot Ankle Clin North Am. 2006;11:531–7.
8. Sammarco GJ, DiRaimondo CV. Surgical treatment of lateral ankle instability syndrome. Am J Sports Med. 1988;16(5):501–11.
9. Pagenstert G, Leumann A, Hintermann B, Valderrabano V. Sports and recreation activity of varus and valgus ankle osteoarthritis before and after realignment surgery. Foot Ankle Int. 2008;29(10):985–93.
10. Burks RT, Morgan J. Anatomy of the lateral ankle ligaments. Am J Sports Med. 1994;22:72–7.
11. Colville MR, Marder RA, Boyle JJ, et al. Strain measurement in lateral ankle ligaments. Am J Sports Med. 1990;18:196–200.
12. Garrick JG. The Frequency of injury, mechanism of injury and epidemiology of ankle sprains. Am J Sports Med. 1977;5:241–2.
13. Espinosa N, Smerek J, Kadaka AR, Myerson MS. Operative management of ankle instability: reconstruction with open and percutaneous methods. Foot Ankle Clin North Am. 2006;11:547–65.
14. Kerkhoffs GM, Rowe BH, Assendelft WJ, Kelly K, Struijs PA, van Dijk CN. Immobilization and functional treatment for acute lateral ankle ligament injuries in adults. Cochrane Database Syst Rev. 2002;(3):CD003762.
15. Pijnenburg AC, Bogaard K, Krips R, Marti RK, Bossuyt PM, Dijk CN. Operative and functional treatment of rupture of the lateral ligament of the ankle: a randomized prospective trial. J Bone Joint Surg Br. 2003;85:525–30.
16. Brostrom L, Sprained ankles VI. Surgical treatment of "chronic" ligament ruptures. Acta Chir Scand. 1966;132(5):551–65.
17. Gould N, Seligson D, Gasman J. Early and late repair of the lateral ligament of the ankle. Foot Ankle. 1980;1(2):84–9.
18. McBride DJ, Ramamurthy C. Chronic ankle instability: management of chronlic lateral ligamentous dysfunction and the varus tibiotalar joint. Foot Ankle Clin North Am. 2006;11:607–23.
19. Boyer DS, Younger ASE. Anatomic reconstruction of the lateral ligamentous complex of the ankle using gracilis autograft. Foot Ankle Clin North Am. 2006;11:585–95.

20. Colville MR, Grondel RJ. Anatomic reconstruction of the lateral ankle ligaments using a split peroneus brevis tendon graft. Am J Sports Med. 1995;23(2):210–3.
21. Sammarco GJ, Idusuyi OB. Reconstruction of the lateral ankle ligaments using a split peroneus brevis tendon graft. Foot Ankle Int. 1999;20(2):97–103.
22. Berlet GC, Saar WE, Ryan A, Lee TH. Thermal-assisted capsular modification for functional ankle instability. Foot Ankle Clin. 2002;7:567–76.
23. Messer TM, Cummins CA, Ahn J, Kelikian AS. Outcome of the modified Broström procedure for chronic lateral ankle instability using suture anchors. Foot Ankle Int. 2000;21(12):996–1003.
24. Snook GA, Chrisman OD, Wilson TC. Long-term results of the Chrisman-Snook operation for reconstruction of the lateral ligaments of the ankle. J Bone Joint Surg Am. 1985;67(1):1–7.
25. Bell SJ, Mologne TS, Sitler DF, Cox JS. Twenty-six-year results after Broström procedure for chronic lateral ankle instability. Am J Sports Med. 2006;34(6):975–8.
26. Karlsson J, Bergsten T, Lansinger O, Peterson L. Reconstruction of the lateral ligaments of the ankle for chronic ankle instability. J Bone Joint Surg Am. 1988;70:581–8.
27. Sugimoto K, Takakura Y, Akiyama K, Kamei S, Kitada C, Kumai T. Long-term results of Watson-Jones tenodesis of the ankle: clinical and radiographic findings after ten to eighteen years of follow-up. J Bone Joint Surg Am. 1998;80:1587–96.
28. Kaikkonen A, Lehtonen H, Kannus P, Jarvinen M. Long-term functional outcome after surgery of chronic ankle instability: a 5 year follow-up of the modified Evans procedure. Scand J Med Sci Sports. 1999;9:239–44.
29. Espinosa N, Smerek JP, Myerson MS. Acute and chronic syndesmotic injuries: pathomechanisms, diagnosis and management. Foot Ankle Clin North Am. 2006;11:639–57.
30. Williams GN, Jones MH, Amendola A. Syndesmotic ankle sprains in athletes. Am J Sports Med. 2007;35(7):1197–207.
31. Xenos JS, Hopkinson WJ, Mulligan ME, Olson EJ, Popovic NA. The tibofibular syndesmosis: evaluation of the ligamentous structures, methods of fixation, and radiographic assessment. J Bone Joint Surg Am. 1995;77:847–56.
32. Hopkinson WJ, St Pierre P, Ryan JB, Wheeler JH. Syndesmosis sprains of the ankle. Foot Ankle. 1990;10:156–60.
33. Zalavras C, Thordarson DB. Ankle syndesmotic injury. J Am Acad Orthop Surg. 2007;15:330–9.
34. Forsythe K, Freedman KB, Stover MD, Patwardhan AG. Comparison of a novel FiberWire-button construct versus metallic screw fixation in a syndesmotic injury model. Foot Ankle Int. 2008;29(1):49–54.
35. Hintermann B, Knupp M, Pagenstert GI. Deltoid ligament injuries: diagnosis and management. Foot Ankle Clin. 2006;11(3):625–37.
36. Close JR. Some applications of the functional anatomy of the ankle joint. J Bone Joint Surg Am. 1956;38:761–81.
37. Buman EM, Khazen G, Haraguchi N. Minimally invasive deltoid ligament reconstruction: a comparison of 3 techniques. Presented at: the annual meeting specialty day AOFAS, 25 March, 2006; Chicago.
38. Deland JT, de Asla RJ, Segal A. Reconstruction of the chronically failed deltoid ligament: a new technique. Foot Ankle Int. 2004;25(11):795–9.

Chapter 14
Insertional and Midsubstance Achilles Tendinopathy

Amol Saxena, Umile Giuseppe Longo, Vincenzo Denaro, and Nicola Maffulli

14.1 Introduction

Achilles tendinopathy is characterized by pain, impaired performance, and swelling in and around the tendon.[1] It can be categorized as insertional and noninsertional, two distinct disorders with different underlying pathophysiologies and management options.[2] Other terms used as synonymous of noninsertional tendinopathy include tendinopathy of the main body of the Achilles tendon (AT) and mid-portion Achilles tendinopathy. In this chapter, we give a detailed overview of insertional tendinopathy of the AT and tendinopathy of the main body of the AT.

14.2 Anatomy

The AT attaches to the middle and inferior aspects of the posterior calcaneus. The inferior AT fibers blend with the proximal attachment of the plantar fascia. The medial and lateral aspects of the tendon insertion have an expansion to these regions of the calcaneus. The medial aspect of the AT expansion is thicker. This expansion is important as it keeps the tendon from migrating proximally when significant

A. Saxena, D.P.M. (✉)
Department of Sports Medicine, PAFMG-Palo Alto Division,
Clark Bldg., 3rd Flr, 795 El Camino Real, Palo Alto, CA 94301, USA
e-mail: heysax@aol.com

U.G. Longo, M.D. • V. Denaro, M.D.
Department of Trauma and Orthopaedic Surgery, University Campus Bio-Medico of Rome,
Rome, Italy

N. Maffulli, M.D., M.S., Ph.D., F.R.C.S (Orth).
Barts and The London School of Medicine and Dentistry, Centre for Sports and Exercise
Medicine, Mile End Hospital, Queen Mary University of London,
London E1 4DG, UK

A. Saxena (ed.), *Sports Medicine and Arthroscopic Surgery of the Foot and Ankle*,   167
DOI 10.1007/978-1-4471-4106-8_14, © Springer-Verlag London 2013

surgical debridement and detachment is needed.[3,4] Calcifications of the tendon in this region arise from micro-trauma and physiological changes causing calcium to precipitate in a lower pH environment. There is an anatomically occurring retrocalcaneal bursa that is adjacent to the superior posterior calcaneus, anterior to the tendon just prior to its insertion. This upper portion of the calcaneus has smooth fibro-cartilage surface in this region. A secondary "adventitious" bursa may occur in areas with more pressure on the tendon, often from constant shoe contact. These bursae occur within the subcutaneous tissue superficial to the AT.

14.3   Insertional Achilles Tendinopathy

Ever since Haglund first described pathology with the Achilles insertion in relation to the posterior calcaneus,[5] many authors have described surgical solutions for the approximately 10% of patients with recalcitrant symptoms.[3,6-10] Nonsurgical management of posterior insertional Achilles tendinopathy such as calcific tendinopathy, retrocalcaneal exostoses, and bursitis is successful in approximately 90% of cases.[11,12] Nonsurgical management often consists of a combination of the following: rest, heel and foot inserts, physical therapy including rehabilitation exercises such as eccentric strengthening, stretching, night splints and immobilization, along with pharmacological methods though injections should be avoided and the benefits of anti-inflammatories may only be useful in acute situations and in patients with inflammatory conditions. Surgical solutions often consist of resection of the offending exostoses and calcification, degenerated tendon along with reattachment of the AT.[3,6,8,12,13]

14.3.1   Clinical Findings

Typical complaints consist of pain from the posterior aspect of the heel, within and around the AT attachment. The posterior heel may be prominent and the insertion "boggy." Swelling posterior laterally may be termed a "pump bump." Bouché and McInnes make a point of outlining the exact area of patient's pain with a "tic-tac-toe" grid so all anatomical structures potentially associated with pathology are considered. In practice, a patient may have a prominent posterolateral bursa but also have symptoms superomedially.[3] Patients may have pain on single-legged heel raise, and some may even have an avulsion due to chronic degeneration. Acute avulsion may require more immediate surgical treatment. Symptoms include pain with activity and rest, along with redness and swelling when experiencing bursitis. Laboratory investigations to rule out inflammatory arthropathies, particularly seronegative enthesopathies, are undertaken with prolonged bursitis.[14] Rheumatological consultation is obtained in patients in whom inflammatory conditions are suspected, especially if surgery is still being considered. Generally, when considering surgical intervention, symptoms are getting progressively worse with activity, despite a significant period of rest. In fact, consideration of rest for a period similar to the postoperative recovery is recommended prior to considering surgery for chronic cases.[15]

14.3.2 Diagnosis

Radiographic studies are helpful. Plain film lateral and 0°-axial radiographs are most commonly ordered[3] (Fig. 14.1). Calcaneal prominence along with tendon calcification is visible. In patients with inflammatory arthropathy, erosions of the posterior and inferior calcaneus are noted.[14] MRI examination can further reveal tendon degeneration, bursitis, and cystic changes of the calcaneus, along with ruling out stress fracture (Fig. 14.2). Diagnostic ultrasound may be helpful in identifying bursitis and tendon degeneration. Various types (cavus, planus, and rectus) of foot morphology have been found with insertional Achilles tendinopathy.[9] Decreased ankle flexibility has also been cited as a cause, but none of these associations have been scientifically validated. Surgical treatment currently has at best Level IV evidence, and primarily includes retrocalcaneal prominence resection with calcific tendon debridement, and reattachment of the AT with soft tissue anchors.[3,6,8,9,12,15] Endoscopic resection of Haglund's prominence has also been described, but indications for isolated superior calcaneal exostectomy alone are, in the authors' opinion, currently limited.[16]

14.3.3 Surgical Technique of Insertional Repair/Retrocalcaneal Exostectomy

Surgical treatment involves removal of the exostoses, pathological bursae, remodeling of the posterior heel, excision of the insertional calcification (if present), and tenodesis of the AT with soft tissue anchors. The patient is placed in the prone position. Typically local anesthesia is used, often in conjunction with intra-venous sedation, but general and spinal anesthesia may be utilized. A tourniquet is typically not used but may be placed on the thigh or on the calf.

The incision is curvilinear from superomedial adjacent to the AT just above the superior calcaneus, inferiorly, across the posterior heel, staying within skin lines as much as possible, ending infero-lateral above the plantar skin lines (Fig. 14.3). The incision is deepened, and pathological bursae and the degenerated AT is excised. An inverted "T" approach to go "through" the AT insertion is used, exposing the superior calcaneus and any insertional calcification within the tendon insertion. The insertion calcification, if present, is excised (often with an osteotome), maintaining as much as the tendon expansion as possible. The superior calcaneus is further exposed after excising the retrocalcaneal bursa. This is resected with a curved osteotome from medial to lateral in both cases of retrocalcaneal exostoses

Fig. 14.1 (**a**) Retrocalcaneal exostosis lateral view. (**b**) "Zero degree" axial view showing lateral calcification. (**c**) Insertional tendocalcinosis

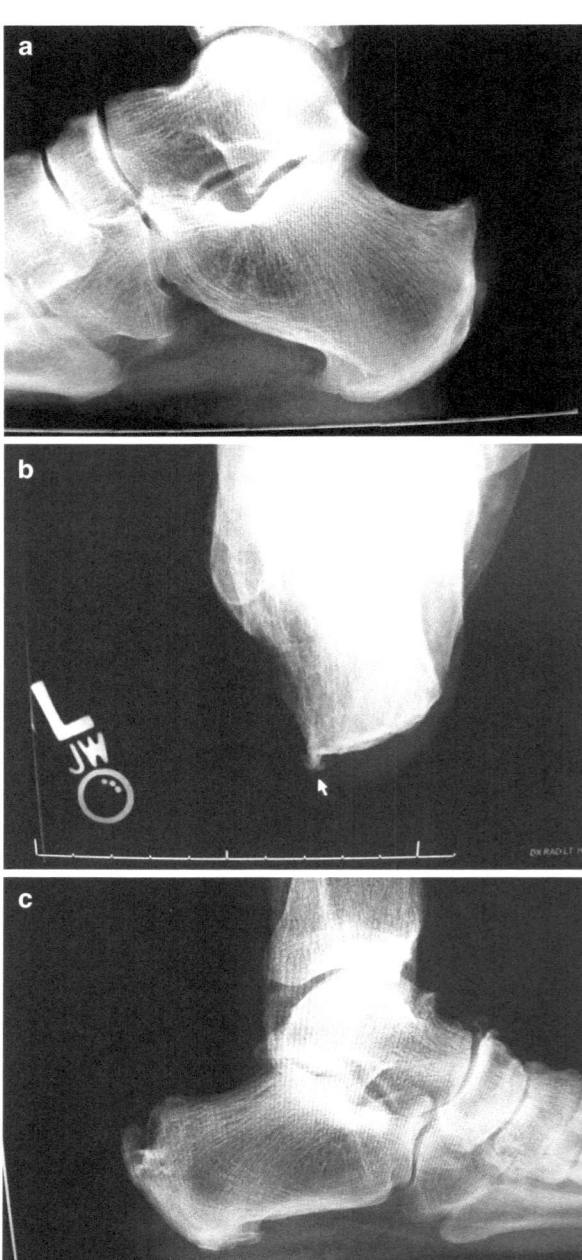

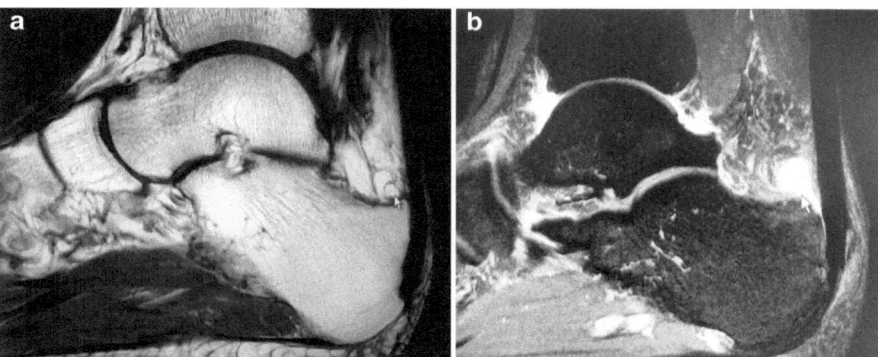

Fig. 14.2 (**a**) T1 MRI showing retrocalcaneal exostosis. (**b**) T2 MRI revealing bursitis

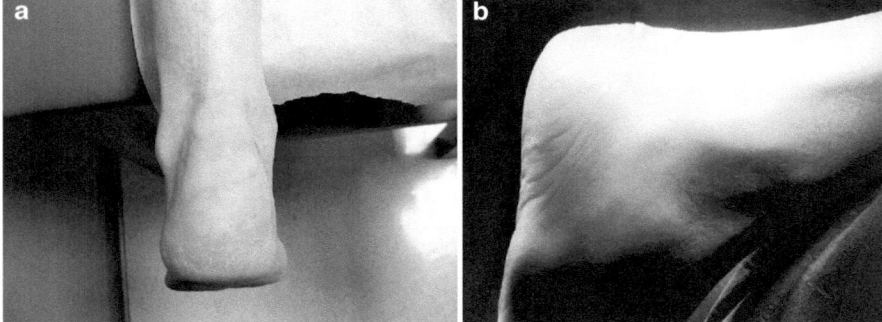

Fig. 14.3 Postoperative incisions showing (**a**) superomedial to infero-lateral approach and (**b**) transverse

(aka "pump bump") and insertional calcification (aka "AITC"). A reciprocating rasp is helpful in smoothing off the rough edges and making a smooth rounded remodeled calcaneus (Fig. 14.4). After copious irrigation, bone wax can be placed on the superior surfaces from medial to lateral to help prevent ectopic bone formation (though this occurs in less than 5% of patients 4 or more years postoperatively).[17]

The AT is reattached with suture anchors. Generally the number of anchors used ranges from 1 to 4[3,6,8,9] (Fig. 14.5). More anchors are used when more of the insertion needs to be reattached. Absorbable anchors superiorly may be helpful, in case re-resection is needed.[9,15] Care should be taken to place the suture knots in non-irritating regions. Irritation and granulomas from suture has recently been noted to occur in about 3% of AT surgeries in general.[13] This can occur with both absorbable and nonabsorbable materials. The tendon proximally is repaired first, particularly in cases where tendon débridement is needed. After inferior reattachment with

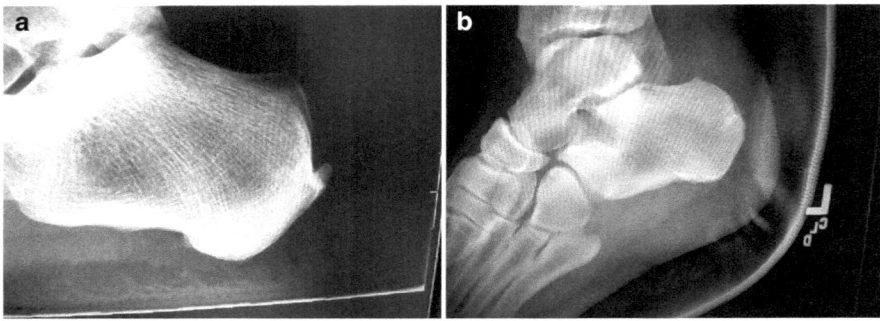

Fig. 14.4 (**a**) Preoperative and (**b**) postoperative Achilles insertional repair with retrocalcaneal exostectomy/bursectomy

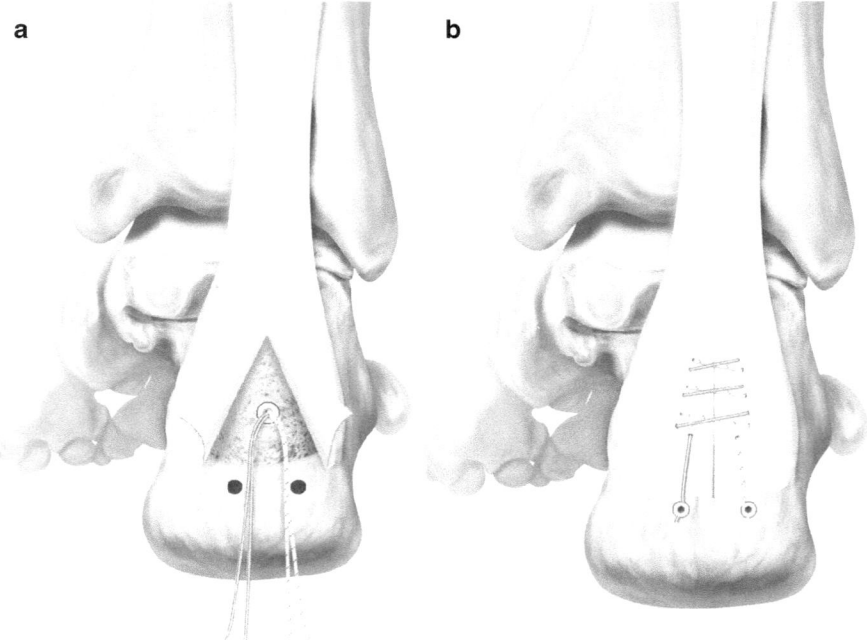

Fig. 14.5 (**a**, **b**) Suture anchors for Achilles tenodesis (Courtesy Arthrex, Inc., used with permission)

additional locking sutures, subcutaneous sutures with absorbable material are used. The skin is re-approximated with 3–0 nylon. A sterile compression dressing is applied, and the patient is placed in a splint or below-knee cast boot in slight equinus. Patients are seen within the first postoperatively week.

14.3.4 Postoperative Care

Patients are usually immobilized in a below-knee cast/boot non-weight bearing, for 4 weeks, followed by a weight-bearing period for an additional 6 weeks.[3,9,15] Sutures are removed at 2 weeks. Patients are advised to take an oral anti-inflammatory (such as indomethocin 75 mg BID or naproxen sodium 500 mg BID) for 2 weeks post-surgery to prevent ectopic bone formation. Patients are advised to continue elevating and icing the limb for the entire postoperative recovery period. Active ROM is allowed at 3 weeks working on plantar flexion and inversion/eversion with a towel. Formal physical therapy is initiated around 8–10 weeks, though cross-training on a stationary bike is allowed with the boot/cast (again with the heel on the pedal) one week post-surgery while still in a cast/boot. Swimming is allowed (without flip-turns) at 6 weeks. Physical therapy includes progressive strengthening (initially with surgical tubing and/or a towel at 3 weeks) including single-legged heel raises. Return to daily activities occurs around 12 weeks; weight-bearing sport activities can take 16 or more weeks.[9,15,18] Prior to using these surgical techniques, soft tissue anchors, and recommended period of immobilization, the results of this type of surgery were not as good as currently reported.

14.3.5 Conclusions

Retrocalcaneal Achilles insertional pathology can be relieved by surgery. Repair of the tendon insertion after debridement and calcaneal resection with soft tissue anchors appears to improve results. Patients should be advised of variability in post-operative convalescence.

14.4 Midsubstance Achilles Tendinopathy

Although scientifically sound epidemiological data are lacking, tendinopathy of the main body of the AT is common in athletes, accounting for 6–17% of all running injuries.[19,20] However, it does present in middle-aged overweight nonathletic patients without history of increased physical activity.[21,22] To date, no data are available to establish the incidence and prevalence of Achilles tendinopathy in other populations, even though the conditions has been correlated with seronegative arthropathies (e.g., ankylosing spondylitis).[23]

The essence of tendinopathy is a failed healing response, with degeneration and haphazard proliferation of tenocytes, disruption of collagen fibers, and subsequent increase in non-collagenous matrix.[24] Tendinopathic lesions affect both collagen matrix and tenocytes. The parallel orientation of collagen fibers is lost; collagen fiber diameter and overall collagen density are decreased.

14.4.1 Diagnosis

The diagnosis of Achilles tendinopathy is mainly based on history and clinical examination. Pain is the pivotal symptom. A common symptom is morning stiffness or stiffness after a period of inactivity, and a gradual onset of pain during activity. In athletes, it occurs at the beginning and end of a training session, with a period of diminished discomfort in between. As the condition progresses, pain may occur during exercise and it may interfere with activities of daily living. In severe cases, pain occurs at rest. In the acute phase, the tendon is diffusely swollen and edematous, and tenderness is usually greatest 2–6 cm proximal to the tendon insertion. A tender, nodular swelling is usually present in chronic cases.

Clinical examination is the best diagnostic tool. Both legs are exposed from above the knees, and the patient examined while standing and prone. The AT should be palpated for tenderness, heat, thickening, nodule, and crepitation.[25] The "painful arc" sign helps to distinguish between tendon and paratenon lesions. In paratendinopathy, the area of maximum thickening and tenderness remains fixed in relation to the malleoli from full dorsiflexion to plantar flexion; lesions within the tendon move with ankle motion. There is often a discrete nodule, whose tenderness markedly decreases or disappears when the tendon is put under tension.[26] In the Royal London Hospital test, the clinician elicits local tenderness by palpating the tendon with the ankle in neutral position or slightly plantar flexed. The tenderness significantly decreases or totally disappears when the ankle is dorsiflexed.[26]

The clinical diagnosis of Achilles tendinopathy, even in experienced hands, is not straightforward, and experienced examiners may have problems in reproducing the results of clinical examination based on simple tests. If a patient presents with tendinopathy of the AT with a tender area of intratendinous swelling that moves with the tendon and whose tenderness significantly decreases or disappears when the tendon is put under tension, a clinical diagnosis of tendinopathy can be formulated, with a high positive predictive chance that the tendon will show ultrasonographic and histologic features of tendinopathy.[26] In this instance, further imaging is indicated only for confirmatory, not diagnostic, purposes, as it is unlikely to change the management of the patient.[26]

14.4.1.1   VISA-A

The Victorian Institute of Sports Assessment – Achilles (VISA-A) questionnaire specifically measures the severity of Achilles tendinopathy.[27] It covers the domains of pain, function, and activity. Scores are summed to give a total out of 100. An asymptomatic person would score 100. In clinical care, the VISA-A questionnaire provides a valid, reliable, and user-friendly index of the severity of Achilles tendinopathy. The VISA-A-S questionnaire showed good responsiveness in a randomized controlled trial (it was sensitive for clinically important changes over time with treatment, easy for the patients to fill out, and the data were easily handled).[28] It has been cross-culturally adapted to Swedish,[29] Italian,[30] and Turkish.[31]

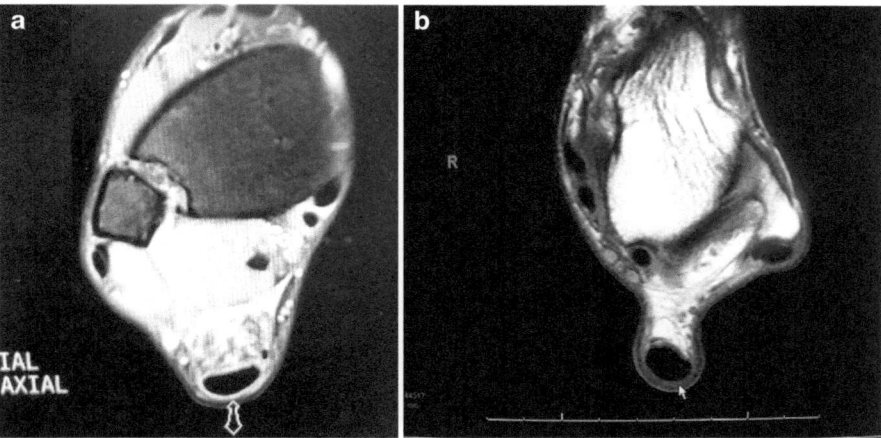

Fig. 14.6 (**a**) T2 and (**b**) T1 MRI showing paratendinosis with "halo-sign" (thickened paratenon)

14.4.1.2   Imaging

Radiographs may be useful in diagnosing associated or incidental bony abnormalities. Radiographs are routinely obtained on patients with symptoms lasting longer than six weeks to rule out bony abnormalities, and identify the possible presence of intratendinous calcific deposits and ossification.

Ultrasonography, though operator-dependent, correlates well with histopathologic finding,[32] and, especially in Europe, it is regarded as the primary imaging method. Only if ultrasonography remains unclear, MR imaging should be performed.[33] A major advantage of ultrasonography over other imaging modalities is its interactive capability.[34-36] Gray scale ultrasonography is associated with color or power Doppler to detect neovascularity.[36]

Magnetic resonance imaging (MRI) provides extensive information about the internal morphology of tendon and surrounding bone as well as other soft tissues. It allows to differentiate between paratendinopathy and tendinopathy of the main body of the tendon (Fig. 14.6). MRI is superior to ultrasound (US) in detecting incomplete tendon ruptures. However, given the high sensitivity of MRI, the data should be interpreted with caution, and correlated to the patient symptoms before making any recommendations.[37]

14.4.2   Management

The management of Achilles tendinopathy lacks evidence-based support, and tendinopathy sufferers are at risk of long-term morbidity with unpredictable clinical outcome.[38] The appropriate moment to switch from conservative to operative therapy remains unknown, as no solid data exist on the natural course of recovery. Nonoperative care should be in general a minimum of 3–6 months prior to considering surgery, since this condition has a good change of resolution. However, each patient should be evaluated independently.

14.4.2.1 Conservative Management

Several therapeutic options lack hard scientific background.[39,40]

Nonsteroidal Anti-inflammatory Drugs (NSAIDs)

Pharmacologic management strategies are essentially based on empirical evidence. Even though tendon biopsies show an absence of inflammatory cell infiltration, anti-inflammatory agents (nonsteroidal anti-inflammatory drugs and corticosteroids) are commonly used.[41] What may appear clinically as an "acute tendinopathy" is actually a well-advanced failure of a chronic healing response in which there is neither histological nor biochemical evidence of inflammation.[42] Ironically, the analgesic effect of NSAIDs[43] allows patients to ignore early symptoms, possibly imposing further damage on the affected tendon and delaying definitive healing.[44] NSAIDs appear to be effective, to some extent, for pain control. Early NSAIDs administration after an injury may have a deleterious effect on long-term tendon healing. Clearly there is a controversy on whether NSAIDs help or hinder the healing process.

Cryotherapy

Cryotherapy has been regarded as a useful intervention in the acute phase of Achilles tendinopathy, as it has an analgesic effect, reduces the metabolic rate of the tendon, and decreases the extravasation of blood and protein from new capillaries found in tendon injuries.[45] However, recent evidence in upper limb tendinopathy indicates that the addition of ice did not offer any advantage over an exercise program consisting of eccentric and static stretching exercises.[46]

Eccentric Exercise

A program of eccentric exercise has been proposed to counteract the failed healing response which apparently underlies tendinopathy, by promoting collagen fiber cross-linkage formation within the tendon, thereby facilitating tendon remodeling.[44] Although evidence of actual histological adaptations following a program of eccentric exercise is lacking, and the mechanisms by which a program of eccentric exercise may help to resolve the pain of tendinopathy remain unclear,[47] clinical results following such exercise program appear promising.[44,48] Though effective in Scandinavian population,[48,49] the results of eccentric exercises observed from other study groups[50,51] are less convincing than those reported from Scandinavia, with a

50–60% of good outcome after a regime of eccentric training both in athletic and sedentary patients. In general, the overall trend suggested a positive effect of an exercise program, with no study reporting adverse effects. Due to the lack of high-quality studies with clinically significant results, no strong conclusions can be made regarding the effectiveness of eccentric training (compared to control interventions) in relieving pain, improving function, or achieving patient satisfaction.[39,47]

In a randomized controlled trial[51] the efficacy of three protocols – a "wait-and-see" approach, repetitive low-energy shock wave therapy, and eccentric calf strengthening – for the management of chronic tendinopathy of the main body of the tendo Achillis was compared. Spontaneous recovery after more than 6 months of symptoms of tendinopathy of the main body of the tendo Achillis was unlikely in the majority of patients. The likelihood of recovery after 4 months was comparable after both eccentric loading and shock wave therapy, as applied. Success rates were in the region of 60% with either of these management modalities.

Combined management strategies (eccentric training and shock wave therapy) resulted in higher success rates compared to eccentric loading alone or shock wave therapy alone in a recent randomized controlled trial.[52] Eccentric training plus shock wave therapy should be offered to patients with chronic recalcitrant tendinopathy of the main body of the AT.[52]

Nitric Oxide

Nitric oxide is a small free radical generated by a family of enzymes, the nitric oxide synthases.[53] Recently, a prospective, randomized, double-blinded, placebo-controlled clinical trial was performed in patients with tendinopathy of the main body of the Achilles to evaluate the efficacy of nitric oxide administration via an adhesive patch.[54] Topical glyceryl trinitrate demonstrated efficacy in chronic noninsertional Achilles tendinopathy, and the treatment benefits continue at 3 years.[55] However, a recent study from England[56] failed to support the clinical benefit of topical glyceryl trinitrate patches.

14.4.2.2 Physical Modalities

The role of physical modalities in the management of tendinopathies remains unclear, and it is not possible to draw firm, evidence-based conclusions on their effectiveness.

The rationale for the clinical use of low-energy shock wave therapy to address the failed healing response of a tendon is the stimulation of soft tissue healing and the inhibition of pain receptors.[51] Low-energy shock wave therapy and eccentric training produced comparable results in a randomized controlled trial,[51] and both management modalities showed outcomes superior to the wait-and-see policy. The likelihood of recovery after 4 months was comparable after both eccentric loading and shock wave therapy, but success rates were 50–60%.

Hyperthermia induced by microwave diathermy raises the temperature of deep tissues to 41–45°C using electromagnetic power.[57] Hyperthermia induced into tissue by microwave diathermy can stimulate repair processes, increase drug activity, allow more efficient relief from pain, help removal toxic wastes, increase tendon extensibility and reduce muscle and joint stiffness.[57]

Ultrasound therapy is a widely available and frequently used electrophysical agent in sports medicine. However, systematic reviews and meta-analyses have repeatedly concluded that there is insufficient evidence to support a beneficial effect of ultrasound at dosages currently being introduced clinically. A new direction for ultrasound therapy in sports medicine has been proposed by research demonstrating that ultrasound can have clinically significant beneficial effects on injured tissue when low-intensity pulsed ultrasound is used.[58]

14.4.2.3 Intratendinous Injection

Sonographically guided intratendinous injection of hyperosmolar dextrose yielded a good clinical response in patients with chronic tendinopathy of the tendo Achillis.[59,60]

14.4.2.4 Sclerosing Injections and Neovascularization

In patients with chronic painful tendinopathy of tendo Achillis, but not in normal pain-free tendons, there is neovascularization outside and inside the ventral part of the tendinopathic area.[61,62] The good clinical effects with eccentric training may be due to the action on the neovessels and accompanying nerves. Also, local anesthetic injected in the area of neovascularization outside the tendon resulted in a pain-free tendon, indicating that this area is involved in pain generation. These are the bases for the injection of sclerosing substance polidocanol under ultrasound and color Doppler-guidance in the area with neovessels and nerves outside the tendon.

14.4.2.5 High Volume Ultrasound Guided Injections

High volume ultrasound guided injections aim to produce local mechanical effects causing neovessels to stretch, break, or occlude.[63] By occluding and possibly breaking these neovessels, the accompanying nerve supply would also be damaged either by trauma or ischemia, therefore decreasing the pain in patients with resistant Achilles tendinopathy. In a pilot study,[63] high volume image guided tendo Achilles injection of normal saline in patients with resistant Achilles tendinopathy decreased the amount of pain perceived by patients, while at the same time improving daily functional ankle and Achilles movements in the short- and long-term.

14.4.3 Surgery

14.4.3.1 Surgical Management of Tendinopathy of the Main Body of the AT

In 24–45.5% of patients with Achilles tendinopathy, conservative management is unsuccessful, and surgery is recommended after exhausting conservative methods of management, often tried for at least 6 months.[64,65] There is a lack of trials on surgical management of Achilles tendinopathy, and therefore the high success rate needs to be interpreted with caution. Surgical options range from simple percutaneous tenotomy[66,67] (possibly ultrasound-guided[68]), to minimally invasive stripping of the tendon,[69] to open procedures (Fig. 14.7).

The classical aim of open surgery is to excise fibrotic adhesions, remove areas of failed healing and make multiple longitudinal incisions in the tendon to detect intratendinous lesions and to restore vascularity and possibly stimulate the remaining viable cells to initiate cell matrix response and healing[45] (Fig 14.8). However, there is no level I evidence that fibrotic adhesions should be removed, and the areas of failed healing should be excised,[66-68] at least if the pathology does not involve the paratenon. Multiple longitudinal tenotomies trigger well-ordered neoangiogenesis of the AT[70] (Fig. 14.9). This would result in improved nutrition and a more favorable environment for healing.

A more recent approach targets not the tendinous lesion itself, but the neo-innervation which accompanies the neovessels. New minimally invasive stripping techniques[69] of neovessels from the Kager's triangle of the AT for patients with tendinopathy allow to achieve safe and secure disruption of neovessels and the accompanying nerve supply, producing a denervation effect. During open procedure, if more than 50% of the tendon is debrided, consideration could be given to a tendon augmentation or transfer.[64]

14.4.3.2 Minimally Invasive Stripping

We have developed a novel management modality whereby a minimal invasive technique of stripping of neovessels from the Kager's triangle of the AT is performed.[69] This achieves safe and secure breaking of neovessels and the accompanying nerve supply.

Under local or general anesthesia, the patient is positioned prone with a calf tourniquet which is inflated to 250 mmHg after exsanguination. Four skin incisions are made. The first two incisions are 0.5-cm longitudinal incisions at the proximal origin of the AT, just medial and lateral to the origin of the tendon. The other two incisions are also 0.5-cm long and longitudinal, but 1 cm distal to the distal end of the tendon insertion on the calcaneus.

A mosquito or a tendon passer is inserted in the proximal incisions, and the AT is freed of the peritendinous adhesions. A Number 1 unmounted Ethibond (Ethicon,

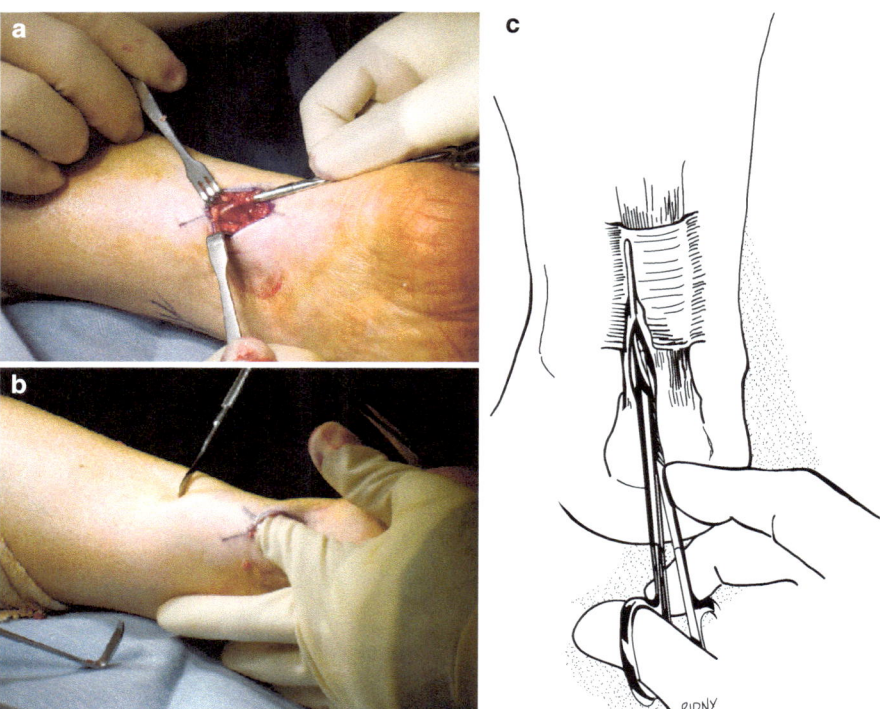

Fig. 14.7 (**a–c**) Intraoperative views and diagram of Achilles peritenolysis/decompression. Note thickened "watershed band." Key to success of the procedure is to make sure all the constricting paratenon is removed. When passively dorsiflexing the ankle, there should be no "tenting" over the Achilles tendon in the watershed region

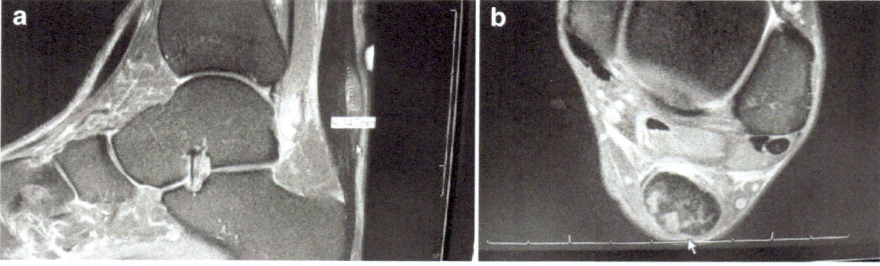

Fig. 14.8 (**a**) lateral T2 and (**b**) axial T2. Preoperative MRI showing significant longitudinal tearing of Achilles tendon in a pole-vaulter with symptoms for 2+ years

Somerville, NJ) suture thread is inserted proximally, passing through the two proximal incisions. The Ethibond is retrieved from the distal incisions, over the posterior aspect of the AT. Using a gentle see-saw motion, similar to using a Gigli saw, the Ethibond suture thread is made to slide posterior to the tendon, which is stripped and freed from the fat of Kager's triangle.

Fig. 14.9 Intraoperative view of Achilles post-débridement and longitudinal tenotomy in patient from Fig. 14.8. Because she was a high-level athlete, the tendon was repaired

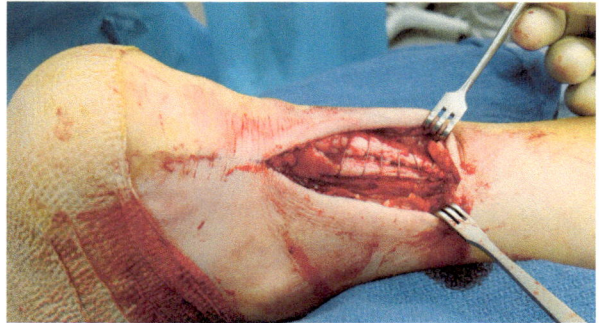

This minimal invasive technique reduces the risks of infection, is technically easy to master, and inexpensive. It may provide greater potential for the management of recalcitrant AT by breaking neovessels and the accompanying nerve supply to the tendon. It can be associated with other minimally invasive procedures to optimize results.

14.4.3.3 Outcome of Surgery

Most authorities anecdotally report excellent or good results in up to 85% of cases. In a systematic review,[71] most of the articles on surgical success rates reported successful results in over 70% of cases. However, this relatively high success rate is not always observed in clinical practice. The articles that reported success rates higher than 70% had poorer methods scores. Surgery appears to work better for athletes[72,73] and males.[74] There is little information on tendon transfers for chronic Achilles tendon ruptures, so one should reserve these procedures for resistant cases where there is no other viable option.[9] Even less is known about artificial tendon materials to supplement the Achilles tendon. Given that granuloma formation is common even with standard absorbable and non-absorbable suture, one should proceed with caution until longer-term studies occur.[13]

14.4.4 Postoperative Care

Rehabilitation is focused on early motion and avoidance of overloading the tendon in the initial healing phase. A period of initial splinting and crutch walking is generally used to allow pain and swelling to subside. After 14 days, patients are encouraged to start daily active and passive ankle range-of-motion exercises. The use of a removable walker boot can be helpful during this phase. Weight bearing is not limited according to the degree of debridement needed at surgery, and encourage early weight bearing. However, extensive debridements and tendon transfers may require protected weight bearing for 4–6 weeks postoperatively. After 6–8 weeks of mostly range-of-motion and light resistive exercises, initial tendon healing would have completed. More intensive strengthening exercises are started, gradually progressing to plyometrics and eventually running and jumping. Chapter 18 details typical rehabilitation post-Achilles surgery.

14.5 Conclusions

Achilles tendinopathy gives rise to significant morbidity, and, at present, only limited scientifically proven management modalities exist. The management of this condition remains a challenge, especially in athletes, in whom the physician often tries to be innovative. In many instances, this carries with it an unquantifiable risk.[75] A better understanding of tendon function and healing will allow specific management strategies to be developed.[76-78] Many interesting techniques are being pioneered.[79-82] Although these emerging technologies may develop into substantial clinical management options, their full impact needs to be evaluated critically in a scientific fashion. Soundwave/ESWT shows good promise while plasma-rich/PRP shows disappointing results in clinical studies, including randomized, prospective placebo controlled trials for Achilles tendinopathy.[83-86] Future trials should use validated functional and clinical outcomes, adequate methodology, and be sufficiently powered. Clearly, studies of high levels of evidence, for instance, large randomized trials, should be conducted to help answer many of the unsolved questions in this field.

References

1. Longo UG, Ronga M, Maffulli N. Achilles tendinopathy. Sports Med Arthrosc. 2009;17: 112–26.
2. Clain MR, Baxter DE. Achilles tendinitis. Foot Ankle. 1992;13:482–7.
3. Bouché R, McInnes B. Posterior heel pain: Haglund's deformity, pump bump deformity amd Achilles insertional calcific tendonitis (AITC). In: Chang T, editor. The foot and ankle. Philadelphia: Lippincott; 2005. p. 265–77.
4. Kolodziej P, Glisson RR, Nunley JA. Risk of avulsion of the Achilles tendon after partial excision for treatment of insertional tendonitis and Haglund's deformity: a biomechanical study. Foot Ankle Int. 1999;20:433–7.
5. Haglund P. Contribution to the diseased conditions of the tendo Achilles. Acta Chir Scand. 1928;63:292–4.
6. Carmont MR, Maffulli N. Management of insertional Achilles tendinopathy through a Cincinnati incision. BMC Musculoskelet Disord. 2007;8:82.
7. Leach RE, Schepsis AA, Takai H. Long-term results of surgical management of Achilles tendinitis in runners. Clin Orthop Relat Res. September 1992;282:208–12.
8. Maffulli N, Testa V, Capasso G, Sullo A. Calcific insertional Achilles tendinopathy: reattachment with bone anchors. Am J Sports Med. 2004;32:174–82.
9. Saxena A, Cheung S. Surgery for chronic Achilles tendinopathy. Review of 91 procedures over 10 years. J Am Podiatr Med Assoc. 2003;93:283–91.

10. Sella EJ, Caminear DS, McLarney EA. Haglund's syndrome. J Foot Ankle Surg. 1998;37:110–4. discussion 173.
11. Johnston E, Scranton P Jr, Pfeffer GB. Chronic disorders of the Achilles tendon: results of conservative and surgical treatments. Foot Ankle Int. 1997;18:570–4.
12. Krishna Sayana M, Maffulli N. Insertional Achilles tendinopathy. Foot Ankle Clin. 2005;10:309–20.
13. Saxena A, Maffulli N, Nguyen A, Li A. Wound complications from surgeries pertaining to the Achilles tendon: an analysis of 219 surgeries. J Am Podiatr Med Assoc. 2008;98:95–101.
14. Malay S, Duggar G. Heel surgery. In: Dalton McGlamry E, editor. Comprehensive textbook of foot surgery. Baltimore: Williams & Wilkins; 1987. p. 268–83.
15. Saxena A. Results of chronic Achilles tendinopathy surgery on elite and nonelite track athletes. Foot Ankle Int. 2003;24:712–20.
16. Leitze Z, Sella EJ, Aversa JM. Endoscopic decompression of the retrocalcaneal space. J Bone Joint Surg Am. 2003;85-A:1488–96.
17. Tozun R, Pinar H, Yesiller E, Hamzaoglu A. Indomethacin for prevention of heterotopic ossification after total hip arthroplasty. J Arthroplasty. 1992;7:57–61.
18. Saxena A. Return to athletic activity after foot and ankle surgery: a preliminary report on select procedures. J Foot Ankle Surg. 2000;39:114–9.
19. Maffulli N, Binfield PM, King JB. Tendon problems in athletic individuals. J Bone Joint Surg Am. 1998;80:142–4.
20. McLauchlan GJ, Handoll HH. Interventions for treating acute and chronic Achilles tendinitis. Cochrane Database Syst Rev. 2001:CD000232.
21. Astrom M. Partial rupture in chronic Achilles tendinopathy. A retrospective analysis of 342 cases. Acta Orthop Scand. 1998;69:404–7.
22. Maffulli N, Khan KM, Puddu G. Overuse tendon conditions: time to change a confusing terminology. Arthroscopy. 1998;14:840–3.
23. Ames PR, Longo UG, Denaro V, Maffulli N. Achilles tendon problems: not just an orthopaedic issue. Disabil Rehabil. 2008;30:1646–50.
24. Maffulli N, Barrass V, Ewen SW. Light microscopic histology of Achilles tendon ruptures. A comparison with unruptured tendons. Am J Sports Med. 2000;28:857–63.
25. Teitz CC, Garrett WE Jr, Miniaci A, Lee MH, Mann RA. Tendon problems in athletic individuals. Instr Course Lect. 1997;46:569–82.
26. Maffulli N, Kenward MG, Testa V, Capasso G, Regine R, King JB. Clinical diagnosis of Achilles tendinopathy with tendinosis. Clin J Sport Med. 2003;13:11–5.
27. Robinson JM, Cook JL, Purdam C, et al. The VISA-A questionnaire: a valid and reliable index of the clinical severity of Achilles tendinopathy. Br J Sports Med. 2001;35:335–41.
28. Silbernagel KG, Thomee R, Eriksson BI, Karlsson J. Continued sports activity, using a pain-monitoring model, during rehabilitation in patients with Achilles tendinopathy: a randomized controlled study. Am J Sports Med. 2007;35:897–906.
29. Silbernagel KG, Thomee R, Karlsson J. Cross-cultural adaptation of the VISA-A questionnaire, an index of clinical severity for patients with Achilles tendinopathy, with reliability, validity and structure evaluations. BMC Musculoskelet Disord. 2005;6:12.
30. Maffulli N, Longo UG, Testa V, Oliva F, Capasso G, Denaro V. Italian translation of the VISA-A score for tendinopathy of the main body of the Achilles tendon. Disabil Rehabil. 2008;30:1635–9.
31. Dogramaci Y, Kalacy A, Kucukkubathorn N, Ynandy T, Esen E, Yanat AN, Khan K. Validation of the VISA-A questionnaire for Turkish language: the VISA-A-Tr study. Br J Sports Med. 2011;45(5):453–5.
32. Rolf C, Movin T. Etiology, histopathology, and outcome of surgery in achillodynia. Foot Ankle Int. 1997;18:565–9.
33. Neuhold A, Stiskal M, Kainberger F, Schwaighofer B. Degenerative Achilles tendon disease: assessment by magnetic resonance and ultrasonography. Eur J Radiol. 1992;14:213–20.
34. Gibbon WW. Musculoskeletal ultrasound. Baillières Clin Rheumatol. 1996;10:561–88.
35. Khan KM, Maffulli N. Tendinopathy: an Achilles' heel for athletes and clinicians. Clin J Sport Med. 1998;8:151–4.

36. Malliaras P, Richards PJ, Garau G, Maffulli N. Achilles tendon Doppler flow may be associated with mechanical load among active athletes. Am J Sports Med. 2008;36(11):2210–5.
37. Leadbetter WB. Cell-matrix response in tendon injury. Clin Sports Med. 1992;11:533–78.
38. Kader D, Saxena A, Movin T, Maffulli N. Achilles tendinopathy: some aspects of basic science and clinical management. Br J Sports Med. 2002;36:239–49.
39. Maffulli N, Longo UG. Conservative management for tendinopathy: is there enough scientific evidence? Rheumatology (Oxford). 2008;47:390–1.
40. Rompe JD, Furia JP, Maffulli N. Mid-portion achilles tendinopathy – current options for treatment. Disabil Rehabil. 2008;30(20–22):1666–76.
41. Leadbetter WB. Anti-inflammatory therapy and sports injury: the role of non-steroidal drugs and corticosteroid injection. Clin Sports Med. 1995;14:353–410.
42. Vane JR. Introduction: mechanism of action of NSAIDs. Br J Rheumatol. 1996;35:1–3.
43. Almekinders LC. The efficacy of non-steroidal anti-inflammatory drugs in the treatment of ligament injuries. Sports Med. 1990;9:137–42.
44. Mafi N, Lorentzon R, Alfredson H. Superior short-term results with eccentric calf muscle training compared to concentric training in a randomized prospective multicenter study on patients with chronic Achilles tendinosis. Knee Surg Sports Traumatol Arthrosc. 2001;9:42–7.
45. Kannus P, Jozsa L. Histopathological changes preceding spontaneous rupture of a tendon. A controlled study of 891 patients. J Bone Joint Surg Am. 1991;73-A:1507–25.
46. Manias P, Stasinopoulos D. A controlled clinical pilot trial to study the effectiveness of ice as a supplement to the exercise programme for the management of lateral elbow tendinopathy. Br J Sports Med. 2006;40:81–5.
47. Maffulli N, Longo UG. How do eccentric exercises work in tendinopathy? Rheumatology (Oxford). 2008;47:1444–5.
48. Roos EM, Engstrom M, Lagerquist A, Soderberg B. Clinical improvement after 6 weeks of eccentric exercise in patients with mid-portion Achilles tendinopathy – a randomized trial with 1-year follow-up. Scand J Med Sci Sports. 2004;14:286–95.
49. Sayana MK, Maffulli N. Eccentric calf muscle training in non-athletic patients with Achilles tendinopathy. J Sci Med Sport. 2007;10:52–8.
50. Murrell GA. Oxygen free radicals and tendon healing. J Shoulder Elbow Surg. 2007;16:S208–14.
51. Rompe JD, Nafe B, Furia JP, Maffulli N. Eccentric loading, shock-wave treatment, or a wait-and-see policy for tendinopathy of the main body of tendo Achillis: a randomized controlled trial. Am J Sports Med. 2007;35:374–83.
52. Rompe JD, Furia J, Maffulli N. Eccentric loading versus eccentric loading plus shock-wave treatment for midportion Achilles tendinopathy: a randomized controlled trial. Am J Sports Med. 2009;37:463–70.
53. Longo UG, Olivia F, Denaro V, Maffulli N. Oxygen species and overuse tendinopathy in athletes. Disabil Rehabil. 2008;30:1563–71.
54. Paoloni JA, Appleyard RC, Nelson J, Murrell GA. Topical glyceryl trinitrate treatment of chronic noninsertional Achilles tendinopathy. A randomized, double-blind, placebo-controlled trial. J Bone Joint Surg Am. 2004;86-A:916–22.
55. Paoloni JA, Murrell GA. Three-year followup study of topical glyceryl trinitrate treatment of chronic noninsertional Achilles tendinopathy. Foot Ankle Int. 2007;28:1064–8.
56. Kane TP, Ismail M, Calder JD. Topical glyceryl trinitrate and noninsertional Achilles tendinopathy: a clinical and cellular investigation. Am J Sports Med. 2008;36:1160–3.
57. Giombini A, Giovannini V, Di Cesare A, et al. Hyperthermia induced by microwave diathermy in the management of muscle and tendon injuries. Br Med Bull. 2007;83:379–96.
58. Warden SJ. A new direction for ultrasound therapy in sports medicine. Sports Med. 2003;33:95–107.
59. Hoksrud A, Ohberg L, Alfredson H, Bahr R. Ultrasound-guided sclerosis of neovessels in painful chronic patellar tendinopathy: a randomized controlled trial. Am J Sports Med. 2006;34:1738–46.

60. Maxwell NJ, Ryan MB, Taunton JE, Gillies JH, Wong AD. Sonographically guided intratendinous injection of hyperosmolar dextrose to treat chronic tendinosis of the Achilles tendon: a pilot study. AJR Am J Roentgenol. 2007;189:W215-20.
61. Knobloch K, Schreibmueller L, Longo UG, Vogt PM. Eccentric exercises for the management of tendinopathy of the main body of the achilles tendon with or without an airHeeltrade mark brace. A randomized controlled trial. B: effects of compliance. Disabil Rehabil. 2008;30(20-22):1692–6.
62. Knobloch K, Schreibmueller L, Longo UG, Vogt PM. Eccentric exercises for the management of tendinopathy of the main body of the achilles tendon with or without the airheeltrade mark brace. A randomized controlled trial. A: effects on pain and microcirculation. Disabil Rehabil. 2008;30(20–22):1685–91.
63. Chan O, O'Dowd D, Padhiar N, et al. High volume image guided injections in chronic Achilles tendinopathy. Disabil Rehabil. 2008;30:1697–708.
64. Maffulli N, Kader D. Tendinopathy of tendo achillis. J Bone Joint Surg Br. 2002;84:1–8.
65. Paavola M, Kannus P, Järvinen TAH, Khan K, Józsa L, Järvinen M. Achilles tendinopathy. J Bone Joint Surg Am. 2002;84-A:2062–76.
66. Maffulli N, Testa V, Capasso G, Bifulco G, Binfield PM. Results of percutaneous longitudinal tenotomy for Achilles tendinopathy in middle- and long-distance runners. Am J Sports Med. 1997;25:835–40.
67. Testa V, Maffulli N, Capasso G, Bifulco G. Percutaneous longitudinal tenotomy in chronic Achilles tendonitis. Bull Hosp Jt Dis. 1996;54:241–4.
68. Testa V, Capasso G, Benazzo F, Maffulli N. Management of Achilles tendinopathy by ultrasound-guided percutaneous tenotomy. Med Sci Sports Exerc. 2002;34:573–80.
69. Longo UG, Ramamurthy C, Denaro V, Maffulli N. Minimally invasive stripping for chronic Achilles tendinopathy. Disabil Rehabil. 2008;30:1709–13.
70. Maffulli N. Re: etiologic factors associated with symptomatic Achilles tendinopathy. Foot Ankle Int. 2007;28:660, author reply 660–1.
71. Tallon C, Coleman BD, Khan KM, Maffulli N. Outcome of surgery for chronic Achilles tendinopathy. A critical review. Am J Sports Med. 2001;29:315–20.
72. Glaser T, Poddar S, Tweed B, Webb CW. Clinical inquiries. What's the best way to treat Achilles tendonopathy? J Fam Pract. 2008;57:261–3.
73. Maffulli N, Testa V, Capasso G, et al. Surgery for chronic Achilles tendinopathy yields worse results in nonathletic patients. Clin J Sport Med. 2006;16:123–8.
74. Maffulli N, Testa V, Capasso G, et al. Surgery for chronic Achilles tendinopathy produces worse results in women. Disabil Rehabil. 2008;30:1714–20.
75. Hamilton B, Remedios D, Loosemore M, Maffulli N. Achilles tendon rupture in an elite athlete following multiple injection therapies. J Sci Med Sport. 2008;11(6):566–8.
76. Movin T, Ryberg A, McBride DJ, Maffulli N. Acute rupture of the Achilles tendon. Foot Ankle Clin. 2005;10:331–56.
77. Sharma P, Maffulli N. Basic biology of tendon injury and healing. Surgeon. 2005;3:309–16.
78. Sharma P, Maffulli N. The future: rehabilitation, gene therapy, optimization of healing. Foot Ankle Clin. 2005;10:383–97.
79. Sharma P, Maffulli N. Biology of tendon injury: healing, modeling and remodeling. J Musculoskelet Neuronal Interact. 2006;6:181–90.
80. Sharma P, Maffulli N. Tendinopathy and tendon injury: the future. Disabil Rehabil. 2008; 30(20-22):1733–45.
81. Sharma P, Maffulli N. Tendon injury and tendinopathy: healing and repair. J Bone Joint Surg Am. 2005;87:187–202.
82. Sharma P, Maffulli N. Understanding and managing Achilles tendinopathy. Br J Hosp Med (Lond). 2006;67:64–7.
83. Rompe JD, Nafe B, Furia J, Maffulli N. Eccentric loading, shock-wave treatment or a wait-and-see policy for tendinopathy of the main body of tendo-Achillis: a randomized controlled trial. Am J Sports Med. 2007;35:374–83.

84. Saxena A, Ramdath S, O'Halloran P, Gerdesmeyer L, Gollwitzer H. Extra-corporeal pulsed-activated Therapy ("EPAT" Sound Wave) for Achilles tendinopathy: a prospective study. J Foot Ankle Surg. 2011; 50(3):315–19.
85. de Vos RJ, Weir A, Tol JL, Verhaar JA, Weinans H, van Schie HT. http://pubmed/21047840. No effects of PRP on ultrasonographic tendon structure and neovascularisation in chronic midportion Achilles tendinopathy. Br J Sports Med. 2011;45(5):387–92.
86. de Vos RJ, Weir A, van Schie HT, Bierma-Zeinstra SM, Verhaar JA, Weinans H, Tol JL. http://pubmed/20068208. Platelet-rich plasma injection for chronic Achilles tendinopathy: a randomized controlled trial. JAMA. 2010;303(2):144–9.

Chapter 15
Peroneal Tendinopathy

Francesco Oliva, Amol Saxena, Nicholas Antonio Ferran, and Nicola Maffulli

15.1 Surgical Techniques for Peroneal Tendons Subluxation

15.1.1 Introduction

Peroneal tendons dislocation is an uncommon sports-related injury. The first case was described by Monteggia in 1803 in a ballet dancer.[1] The injury is frequently associated with sports with cutting maneuvers such as judo, gymnastics, soccer, rugby, basketball, ice skating, skiing, water skiing, and mountaineering.[2] No specific age range is associated with the condition, but it clearly appears from the reported series that there is a relationship between dislocation of peroneal tendons and sport active people and road accidents.

Acute traumatic subluxation of the peroneal tendons is uncommon.[3] Acute injuries to the superior peroneal retinaculum can be initially managed conservatively with immobilization in a non-weight-bearing cast; this has a success rate of approximately 50%,[3,4] with preadolescent patients showing high rates of resolution after conservative management.[5]

F. Oliva, M.D., Ph.D.
Department of Trauma and Orthopaedic Surgery, University of Rome "Tor Vergata", Rome, Italy

A. Saxena, D.P.M. (✉)
Department of Sports Medicine, PAFMG-Palo Alto Division,
Clark Bldg., 3rd Flr, 795 El Camino Real, Palo Alto, CA 94301, USA
e-mail: heysax@aol.com

N.A. Ferran, M.B.B.S., M.R.C.S.Ed.
Department of Trauma and Orthopaedics, Lincoln County Hospital, Lincoln, Lincolnshire, UK

N. Maffulli, M.D., M.S., Ph.D., F.R.C.S (Orth).
Barts and The London School of Medicine and Dentistry, Centre for Sports and Exercise Medicine, Mile End Hospital, Queen Mary University of London,
London, E1 4DG, UK

A. Saxena (ed.), *Sports Medicine and Arthroscopic Surgery of the Foot and Ankle*, 187
DOI 10.1007/978-1-4471-4106-8_15, © Springer-Verlag London 2013

In chronic subluxation, patients often report previous ankle injuries that, in some cases, may have been misdiagnosed as a sprain. An unstable ankle that gives way or is associated with a popping or snapping sensation is another common complaint. Chronic subluxation of the peroneal tendons may be traumatic or habitual and voluntary. In the latter case, congenital deficiency of the superior peroneal retinaculum (SPR) and a shallow fibular groove may play a role.[6] In traumatic chronic subluxation, there is little to be gained with conservative management, and surgical management is generally advocated.[4,6-12] Often the clinical diagnosis can be difficult, and some authors report a 60% diagnostic capability at first clinical evaluation.[13]

15.1.2   Anatomy

The peroneal muscles lie in the lateral compartment of the leg. They are innervated by the superficial peroneal nerve and supplied by the posterior peroneal artery and branches of the medial tarsal artery. The peroneus longus muscle originates from the head and upper two-thirds of the peroneal surface of the fibula, and from the intermuscular septa. In 20% of Caucasians, a sesamoid bone, the *os peroneum*, can be observed close to the calcaneocuboid joint. The peroneus brevis muscle originates from the lower two-thirds of the fibula in front of that of the peroneus longus. The two peroneal tendons enter together in a common synovial sheath 4 cm above of the lateral malleolus, going through a fibro-osseous tunnel, the retromalleolar groove. The peroneus longus tendon lies posterior and lateral to the peroneus brevis tendon.

The peroneus tertius muscle, normally absent in 10.5% of dissected limbs, arises from the distal third of the anterior aspect of the fibula. The muscle belly, usually not separated from the extensor digitorum longus muscle, ends proximal to the inferior extensor retinaculum.[14] This anatomical variant can rarely cause antero-lateral pain and snapping ankle.[15]

Another anatomical variant of the peroneal tendons is the rare peroneus quartus, which, with a number of different attachments, is present in 6.6% of the dissected legs.[16] This tendon is as important as the peroneus tertius in the differential diagnosis with peroneal tendons subluxation and posterolateral ankle pain.

The retrofibular (also called retromalleolar) groove is formed not by the concavity of the fibula itself, but by a relatively pronounced ridge of collagenous soft tissue blended with the periosteum that extends along the posterolateral lip of the distal fibula.[17,18] The other component of the retrofibular groove is the SPR posterolaterally, a fibrous band that originates from the distal lateral surface of fibula. The SPR is extremely variable in width, thickness, and insertional patterns. It normally has two bands: The superior band inserts on the Achilles tendon[19]; the inferior band inserts on the peroneal tubercle on the lateral surface of calcaneus.[20]

The peroneus longus passes between the cuboid groove and the long plantar ligament, and inserts onto the plantar surface of 1st metatarsal and the lateral face of medial cuneiform. The sural nerve lies in proximity of the peroneal groove. The sural nerve descends between the medial and lateral heads of the gastrocnemius, pierces of deep fascia proximally in the leg, and is joined by a sural communicating branch of the common peroneal nerve. It descends lateral to the Achilles tendon, near the small saphenous vein, to the region between the lateral malleolus and the calcaneus. It supplies the posterior and lateral skin of the distal third of the leg, proceeding distal to the lateral malleolus along the lateral side of the foot and little toe. It should be preserved at surgery.

The peroneal tendons receive their vascular supply from separate vincula that arise from the posterior peroneal artery and from the medial tarsal artery.[21] There are three distinct avascular zones: one in the peroneus brevis tendon when it curves around the lateral malleolus, and two in the peroneus longus.[22] The first avascular zone in the peroneus longus lies at the curve around the lateral malleolus, and the second occurs where the tendon curves around the cuboid.[22]

The peroneus brevis abducts and everts the foot, and flexes the foot plantarly. The peroneus longus plays the same functions of the peroneus brevis, but it is an important stabilizer of the medial column of the foot during stance. Together, they are dynamic stabilizers of the lateral ankle complex. Their antagonists are the flexor digitorum longus, flexor hallucis longus, and posterior and anterior tibialis.

15.1.3 Physiopathology

An acute peroneal tendons subluxation may occur when the tendons dislocate from the retrofibular groove during tendon loading. The most common mechanism is a sudden, reflexive contraction of the peroneal muscles during acute inversion of the foot with the ankle dorsiflexed, or during forced dorsiflexion of the everted foot.[20] Basset and Speer analyzed the links between the position of the foot and the type of disorders as a result of inversion ankle injuries. Ankle inversion and plantar flexion less than 15° may produce an injury of the SPR. At a plantar flexion angle greater than 25°, the peroneal tendons are protected from injury.[23]

The SPR is the primary restraint of the peroneal tendons: Its integrity is fundamental to avoid a peroneal tendon subluxation.[24] Disruption of the SPR occurs infrequently.[25] Damages of the SPR are associated with lateral ankle instability and inadequate concavity or depth of the retromalleolar groove.[26] Laxity of the SPR can result from a calcaneovalgus foot in neuromuscular diseases. Also, the rare congenital absence of the SPR must be considered as contributor to the mechanism of dislocation.[27-29]

Acute rupture of the SPR with potential subluxation of the peroneal tendons may cause longitudinal tears in the peroneus brevis tendon.[22] In the anatomical area where the peroneus brevis tendon passes through the fibular groove, the tendon is nearly avascular.[22] In cadaveric studies, disruption of the lateral collateral ankle ligaments places considerable strain on the SPR: this explains why the two conditions commonly coexist.[26]

Still poorly studied are non-traumatic subluxations of peroneal tendons, which can be caused by congenital or acquired pathological conditions. Hence, several congenital anatomical abnormalities, as a convex, flat or shallow, or, in rare cases, even absent retrofibular groove, may be present.[25,29] The absence of the SPR may also be congenital.[30] A bifid peroneus brevis has also been reported as a cause of subluxation.[31] A paralytic calcaneovalgus ankle is often associated with laxity of the retinaculum.[32]

Congenital dislocation of the peroneal tendons may be associated with a calcaneoval-gus foot type.[29] Acquired peroneal tendon subluxation is described in patients with neuromuscular diseases such as cerebral palsy,[3] and can also occur when the posterior surface of the lateral fibula is deformed as a consequence of osteochondritis.[33]

15.1.4 Classifications

Peroneal tendons subluxation is due mostly to a damage of the SPR. Eckert and Davis in 1976 distinguished three grades of acute tears. In grade 1, the retinaculum is separated from the collagenous lip and lateral malleolus. In grade 2, the collage-nous lip is elevated with the retinaculum. In grade 3, a thin sliver of bone, visible on radiographs, is avulsed with the collagenous lip and the retinaculum.[25] Ogden in 1987 added a fourth grade, describing it as the SPR torn away from its posterior attachment on the calcaneus.[34] Clinical determination of injury grade is not possible, except for grade 3 injuries, which can be diagnosed on radiographs. Previously, some authors have described an intrasheath peroneal subluxation,[35,36] but only recently Raikin and colleagues[37] proposed as a subgroup of peroneal subluxation an intrasheath subluxation. In this instance, the peroneal tendons switch their relative positions (the longus tendon comes to lie deep and medial to the brevis tendon) within the peroneal groove. An associated tear of the peroneous brevis is described without any lesion of the superior retinaculum. The clinical signs of intrasheath subluxation are very similar to the grade 1 of Eckert and Davis classification, but ultrasonography can help to diagnose these variants. Realistically, it is hard to believe that the SPR remains intact during a switch of the positions of the peroneal tendons. Hence, probably even intrasheath peroneal dislocations should be classified as a grade I injury according to Eckert and Davis (Fig. 15.1).

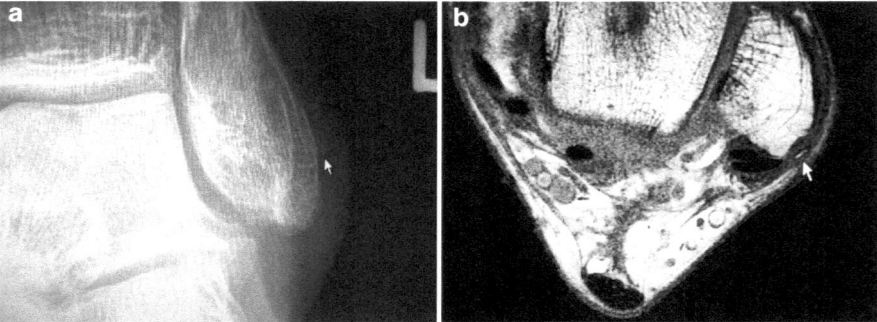

Fig. 15.1 (**a**) Pre-op X-ray showing avulsed peroneal retinaculum. (**b**) MRI showing torn peroneal retinaculum. (**c**) Diagram of the classification of peroneal retinaculum tears. PLT, peroneus longus tendon; PBT, peroneus brevis tendon; SPR, superior peroneal retinaculum

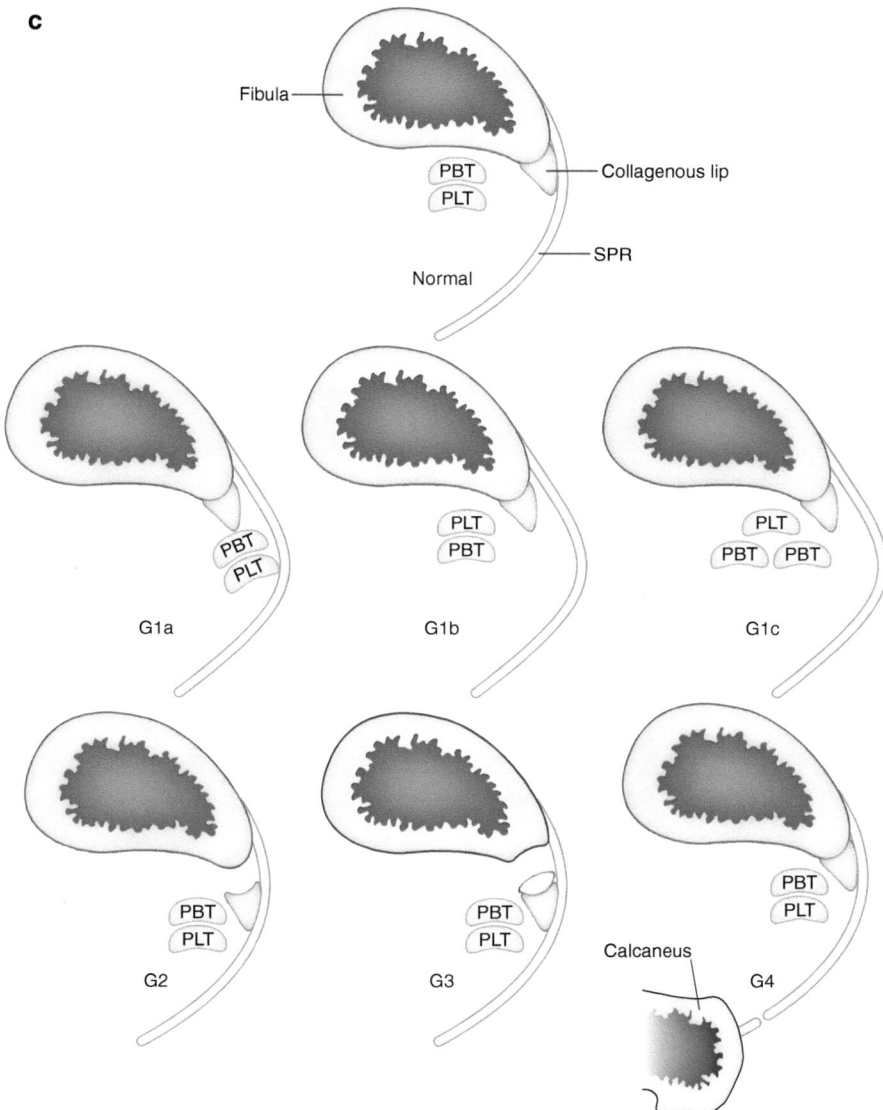

Fig. 15.1 (continued)

15.1.5 Surgical Techniques

Many surgical techniques limited only to case series have been described but only Level IV/Grade C evidence has been produced. No randomized studies have been conducted to determine which procedure is the most successful. (Table 15.1)[38-56]

Table 15.1 Studies and surgical techniques for the management of peroneal tendons subluxation

Authors	Year	Level of evidence	Number of cases	Procedures
Eckert and Davis[25]	1976	IV	73	Anatomical reattachment of SPR
Marti[38]	1977	IV	12	Modified Kelly
Zoellner and Clancy[12]	1979	IV	9	Groove deepening
Escalas et al.[4]	1980	IV	28	Jones procedure
Arrowsmith et al.[39]	1983	IV	6	Anatomical reattachment of SPR plus groove deepening
Poll and Duijfjes[40]	1984	IV	10	Rerouting tendon under CFL
Martens et al.[41]	1986	IV	11	Rerouting tendon under CFL
Micheli et al.[42]	1989	IV	12	Modified kelly
Orthner et al.[43]	1989	IV	23	Anatomical reattachment plus screw
Wirth[44]	1990	IV	15	Modified Viernstein and Kelly
Thomas et al.[45]	1992	IV	31	Modified Ellis-Jones
Steinböck et al.[46]	1994	IV	13	Rerouting tendon under CFL
Mason and Henderson[47]	1996	IV	11	Anatomical reattachment of SPR
Karlsson et al.[48]	1996	IV	15	Soft tissue reconstruction of superior retinaculum
Kollias and Ferkel[49]	1997	IV	12	Groove deepening
Hui et al.[50]	1998	IV	21	Anatomical reattachment of SPR
Mendicino et al.[51]	2001	IV	?	Groove deepening
Shawen et al.[52]	2004	IV	20	Groove deepening
Porter D, McCarrol J et al.[53]	2005	IV	13	Groove deepening
Adachi et al.[54]	2006	IV	20	Anatomical reattachment of SPR
Maffulli et al.[55]	2006	IV	14	Anatomical reattachment of SPR
Ogawa et al.[56]	2007	IV	15	Groove deepening

Studies which reported less than five patients are not listed

Generally, five categories of surgical repair are listed: (1) Anatomic reattachment of the retinaculum; (2) Reinforcement of the superior peroneal retinaculum with local tissue transfers; (3) Rerouting the peroneal tendons behind the calcaneofibular ligament; (4) Bone block procedures; (5) Groove-deepening procedures.

15.1.5.1 Anatomic Reattachment of SPR

The aim of anatomic reattachment of the SPR is the restoration of the primary restraint of the peroneal tendons. Reattachment with sutures brought through drill holes in the distal fibula has been described by several authors.[8,25,38-40,47,48] Alternatively, Beck[6] brought the retinaculum through a slip produced in the distal fibula and fixed this with a screw, reporting on nine patients without complication. Eighteen of 21 patients treated with the "Singapore operation" at 9 years had excellent results. Three patients experienced postoperative pain and neuromas, but no recurrence was noted.[50] Karlsson and colleagues reported 13 patients with good to excellent results associating a groove deepening in conjunction with reattachment of the SPR if the posterior surface of the fibula was flat or convex.[48] Orthner et al.

obtained excellent results for peroneal tendons subluxation suturing side by side the SPR in acute lesions.[43] Adachi et al. proposed retinaculoplasty, opening the false pouch through one incision, and suturing the SPR to the fibula while tensioning it. In this study, the authors reported that 15 of the 18 patients involved in sports activities returned to their previous activities without reducing their activity levels.[54] Recently, an endoscopic technique for the anatomical repair of the SPR has been described.[57] Anatomic reattachment of superior retinaculum seems to be the preferred technique in patients with acute subluxation of peroneal tendons.

15.1.5.2 Reinforcement of SPR with Soft Tissue

Several authors have described procedures to augment or reinforce an attenuated SPR with soft tissue transfer. Ellis-Jones[58] first described restraining the peroneal tendons with a strip of Achilles tendon anchored through a drill hole in the fibula. No recurrences were noted in a long-term follow-up of 15 patients who underwent the Ellis-Jones repair.[4] Thomas et al.[45] described a modification to this procedure that allowed the use of a smaller strip of Achilles tendon, reducing the risk of weakening the Achilles tendon. Use of the tendon of peroneus brevis,[39,59,60] plantaris[61,62] and peroneus quartus[63] have been described for the same purpose. Zoellner and Clancy[12] and Gould[9] used periosteal flaps to restrain the peroneal tendons in a deepened peroneal groove with satisfactory results. In patients treated with a periosteal flap from the retrofibular groove on its own or together with groove deepening, no postoperative complications were noted.[64]

15.1.5.3 Rerouting the Peroneal Tendons Behind the Calcaneofibular Ligament

This surgical technique does not address the issue of restoration of the anatomy of the SPR, but uses the calcaneofibular ligament as the natural alternative restraint. Platzgummer[65] and later Steinbock et al.[46] divided the calcaneofibular ligament, transposed the tendons behind it, and sutured the calcaneofibular ligament back together. The 13 patients operated with this technique showed good or excellent results, with no evidence of recurrence or instability. Sarmiento and Wolf divided the peroneal tendons and re-sutured them after rerouting them behind the calcaneofibular ligament[66]; 11 patients showed no evidence of recurrence or instability at follow-up, although two patients suffered a sural nerve injury. Martens et al. used the same technique of Sarmiento with excellent results at 30-month follow-up in 11 patients.[41] Both methods may potentially weaken the relevant structures. To preserve the integrity of the calcaneofibular ligament, a bone block of the ligamentous insertion on the fibula[67] or the calcaneus[40] can be mobilized, the tendons are transposed, and the bone block is reattached with a screw. Pozzo and Jackson[11] reported no complication and return to full level of activity in a case report. Poll and Duijfjes[40] reported ten patients with no recurrence or instability. Ferroudji et al.

reported their experience with 19 patients, with excellent results in 17 patients. Sports activities were resumed after an average of 3.3 months.[68] This surgical technique should be preferred in patients with chronic luxation of the peroneal tendons in whom the SPR is absent.

15.1.5.4   Bone Block Procedure

These surgical procedures were developed to deepen the retrofibular groove using a bone graft as a physical restraint to the peroneal tendons. In 1920, Kelly[67] described a bone block procedure using screw fixation and later designed a wedge-shaped graft that avoided the use of screws near the ankle joint. Watson-Jones and DuVries[69,70] modified Kelly's technique. Watson-Jones[69] used an osteoperiosteal flap anchored by a soft tissue pedicle, and secured it posteriorly with sutures. DuVries[70] anchored a posteriorly displaced wedge with a screw. Other authors reported on patients with chronic subluxation operated with a modified Kelly technique with no recurrence.[38,44] In 1989, Micheli and colleagues[42] treated 12 patients with an inferiorly displaced fibula bone graft fixed with screws; one patient suffered a traumatic fracture of the graft, and two required exploration for pain; there were no recurrences of the subluxation. Adhesion of the peroneal tendons to the fresh bone wound, fractures of bone grafts, and the need for metalwork are major disadvantages of bone block procedures.[6] This surgical technique seems to be the more exposed to intraoperative and postoperative complications, and should be reserved for selected cases.

15.1.5.5   Groove Deepening

Patients presenting with a flat or convex retrofibular sulcus could be managed with this surgical technique. Zoellner and Clancy[12] elevated an osteoperiosteal flap on the posterior aspect of the distal fibula, and removed cancellous bone with a gouge. The flap was then reduced into the deepened sulcus, and the tendons replaced into this. Their nine patients had excellent results with no recurrence or instability. Hutchinson and Gustafson described a similar method in combination with SPR reattachment. Of 20 patients, three had poor results with recurrence of the subluxation, and one of these developed reflex sympathetic dystrophy.[71] Gould[9] reported a single patient in whom groove deepening was incorporated with restraint of the peroneal tendons by reflection of elevated osteoperiosteal flap. Recently, Ogawa et al. used an indirect fibular groove–deepening technique.[56] Mendicino and colleagues[51] employed intramedullary drilling and cortical impaction to achieve groove deepening. Porter et al. proposed groove deepening associated with an accelerated rehabilitation program. Eight of 13 patients returned to pre-injury sports participation.[53] The depth of the retrofibular sulcus was previously thought to play an important role in restraining the peroneal tendons.[49,52] Recently, however, the need for groove deepening has been questioned. Anatomic studies demonstrate the incidence of a flat or convex sulcus as high as 18%,[72] 28%,[58] and 30%.[73] The low incidence of peroneal tendon subluxation would suggest that the morphology of the groove is not a predisposing factor to subluxation.[72] Histologic studies demonstrating that the peroneal groove is defined by the fibrocartilagenous periosteal cushion and not by the bony sulcus add weight to this argument.

15.1.6 Preferred Surgical Technique

Under general or spinal anesthetic, the patient is placed supine on the operating table with a sandbag under the buttock of the operative side to internally rotate the affected leg. A tourniquet is applied to the thigh, the leg exsanguinated, and the cuff inflated to 250 mmHg. A 5-cm longitudinal incision is made along the course of the peroneal tendons. The incision starts posterior to the tip of the lateral malleolus and progressed proximally, staying well anterior to the sural nerve. The incision is deepened to the peroneal tendon sheath, which is incised longitudinally 3 mm posterior to the posterior border of the fibula. Normally, the SPR itself is thin and deficient, and it was detached from its posterior attachment on the calcaneus in our case series.[55] The peroneal tendons are identified by blunt dissection and protected. Attrition lesions and longitudinal tears of peroneal tendons when found are treated with a very gentle débridement or suturing with absorbable sutures.[74-76] After that, we expose the lateral aspect of the lateral malleolus, and the "pouch" formed between the bony surface of the lateral malleolus and the superior peroneal retinaculum, where the tendons subluxate, becomes visible. The SPR does not heal back to its normal attachment on the posterolateral aspect of the fibula but in an elongated fashion more anteriorly on the lateral aspect of the fibula, creating a pouch on the lateral fibula into which the tendons can subluxate. The bony surface of the lateral malleolus is roughened with a periosteal elevator to produce a bleeding surface, and three or four anchors (Mitek GII, Ethicon Ltd, Edinburgh, Scotland) with 2/0 absorbable sutures (Vicryl, polyglactin 910 braided absorbable suture, Ethicon) are inserted along the posterior border of the lower fibula (Fig. 15.2). After manual testing that the anchors cannot be dislodged, the SPR is reconstructed in a "vest over pants" fashion,[74] making sure that the pouch between the bony surface of the lateral malleolus and the SPR is totally obliterated. The ankle is kept in eversion and slight dorsiflexion so that the peroneal tendons were in the "worst possible position." The strength of the repair is tested moving the ankle through the whole range of motion. The wound is closed in layers with 2/0 Vicryl for the subcutaneous fat, un-dyed 3/0 Vicryl for subcuticular, and Steri-Strips for the skin (3M, Loughborough, United Kingdom). Dressing swabs, dressing, and crepe bandage are applied. A below-the-knee walking cast is applied with the ankle in neutral and slight eversion. Weight bearing is allowed from the day after the operation, and the cast is removed 4 weeks after the procedure, when rehabilitation is started. Gradual return to activities and to sport is allowed during the course of 3–4 months from the procedure.[55,76]

Fig. 15.2 Anatomical reattachment of the superior retinaculum with anchors. (**a**) Diagram and (**b**) X-ray of anchor placement. (**c**) Intraoperative view of suture placement for retinaculum repair

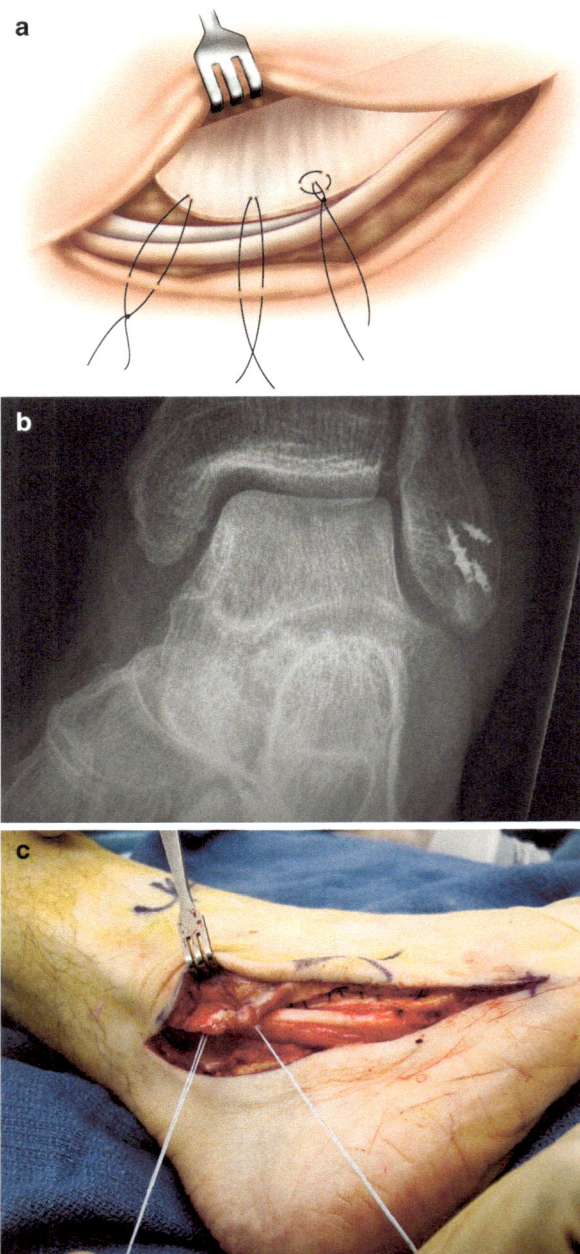

15.1.7   Postoperative Care

Patients are discharged the day after surgery, after having been taught to use crutches by an orthopedic physiotherapist. No thrombo-prophylaxis is used. Patients are allowed to bear weight on the operated leg as tolerated, but are told to keep the leg elevated as much as possible for the first 2 postoperative weeks. Patients are seen on an outpatient basis at the second postoperative week, and the cast is removed 4 weeks from the operation. Patients then mobilize the ankle with physiotherapy guidance. They are allowed to partially weight-bear, and commenced gradual stretching and strengthening exercises over 8–10 weeks after surgery. Cycling and swimming are started 2 weeks after removal of the cast. Patients are allowed to return to their sport on the fifth postoperative month.[55,75,76]

15.2   Surgical Techniques for Peroneal Tendon Tears

15.2.1   Introduction

Peroneal tendon tears were thought to be uncommon and a relatively new entity when reported by Evans in 1966. Peroneal tendon tears were seldom described until the early 1990s, when numerous case reports and moderately sized case series were published.[23,77-89] Peroneal tendon tears are thought to occur from both acute trauma and chronic instability, with and without subluxation. Peroneal retinaculum insufficiency is described in the preceding section. Chronic retinaculum insufficiency has been associated with peroneal tendon tears.[80-82,90,91] As with peroneal retinaculum pathology, tendon tears can often be difficult to recognize immediately. Diagnostic tests and clinical exam are paramount. Sobel and Mizel describe the proximal injuries as "Zone I" and the distal injuries associated with the Os Peroneum as "Zone II." Zone I injuries generally involve tears and dislocations of the tendon of peroneus brevis, while Zone II injuries involve Peroneus Longus pathology often with an Os Peroneum. They coined this condition POPS, Painful Os Peroneum Syndrome.[81] Surgical treatment for both regions is often effective; the current treatment recommendations are based on Level IV & V Evidence.[80]

15.2.2   Anatomy

Much of the pertinent anatomy has been described in the previous section. In addition, the incidence of the Os Peroneum and its association with lateral foot pain should be considered.[79,81] The Os Peroneum is present in 4–26% of individuals, depending on race and ethnicity.[79,92-94] A low-lying muscle from Peroneus Brevis or an anomalous Peroneus Quartus has also been associated with peroneal tendon tears (Fig. 15.3).[16,95,96] Peroneal tubercle hypertrophy has also been noted with peroneal tendon tears.[78-81,89]

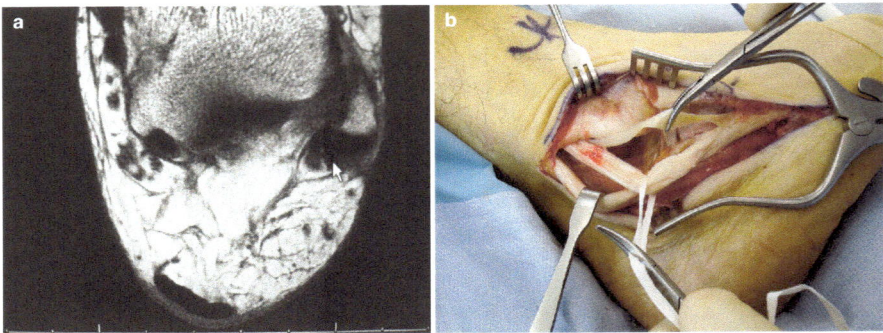

Fig. 15.3 (**a**) MRI showing accessory peroneal (quartus) tendon and peroneal brevis tear. (**b**) Intra-op view showing accessory peroneal (quartus) tendon and peroneal brevis tear

15.2.3   Clinical Findings

Patients with peroneal tendon tears complain of lateral ankle and foot pain. Acute onset of pain can occur with inversion injuries. Patients may state they felt a "pop" and have ankle weakness. Ankle instability was noted as early as 1979 with peroneal tears.[97] Clinically, patients may have noticeable pain with active resistance to the Peronei, and with single-legged weight bearing. Proprioception is altered. Swelling is often present along the peroneal tendons. Cavo-varus foot structure may be present causing a supinated foot structure, thereby putting more strain on the Peroneals. A Coleman block test should be performed to evaluate for a rigidly plantarflexed first ray causing hindfoot varus, versus a calcaneus varus (Fig. 15.4).[80] Weight-bearing plain radiographs should identify ankle varus, degenerative arthritis, accessory ossicles, and exostoses (Fig. 15.5). An Os Peroneum is often present within the Peroneus Longus tendon in either a bony or cartilaginous form. A proximally migrated Os Peroneum indicates rupture of the Peroneus Longus (Fig. 15.6).[80-82,86,88,89,94] Other bony structures can be associated with peroneal tendinopathy. A hypertrophied peroneal tubercle on the lateral calcaneus can often be associated with fraying and even laceration of the adjacent tendons, which is best visualized on MRI (Fig. 15.7).[80-82,86] Subluxation of the Peronei from posterior to the fibula may result in tearing of the Peroneus Brevis in particular, more commonly in older patients (Fig. 15.8). This may be due to long-standing insufficiency.[80,98] Inspection of shoe gear, inserts, and orthoses should also be performed. History of inflammatory arthritis such as rheumatoid arthritis, Gout and Reiter's syndrome, and subsequent testing when indicated should be considered.[99]

Radiographic tests for peroneal tendinopathy also include tenograms and MRI examinations. Tenograms are useful for diagnosing stenosing tenosynovitis (Fig. 15.9). MRI can also indentify this, particularly since fluid is often evident in pathological states of tendons.[27,90] Ultrasound may be used as it shows fluid within the tendon sheath and has high specificity for dislocations and tears, but osteochondral

Fig. 15.4 (**a**) Patient with right-sided peroneus longus tear, with previous repair on left. Note plantarflexed 1st metatarsal. (**b**) Coleman block test showing varus rearfoot when forefoot is on the ground. (**c**) With forefoot suspended off the ground, the rearfoot moves to neutral. This demonstrates that the patient's rearfoot varus deformity is due to the plantarflexed 1st metatarsal

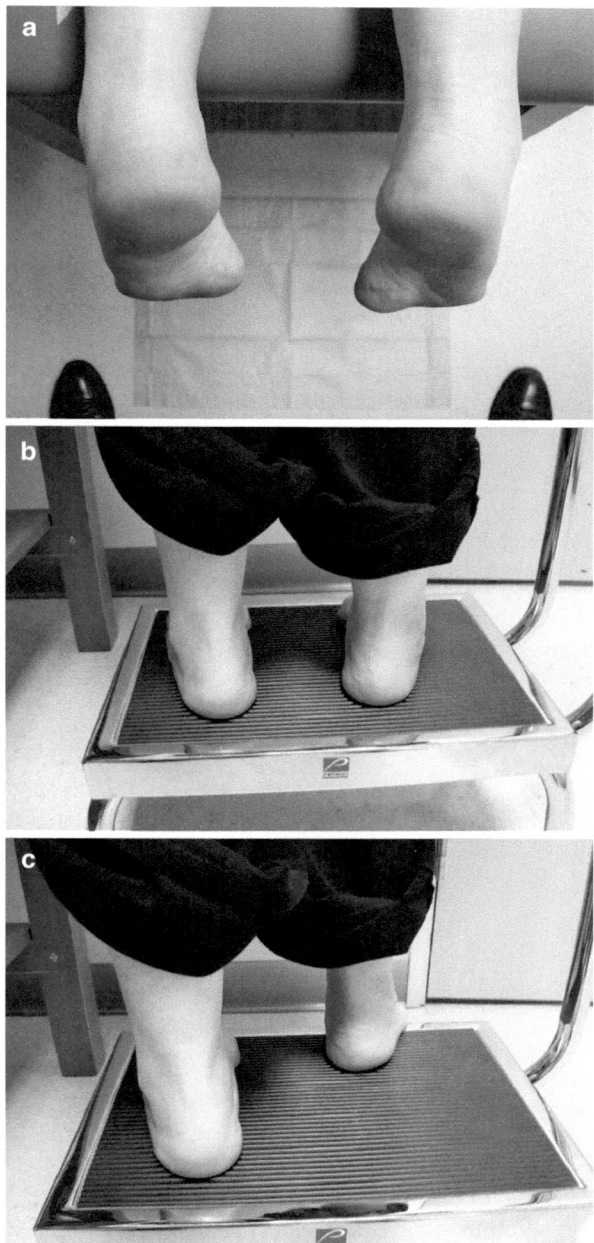

and transchondral defects and accessory ossicles may not be seen with ultrasound.[37,80] Fluid in the peroneal sheath may be indicative of a longitudinal tear, particularly with MRI (Fig. 15.10).[80,86,88,90] MRI has a fairly high sensitivity and

Fig. 15.5 Prominent peroneal tubercle

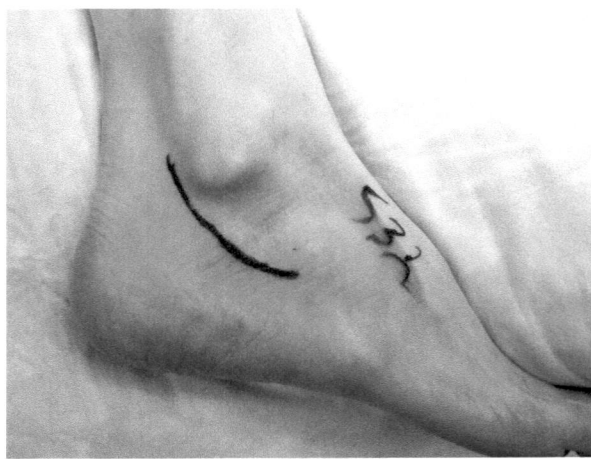

Fig. 15.6 Proximally migrated os peroneum indicating peroneus longus rupture

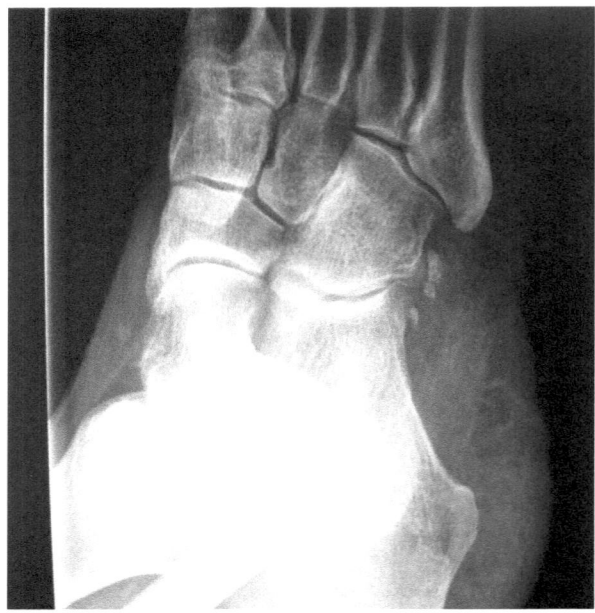

specificity rate, and has become the "gold standard," though false-positives occur very commonly.[80,86,90] The fact that many patients have asymptomatic tears noted on MRI exams points to the critical importance of the clinical exam.

To conclude a patient may have a peroneal tendon tear when suggested on MRI, and it is important in this instance to document peroneal weakness and pain. A diagnostic injection within the peroneal sheath (from proximal to the retinaculum with approximately 2 mL of local anesthetic) providing relief can confirm the

Fig. 15.7 MRI showing hypertrophic peroneal tubercle causing fraying of peroneals

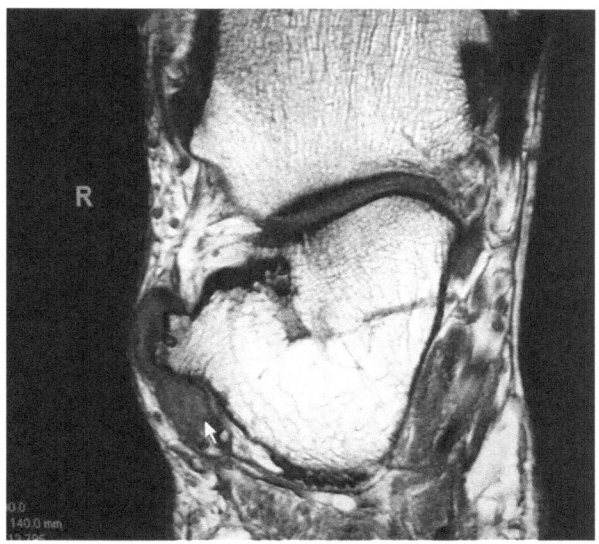

diagnosis, and is recommended in less clear-cut cases.[81] Care should be taken not to anesthetize the local nerves and infiltrate into the ankle or subtalar joint, which can give false relief of symptoms from injecting the wrong structures. Generally, peroneal tenosynovitis without tendon tear responds to nonsurgical treatment. (In fact, the local anesthestic injection, if performed, can produce a volume adhesiotomy and further relieve symptoms.) Typical nonsurgical treatment of peroneal tendinopathy includes bracing, inserts including custom orthoses and/or shoes with lateral (valgus) wedging, physical therapy and immobilization in a below-knee boot or cast, though the long-term results of this can be unsatisfactory. If patients report worsening of symptoms with physical therapy, it is likely due to a peroneal tendon tear becoming aggravated with increased activity. At this point, one should consider surgical intervention. Results of surgical treatment of peroneal tendon tears have been well-documented in case series with good success. Many authors report significant improvement of patients' activity levels and functional scores post-surgery even in the long-term.[13,27,80,82-87,89,91,98,99]

15.2.4 Surgical Technique

Surgical treatment typically involves repair of the torn tendon(s). General anesthesia is typically preferred with a pneumatic thigh tourniquet. Spinal or regional anesthesia may be used. The patient is generally placed in the lateral position on a "bean bag," unless other procedures such as ankle arthroscopy need to be performed. During the surgical portion of the tendon repair, the bean bag is inflated to help lateralize the patient if adequate internal rotation of the lower limb is available.

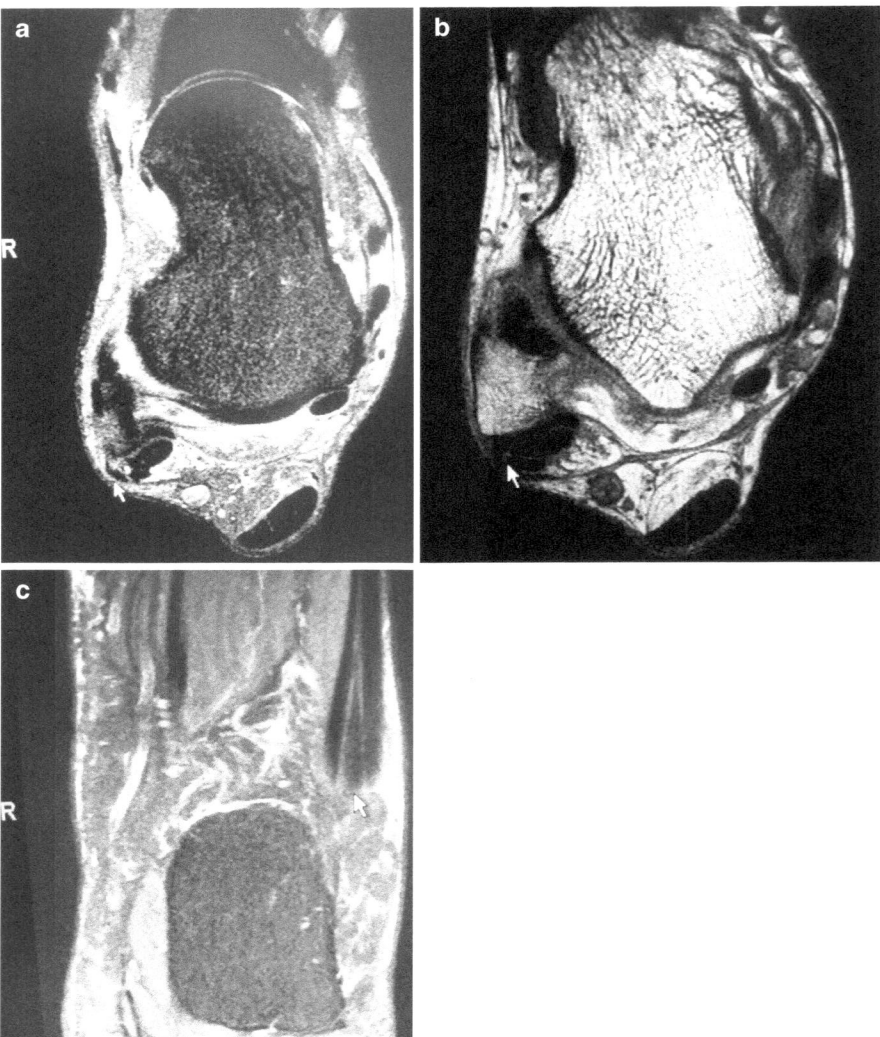

Fig. 15.8 MRI showing avulsed peroneal collangenous lip (**a**), split peroneus brevis (**b**), absent peroneus brevis with empty sheath (**c**)

Otherwise, the patient is re-positioned lateral intraoperatively, and re-prepping and draping is performed. It is helpful to mark the proposed lateral incision sites prior to distending the ankle joint with arthroscopy, if being performed prior to tendon repair.

A lateral incision is typically made along the course of the peronei tendons, in the region of the patient's pain and pathology. The incision may be extended proximally if a retinaculum repair or a more proximal rupture needs to be addressed.

Fig. 15.9 Tenogram of stenosing tenosynovitis

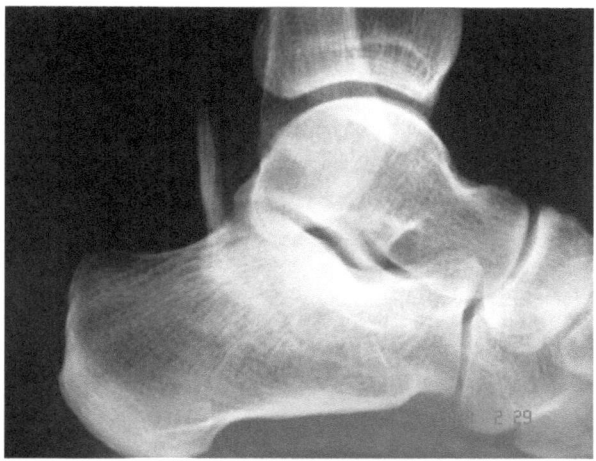

The distal portion of the incision can be directed more dorsally for concomitant ankle stabilization. The common peroneal sheath is incised, the tendons inspected, together with the adjacent bony structures (Fig. 15.11). The tendons can be manipulated with moistened umbilical tape. When an Os Peroneum is excised, the distal and proximal aspects of the Peroneus Longus tendon are tenodesed to the Peroneus Brevis with 2–0 or 3–0 monofilament suture. In North America, nonabsorbable sutures are more commonly used, while in Europe, absorbable sutures are preferred.[75,76,83-89] In patients with chronically degenerated and frayed tendons, excision of the abnormal tendon is performed. Delayed primary repair is commonly performed by tubularizing the torn tendon with nonabsorbable monofilament suture, though other materials have been utilized. (Fig. 15.12) If there is a large gap after débridement of nonviable tissue, the tendon is tenodesed to the adjacent tendon. Some authors recommend tenodesis when greater than 50% of the tendon girth or 2 cm of the length is damaged.[80,82,85,86] Tendon "substitutes" being utilized for tendon repair have been promoted, but no long-term studies exist to date. Often, in chronic cases when both tendons are torn, the Peroneus Longus has retracted proximally, and the distal aspect of the Peroneus Brevis is intact. In such cases, the tendon of peroneus Longus is tenodesed to the base of the 5th metatarsal to maintain eversion of the foot.[81,86] The surgical wound is closed in layers.

If both tendons are severely damaged and not reconstructable, a free tendon graft may be used, such as doubled Plantaris tendon or a transfer of either the Flexor Hallucis or Digitorum Longus can be performed. An interim procedure of inserting a Hunter's Rod as a temporary conduit has been described prior to delayed repair.[80,91,100] A second procedure involving tendon transfer for peroneal reconstruction is performed 3 months later.[27,100]

Surgically, other structural issues may need addressing. Exostoses from the peroneal tubercle or distal fibula should be reduced.[80,81,86] Bone wax can be applied. The surgeon should be prepared in older patients to apply supplemental bone graft/substitute when the peroneal tubercle is resected as often the underlying calcaneus

Fig. 15.10 Fluid in peroneal sheath on MRI with torn peroneals frontal (**a**) and axial (**b**) views

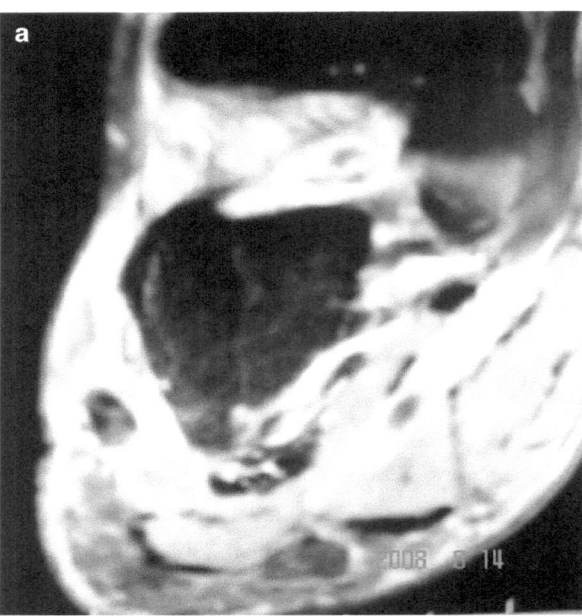

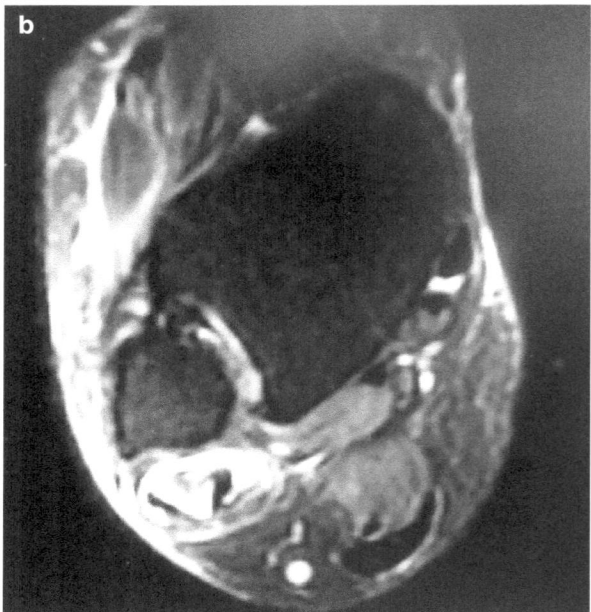

is cystic, particularly in females. Subluxations are surgically corrected with ligament repair, accessory muscle resection, and groove deepening if needed, as described in the section above. Severe rearfoot varus deformity (>10°) generally should be addressed at the time of surgery, though, in highly athletic patients, this

Fig. 15.11 (**a**) Peroneal
sheath opened showing torn
peroneus longus. (**b**) Peroneal
sheath opened showing torn
peroneus brevis. Note
exostoses adjacent to tear (**c**)

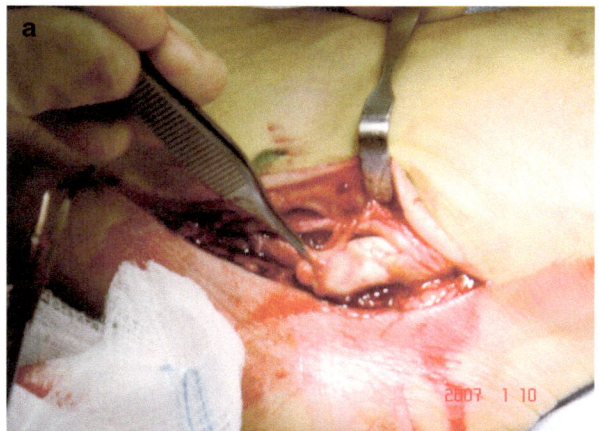

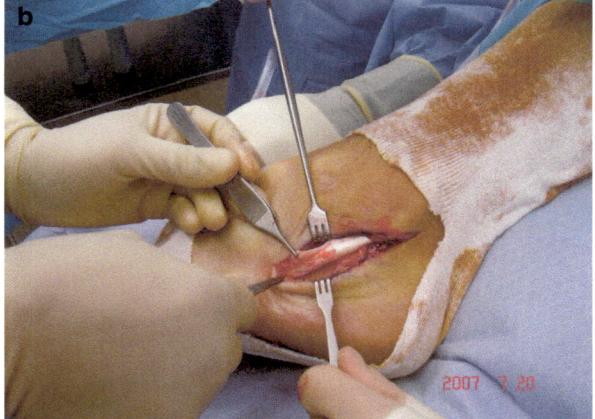

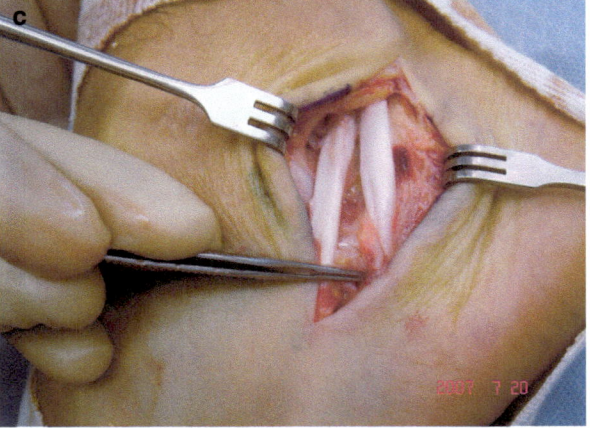

Fig. 15.12 Repaired tendon

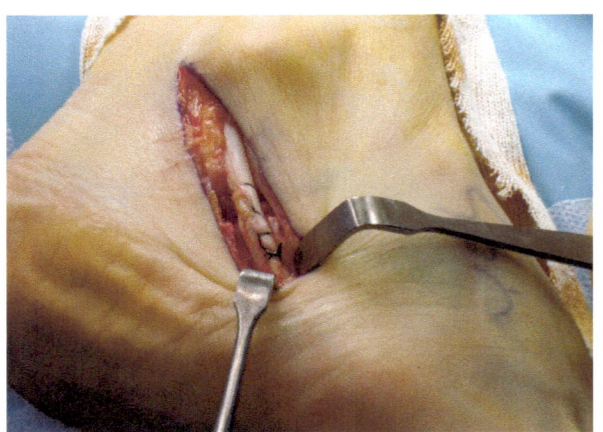

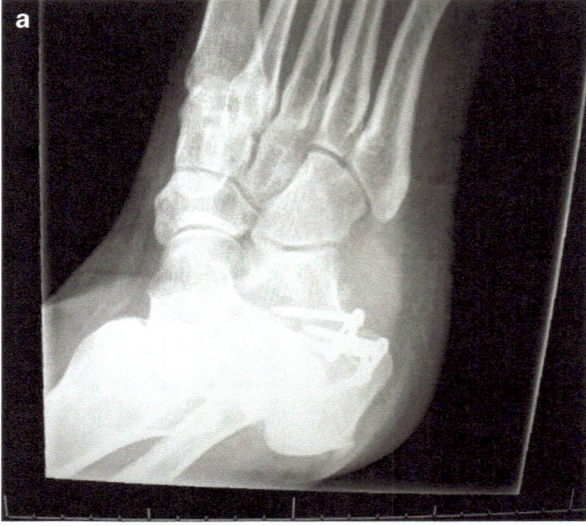

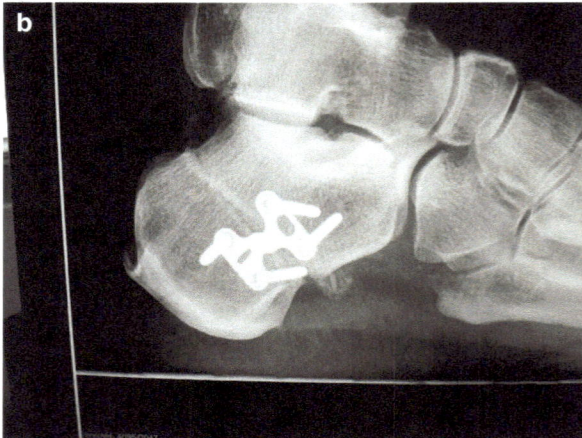

Fig. 15.13 Lateral displacement calcaneal osteotomy in a patient with severe calcaneal varus and both peroneal tendons ruptured, oblique (**a**) and lateral (**b**) X-rays

Fig. 15.14 Elevating 1st
metatarsal osteotomy in a
patient with torn peroneus
brevis and plantarflexed 1st
metatarsal lateral (**a**) and AP
(**b**) X-rays

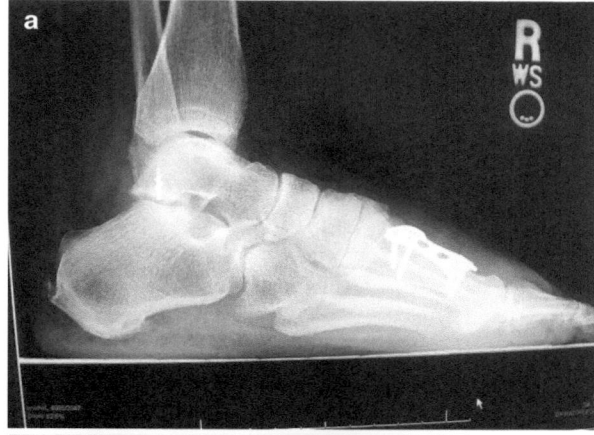

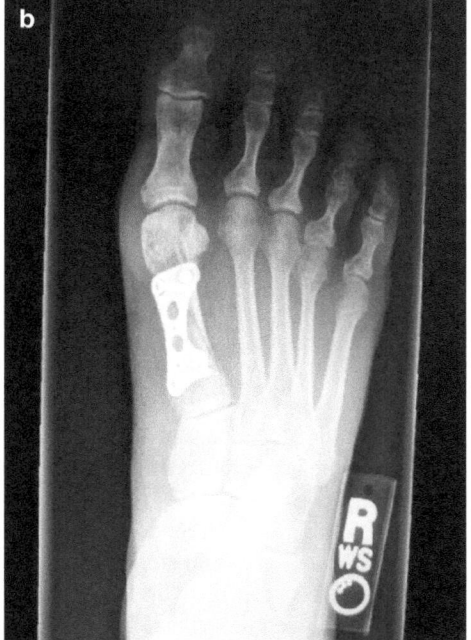

may be deferred.[27,86] For calcaneal varus deformity, a combined lateral displacement and varus reducing osteotomy is performed with either plate or screw fixation (Fig. 15.13). With patients that have a rigidly plantarflexed 1st metatarsal, an osteotomy of the base is performed to elevate it to the level of the 2nd metatarsal. Care should be taken to avoid creating a transfer lesion to the 2nd metatarsal, but this is essentially unavoidable with a short 1st metatarsal. Consideration of prophylactic shortening of an elongated 2nd metatarsal should be done if elevating a short plantarflexed 1st metatarsal. Plate or screw fixation is also used on the 1st metatarsal (Fig. 15.14). Other surgical considerations for severe instability are subtalar arthrodesis (for absent Peroneus Brevis) or calcaneal-cuboid arthrodesis (for absent Peroneus Longus). [27,81] Postoperative complications from peroneal tendon repair can include continued symptoms with activity limitations, re-rupture (particularly if structural deformity is not addressed), and neurovascular compromise.[27,80,85,86]

15.2.5 Postoperative Care

Postoperatively patients with peroneal tendon repair alone are kept non-weight bearing for 3 weeks, generally with a below-knee cast or boot. Stationary biking with the heel on the pedal is permitted with a boot or cast once edema and pain subsides, and swimming is allowed after 4 weeks. Ankle range-of-motion exercises can be begun at 3 weeks. If a calcaneal or 1st metatarsal osteotomy is performed, patients are kept non-weight bearing for 4–6 weeks, depending on bony consolidation. Patients wear a below-knee cast boot for 6–10 weeks until pain-free (the longer time frame is used for patients with osteotomies). Physical therapy is initiated between 5 and 10 weeks. Return to regular activities including sports takes 3–6 months. Consideration of ankle support or taping, and possibly foot orthoses for the first year postoperative should be assessed. Most athletic patients use ankle brace or tape for the first sport season after the surgery.

15.3 Conclusion

Recurrent peroneal tendon subluxation is an uncommon sports- and road-related injury. It occurs when the acute injury is misdiagnosed or not adequately managed. The primary pathology is the damage of the Superior Peroneal Retinaculum, which is the main restraint to the peroneal tendons. Diagnosis relies on clinical suspicion and clinical examination. There is no standardized method to report the severity of the condition, and therefore, it is difficult to compare the various case series. Many surgical techniques have been described, but it is hard to understand from the relatively small series which procedure is the gold standard. In our experience, if an anatomic approach is used, reattachment of the SPR is a most appropriate technique. Rarely, the retinaculum in recurrent cases may not be robust enough to withstand repair, and a different approach to the problem may be required. Randomized controlled trials may be the way forward in determining the best surgical procedure for subluxing peroneals. Repair of torn Peroneal tendons appears more straightforward with tubularization of the tendons involved. Tenodesis to the adjacent peroneal tendon is needed in cases of excision of an Os Peroneum, and where >50% of the tendon girth is lost or more than 2 cm of tendon length is damaged. FHL transfer may be indicated in special cases where reconstruction is not possible. Surgeons should consider other forms of structural pathology such as ankle instability, exostoses, calcaneal varus, and plantarflexed 1st metatarsal.

References

1. Monteggia GB. Instituzini chirurgiche, part III. Stamperia Pirotta Maspero, Milan:1803: 336–41.
2. Mizel MS. Orthopedic knowledge update. Foot and ankle 2. Rosemont: American Academy of Orthopedic Surgeons; 1998.
3. Stover CN, Bryan DR. Traumatic dislocation of the peroneal tendons. Am J Surg. 1962;103: 180–6.
4. Escalas F, Figueras JM, Merino JA. Dislocation of the peroneal tendons. J Bone Joint Surg. 1980;62:451–3.
5. Kojima Y, Kataoka Y, Suzuki Sj, Akagi M. Dislocation of the peroneal tendons in neonates and infants. Clin Orthop Relat Res. 1991;266:180.
6. Beck E. Operative treatment of recurrent dislocation of the peroneal tendons. Arch Orthop Trauma Surg. 1981;98:247–50.
7. Alm A, Lamke L, Liljedahl S. Surgical treatment of dislocation of the peroneal tendons. Injury. 1975;7:14–9.
8. Das DS, Balasubramaniam P. A repair operation for recurrent dislocation of peroneal tendons. J Bone Joint Surg Br. 1985;67:585–7.
9. Gould N. Technique tips: footings, repair of dislocating peroneal tendons. Foot Ankle. 1986;6:208–13.
10. Jones E. Operative treatment of chronic dislocation of the peroneal tendons. J Bone Joint Surg. 1932;4:574–6.
11. Pozzo J, Jackson A. A rerouting operation for dislocation of peroneal tendons: operative technique and case report. Foot Ankle. 1984;5:42–4.
12. Zoellner G, Clancy WJ. Recurrent dislocation of the peroneal tendon. J Bone Joint Surg. 1979;61:292–4.
13. Dombek MF, Lamm BM, Saltrick K, Mendicino RW, Catanzariti AR. Peroneal tendon tears: a retrospective review. J Foot Ankle Surg. 2003;42:250–8.
14. Joshi SD, Joshi SS, Athavale SA. Morphology of peroneus tertius muscle. Clin Anat. 2006;19:611–4.
15. Sammarco GJ, Henning C. Peroneus tertius muscle as a cause of snapping and ankle pain: a case report. Am J Sports Med. 2007;35:1377–9.
16. Zammit J, Singh D. The peroneus quartus muscle. Anatomy and clinical relevance. J Bone Joint Surg Br. 2003;85:1134–7.
17. Molloy R, Tisdel C. Failed treatment of peroneal tendon injuries. Foot Ankle Clin. 2003;8:115–29.
18. Brage ME, Hansen ST Jr. Traumatic subluxation/dislocation of the peroneal tendons. Foot Ankle. 1992;13:423–31.
19. Davis WH, Sobel M, Deland J, Bohne WH, Patel MB. The superior peroneal retinaculum: an anatomic study. Foot Ankle Int. 1994;15:271–5.
20. Kumai T, Benjamin M. The histological structure of the malleolar groove of the fibula in man: its direct bearing on the displacement of peroneal tendons and their surgical repair. J Anat. 2003;203:257–62.
21. Sobel M, Geppert MJ, Hannafin JA, Bohne WH, Arnoczky SP. Microvascular anatomy of the peroneal tendons. Foot Ankle. 1992;13:469–72.
22. Petersen W, Bobka T, Stein V, Tillmann B. Blood supply of the peroneal tendons: injection and immunohistochemical studies of cadaver tendons. Acta Orthop Scand. 2000;71:168–74.

23. Bassett FH 3rd, Speer KP. Longitudinal rupture of the peroneal tendons. Am J Sports Med. 1993;21:354–7.
24. Safran MR, O'Malley D Jr, Fu FH. Peroneal tendon subluxation in athletes: new exam technique, case reports, and review. Med Sci Sports Exerc. 1999;31:487–92.
25. Eckert WR, Davis EA. Acute rupture of the peroneal retinaculum. J Bone Joint Surg. 1976;58A:670–3.
26. Geppert MJ, Sobel M, Bohne WH. Lateral ankle instability as a cause of superior peroneal retinacular laxity: an anatomic and biomechanical study of cadaveric feet. Foot Ankle. 1993;14:330–4.
27. Selmani E, Gjata V, Gjika E. Current concepts review: peroneal tendon disorders. Foot Ankle Int. 2006;27:221–8.
28. Bonnin M, Tavernier T, Bouysset M. Split lesions of the peroneus brevis tendon in chronic ankle laxity. Am J Sports Med. 1997;25:699–703.
29. Purnell ML, Drummond DS, Engber WD, Breed AL. Congenital dislocation of the peroneal tendons in the calcaneovalgus foot. J Bone Joint Surg Br. 1983;65:316–9.
30. Bonnin JG. Injuries of the ankle. Darien: Hafner Publishing Co; 1970. p. 32.
31. Hammerschlag WA, Goldner JL. Chronic peroneal tendon subluxation produced by an anomalous peroneus brevis: case report and literature review. Foot Ankle. 1989;10:45–7.
32. Estor A, Aimes A. La luxation congenitale des tendons des muscles peroniers lateraux. Rev Orthop. 1923;10:1.
33. Harper MC. Subluxation of the peroneal tendons within the peroneal groove: a report of two cases. Foot Ankle Int. 1997;18:369–70.
34. Oden RR. Tendon injuries about the ankle resulting from skiing. Clin Orthop Relat Res. 1987;216:63–9.
35. McConkey JP, Favero KJ. Subluxation of the peroneal tendons within the peroneal tendon sheath. A case report. Am J Sports Med. 1987;15:511–3.
36. Stukenborg-Colsman C, Wirth CJ. Resection of the tendon of the peroneal brevis muscle in "clicking" peroneal tendons – a report of 3 cases. Z Orthop Ihre Grenzgeb. 2000;138:265–8.
37. Raikin SM, Elias I, Nazarian LN. Intrasheath subluxation of the peroneal tendons. J Bone Joint Surg Am. 2008;90:992–9.
38. Marti R. Dislocation of the peroneal tendons. Am J Sports Med. 1977;5:19–22.
39. Arrowsmith SR, Fleming LL, Allman FL. Traumatic dislocations of the peroneal tendons. Am J Sports Med. 1983;11:142–6.
40. Poll RG, Duijfjes F. The treatment of recurrent dislocation of the peroneal tendons. J Bone Joint Surg Br. 1984;66:98–100.
41. Martens MA, Noyez JF, Mulier JC. Recurrent dislocation of the peroneal tendons. Results of rerouting the tendons under the calcaneofibular ligament. Am J Sports Med. 1986;14:148–50.
42. Micheli LJ, Waters PM, Sanders DP. Sliding fibular graft repair for chronic dislocation of the peroneal tendons. Am J Sports Med. 1989;17:68–71.
43. Orthner E, Polcik J, Schabus R. Dislocation of peroneal tendons. Unfallchirurg. 1989;92:589–94.
44. Wirth CJ. A modified Vierstein and Kelly surgical technique for correcting chronic peroneal tendon dislocation. Z Orthop Ihre Grenzgeb. 1990;128:170–3.
45. Thomas JL, Sheridan L, Graviet S. A modification of the Ellis Jones procedure for chronic peroneal subluxation. J Foot Surg. 1992;31:454–8.
46. Steinböck G, Pinsger M. Treatment of peroneal tendon dislocation by transposition under the calcaneofibular ligament. Foot Ankle Int. 1994;15:107–11.
47. Mason RB, Henderson JP. Traumatic peroneal tendon instability. Am J Sports Med. 1996;24:652–8.
48. Karlsson J, Eriksson BI, Sward L. Recurrent dislocation of the peroneal tendons. Scand J Med Sci Sports. 1996;6:242–6.
49. Kollias SL, Ferkel RD. Fibular grooving for recurrent peroneal tendon subluxation. Am J Sports Med. 1997;25:329–35.

50. Hui JH, De Das S, Balasubramaniam P. The Singapore operation for recurrent dislocation of peroneal tendons: long-term results. J Bone Joint Surg Br. 1998;80:325–7.
51. Mendicino RW, Orsini RC, Whitman SE, et al. Fibular groove deepening for recurrent peroneal subluxation. J Foot Ankle Surg. 2001;40:252–63.
52. Shawen SB, Anderson RB. Indirect groove deepening in the management of chronic peroneal tendon dislocation. Tech Foot Ankle Surg. 2004;3:118–25.
53. Porter D, McCarroll J, Knapp E, Torma J. Peroneal tendon subluxation in athletes: fibular groove deepening and retinacular reconstruction. Foot Ankle Int. 2005;26:436–41.
54. Adachi N, Fukuhara K, Tanaka H, Nakasa T, Ochi M. Superior retinaculoplasty for recurrent dislocation of peroneal tendons. Foot Ankle Int. 2006;27:1074–8.
55. Maffulli N, Ferran NA, Oliva F, Testa V. Recurrent subluxation of the peroneal tendons. Am J Sports Med. 2006;34:986–92.
56. Ogawa BK, Thordarson DB, Zalavras C. Peroneal tendon subluxation repair with an indirect fibular groove deepening technique. Foot Ankle Int. 2007;28:1194–7.
57. Lui TH. Endoscopic peroneal retinaculum reconstruction. Knee Surg Sports Traumatol Arthrosc. 2006;14:478–81.
58. Jones E. Operative treatment of chronic dislocation of the peroneal tendons. Bone Joint Surg. 1932;14:574–6.
59. Smith TF, Vito GR. Subluxing peroneal tendons. An anatomic approach. Clin Podiatr Med Surg. 1991;8:555–77.
60. Gurevitz SL. Surgical correction of subluxing peroneal tendons with a case report. J Am Podiatr Assoc. 1979;69:357–63.
61. Miller JW. Dislocation of peroneal tendons, a new operative procedure. A case report. Am J Orthop. 1967;9:136–7.
62. Hansen BH. Reconstruction of the peroneal retinaculum using the plantaris tendon: a case report. Scand J Med Sci Sports. 1996;6:355–8.
63. Mick CA, Lynch F. Reconstruction of the peroneal retinaculum using the peroneus quartus. A case report. J Bone Joint Surg Am. 1987;69:296–7.
64. Lin S, Tan V, Okereke E. Subluxating peroneal tendon: repair of superior peroneal retinaculum using a retrofibular periosteal flap. Tech Foot Ankle Surg. 2003;2:262–7.
65. Platzgummer H. Uber ein einfaches Verfahren zur operativen Behandlung der habituellen Peronaeussehnenluxation. Arch Orthop Unfallchir. 1967;61:144–50.
66. Sarmiento A, Wolf M. Subluxation of peroneal tendons. Case treated by rerouting tendons under calcaneofibular ligament. J Bone Joint Surg Am. 1975;57:115–6.
67. Kelly RE. An operation for the chronic dislocation of the peroneal tendons. Br J Surg. 1920;7:502.
68. Ferroudji M, Spaas F, Martens M. Rerouting operation for recurrent dislocation of the peroneal tendons by the Pöll and Duijfjes procedure. Foot Ankle Surg. 2003;9:103–8.
69. Watson-Jones R. Fractures and joint injuries. 4th ed. Baltimore: Williams &Wilkins; 1956.
70. DuVries HL. Surgery of the foot. 4th ed. St. Louis: C.V. Mosby Co.; 1978.
71. Hutchinson BL, Gustafson LS. Chronic peroneal tendon subluxation. New surgical technique and retrospective analysis. J Am Podiatr Med Assoc. 1994;84:511–7.
72. Edwards ME. The relation of the peroneal tendons to the fibula, calcaneus and cuboideum. Am J Anat. 1928;42:213–53.
73. Mabit C, Salanne PH, Blanchard F, Boncoeur-Martel F. Fiorenza. The retromalleolar groove of the fibula: a radioanatomical study. Foot Ankle Surg. 1999;5:179–86.
74. Oliva F, Ferran N, Maffulli N. Peroneal retinaculoplasty with anchors for peroneal tendon subluxation. Bull Hosp Jt Dis. 2006;63:113–6.
75. Ferran NA, Oliva F, Maffulli N. Recurrent subluxation of the peroneal tendons. Sports Med. 2006;36:839–46.
76. Ferran NA, Oliva F, Maffulli N. Management of recurrent subluxation of the peroneal tendons. Foot Ankle Clin. 2006;11:465–74.
77. Evans JD. Subcutaneous rupture of the tendon of peroneus longus: report of a case. *J Bone Joint Surg Br.* 1966;48:507–9.

78. Sammarco GJ. Peroneal tendon injuries. Orthop Clin North Am. 1994;25:135–45.
79. Sobel M, Geppert M, Olson E, Bohne W, Arnoczky S. The dynamics of peroneous brevis splits: a proposed mechanism, technique of diagnosis, and classification of injury. Foot Ankle. 1992;13:413–22.
80. Heckman DS, Reddy S, Pedowitz D, Wapner KL, Parekh SG. Operative treatment for peroneal tendon disorders. J Bone Joint Surg Am. 2008;90(2):404–18.
81. Sobel M, Mizel M. Peroneal tendon injury in current practice in foot and ankle surgery, vol. 1. New York: Mc-Graw Hill, Inc; 1993. p. 30–56.
82. Squires N, Myerson MS, Gamba C. Surgical treatment of peroneal tendon tears. Foot Ankle Clin. 2007;12(4):675–95.
83. Slater HK. Acute peroneal tendon tears. Foot Ankle Clin. 2007;12(4):659–74.
84. Steel MW, DeOrio JK. Peroneal tendon tears: return to sports after operative treatment. Foot Ankle Int. 2007;28(1):49–54.
85. Redfern D, Myerson M. The management of concomitant tears of the peroneus longus and brevis tendons. Foot Ankle Int. 2004;25(10):695–707.
86. Saxena A, Cassidy A. Peroneal tendon injuries: an evaluation of 49 tears in 41 patients. J Foot Ankle Surg. 2003;42(4):215–20.
87. Cooper ME, Selesnick FH, Murphy BJ. Partial peroneus longus tendon rupture in professional basketball players: a report of 2 cases. Am J Orthop. 2002;31(12):691–4.
88. Brandes C, Smith R. Characterization of patients with primary peroneus longus tendonopathy. Foot Ankle Int. 2000;21:462–8.
89. Saxena A, Pham B. Longitudinal peroneal tendon tears. J Foot Ankle Surg. 1997;36(3):173–9.
90. Kuwada GT. Surgical correlation of preoperative MRI findings of trauma to tendons and ligaments of the foot and ankle. J Am Podiatr Med Assoc. 2008;98(5):370–3.
91. Borton DC, Lucas P, Jomha NM, Cross MJ, Slater K. Operative reconstruction after transverse rupture of the tendons of both peroneus longus and brevis. Surgical reconstruction by transfer of the flexor digitorum longus tendon. J Bone Joint Surg Br. 1998;80(5):781–4.
92. LeMinor JM. Comparative anatomy and significance of the sesamoid bone of the peroneus longus muscle (os peroneum). J Anat. 1987;15:85–99.
93. Muehleman C. Os peroneum: a case of mistaken identity. Clin Anat. 2008;21:741.
94. Sobel M, Pavlov H, Geppert M, Thompson F, DiCarlo E, Davis W. Painful os peroneum syndrome: a spectrum of conditions responsible for plantar lateral foot pain. Foot Ankle Int. 1994;15:112–24.
95. Geller J, Lin S, Cordas D, Vierira P. Relationship of a low-lying muscle belly to tears of the peroneus brevis tendon. Am J Orthop. 2003;32:541–4.
96. Sobel M, Levy M, Bohne W. Congenital variations of the peroneus quartus muscle: an anatomic study. Foot Ankle. 1990;11:81–90.
97. Abraham E, Stimaman J. Neglected rupture of the peroneal tendons causing recurrent sprains of the ankle: case report. J Bone Joint Surg Am. 1979;61:1247–8.
98. Saxena A, Ewen B. Peroneal retinaculum tears: surgical results in 31 athletic patients. Submitted to J Foot Ankle Surg. 2010;49(3):238–41.
99. Lagoutaris E, Adams H, DiDomenico L, Rothenberg R. Longitudinal tears of both peroneal tendons associated with tophaceous gouty infiltration: a case report. J Foot Ankle Surg. 2005;44:222–4.
100. Wapner K, Taras J, Lin S, Chao W. Staged reconstruction for chronic rupture of both peroneal tendons using hunter rod and flexor hallucis longus tendon transfer: a long-term follow-up study. Foot Ankle Int. 2006;27:591–7.

Chapter 16
Advances in Anterior Ankle and Subtalar Arthroscopy

John F. Grady, Amol Saxena, Audra M. Smith, and Yelena Boumendjel

Much advancement has been made in ankle arthroscopy. In 1931, Burman concluded the ankle joint was not appropriate for arthroscopy due to its small size.[1,2] However, Takagi, in 1982, described a routine method to examine the ankle through arthroscopy.[3] Over the years, smaller scopes have been developed that are suitable for the ankle, which has advanced the practice immensely.

Traditional anterior ankle arthroscopy is done using anteromedial and anterolateral portals of entry.[4,5] Some of the most common pathologies addressed with these portals include osteochondral defects (OCD), loose bodies, anterior impingement lesions, chronic synovitis, and intra-articular soft tissue masses.[5-12] Limitations of this approach occur due to the anatomic structure of the talus. The talus is wider anteriorly and has a convex slope from anterior to posterior and is mildly concave from medial to lateral. Also a consideration are the synovial recesses which are evident in the sagittal plane about the talus.[12,13] (Fig. 16.1) Berndt and Hardy classified typical OCD lesions that occur anterior-lateral or posterior-medial; however, if a lesion happens to be posterior medial or midline directly under the malleoli they can be difficult to access.[14] These posterior medial lesions occur as a result of an inverted ankle that is forcefully plantarflexed and they are generally deeper than the typical lesions (Fig. 16.2). The literature suggests performing a medial malleolar osteotomy to reach these defects.[4,15,16] This chapter will discuss new arthroscopic

J.F. Grady, D.P.M.
Department of Surgery, Foot and Ankle Institute of Illinois,
Oak Lawn, IL, USA

A. Saxena, D.P.M. (✉)
Department of Sports Medicine, PAFMG-Palo Alto Division,
Clark Bldg., 3rd Flr, 795 El Camino Real, Palo Alto, CA 94301, USA
e-mail: heysax@aol.com

A.M. Smith, D.P.M. • Y. Boumendjel, D.P.M.
Department of Podiatry, Jesse Brown VA Medical Center,
Chicago, IL, USA

A. Saxena (ed.), *Sports Medicine and Arthroscopic Surgery of the Foot and Ankle*,
DOI 10.1007/978-1-4471-4106-8_16, © Springer-Verlag London 2013

Fig. 16.1 (**a**) Diagram
showing talar configuration
which is wider anteriorly;
(**b**) synovial recesses of the
ankle and subtalar joints

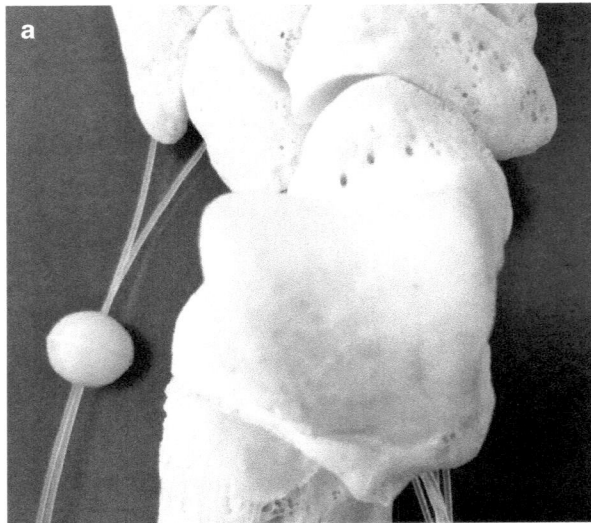

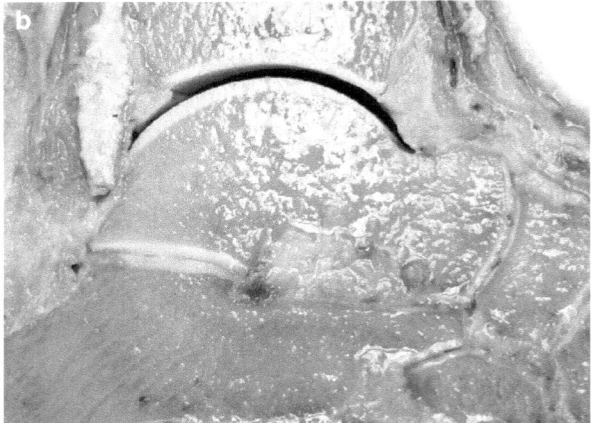

techniques to reach the entire medial talar joint surface without having to osteoto-
mize the medial malleolus and arthroscopic arthrodesis of the ankle and subtalar
joints. Posterior ankle arthroscopy is discussed in Chap. 17.

Like with any surgical planning, the initial assessment and appropriate
diagnosis of pathology is most important when deciding on the procedure to perform. Clinicians commonly will use MRI and high resolution CT imaging to help
confirm or rule out defects to the talar dome and within the ankle joint.[17-20] These
imaging modalities are more sensitive than standard radiographs. If arthroscopy
is the procedure of choice for a medial osteochondral lesion, then the following
surgical technique using a Micro Vector™ (Smith Nephew, Andover, MA, USA)
or Arthrex ankle (Arthrex™, Naples, FL, USA) drill guide can be used to better
access the joint (Fig. 16.3).

Fig. 16.2 MRI showing posteromedial lesion

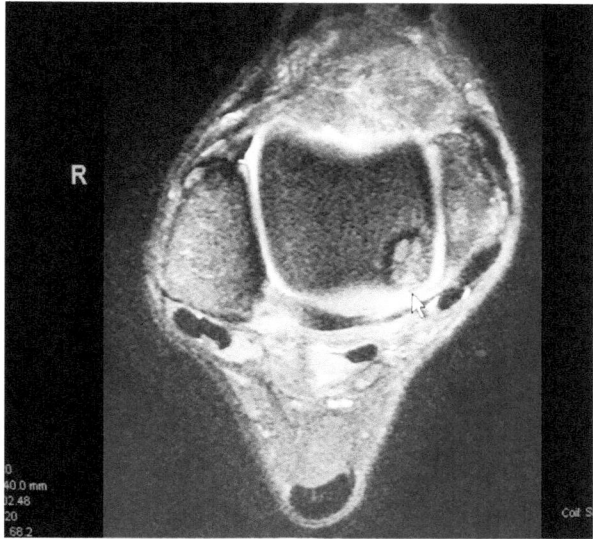

Fig. 16.3 Arthrex™ drill guide

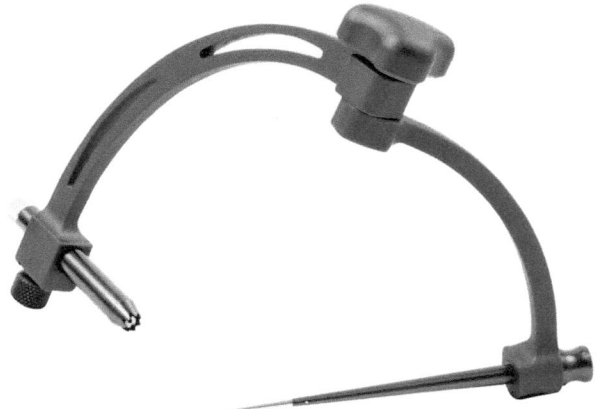

16.1   Surgical Technique

First, the ankle is anesthetized. Using approximately 5 cc of lidocaine (plain or with epinephrine) anesthetize the traditional portal areas. Then insert an 18 gauge needle through one of the portals past the ankle joint capsule and inject approximately 5–6 cc of local anesthetic. This will provide both anesthesia and distention of the ankle joint. An additional 15 cc of normal saline is then injected for further distention of the joint. If general anesthesia is used, a thigh tourniquet can be utilized and inflated to 350–400 mmHg. When local anesthesia is used, a high ankle tourniquet can be applied and inflated to 250–300 mmHg.[4] Some surgeons prefer not to place local

Fig. 16.4 Anteromedial
portal

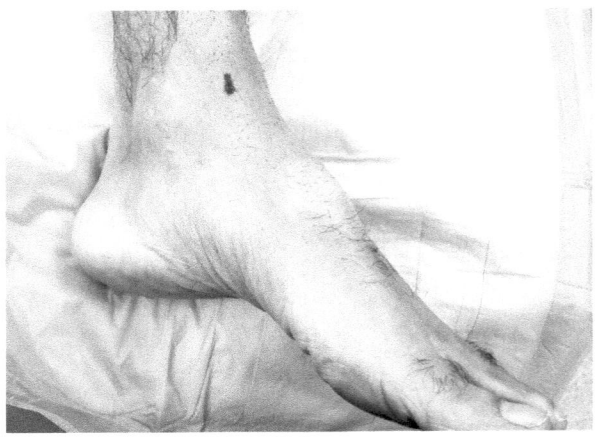

anesthetic within the joint pre-operatively, but rather, anesthetize the joint proximally. This is due to the fact some prefer not to use a tourniquet in order to verify bleeding during marrow stimulation techniques, i.e., microfracture. An arthroscopic "Dual Wave™" pump (Arthrex, Inc, Naples, FL USA) is preferred to maintain joint distraction (usually at 35 mmHg) and is an alternative to a tourniquet.

Using a noninvasive technique, distract the ankle joint.[21,22] The first portal is anterior at the ankle level, lateral to the anterior lip of the medial malleolus, and medial to the tibialis anterior. It should be made midway between these two structures (Fig. 16.4). Make a 6-mm incision right at the anterior aspect of the joint and use a mosquito hemostat to bluntly dissect down to the capsule. The subcutaneous tissue is examined for neurovascular structures. Seeing none, the incision is deepened through the capsule and immediately fluid should be noted. Next insert the obturator and cannula (Fig. 16.5). At this time the obturator is removed, and the arthroscope is inserted through the cannula and connected to irrigation (ingress). Keeping the foot dorsiflexed while inserting instruments during anterior arthroscopy helps protect the articular surfaces. One should have a constant ingress and egress of fluid (often through another portal or attached to a shaver to allow for suction) to ensure the joint is distracted at all times while the arthroscope is in place; this will avoid damage to the cartilage surfaces, while allowing clearing of debris.[4,5,23] Then we rotate the arthroscope laterally at the anterior aspect of the joint until visualization is made of the two branches of the superficial peroneal nerve, the intermediate dorsal cutaneous nerve, and the medial dorsal cutaneous nerve (Fig. 16.6). With the light shining from beneath (transillumination), a lateral incision is made between the two branches, which should be just lateral to the extensor digitorum longus tendon but medial to the anterior lip of the fibular malleolus right at the ankle level (Fig. 16.6). Next a 6-mm incision is made here and deepened using blunt dissection with a hemostat. The area is examined for any possibility of neurovascular structures which might be damaged when inserting the cannula. Next, an obturator and cannula are inserted until fluid return is noted

Fig. 16.5 Inserting
obturator/cannula

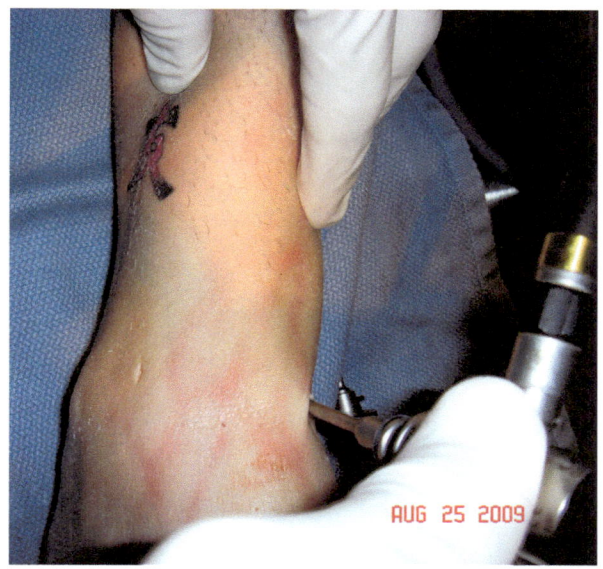

Fig. 16.6 Transillumination
to create anterolateral portal

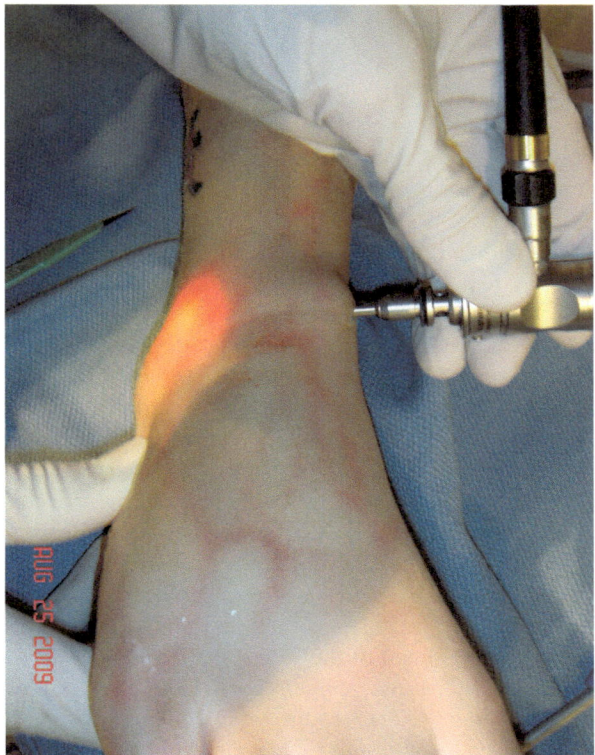

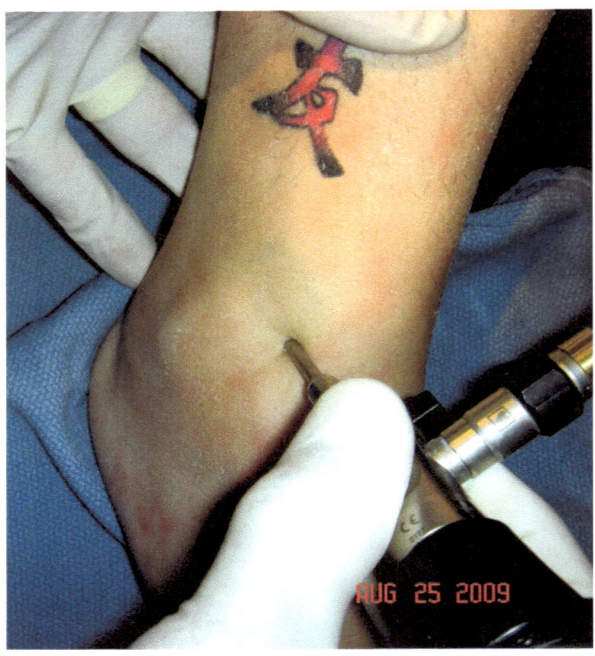

after puncturing the synovial membrane. The arthroscope is then removed from the medial portal leaving cannula intact. The arthroscope is now inserted laterally, and examination of the joint can proceed (Fig. 16.7). At this stage, it is important to examine the area in front first which is the lateral shoulder and gutter (Fig. 16.8). Next, we focus our attention medially, going across the joint into the medial shoulder and then the medial gutter (Fig. 16.9). For better visualization, the arthroscope is now removed with the cannula left intact laterally and the arthroscope is now inserted into the medial cannula and examination of the medial gutter and then the posterior aspect of the joint can take place (Fig. 16.10). Once the arthroscope is in position and proper ingress and egress of fluid is established, use the full radius 3.5-mm shaver to clear away any hypertrophic synovium to get a better view of the talar defect. The lesion can then be treated via subchondral drilling, microfracture, curettage, or abrading the base.[4,24]

A technique to access difficult-to-visualize (and instrument) lesions was described by Grady and Hughes.[25] If the defect is noted to be located within the posterior medial half of the talar dome and cannot be adequately accessed, a Micro Vector drill guide can be used to create an additional portal through the medial malleolus.[25] (Fig. 16.11) The guide is made up of two curved articulating arms at 170° with constant alignment of the probe and guide regardless of the arm position. A 0.45, 0.62, or 0.125 k-wire guide is available with serrated tip to maintain bone position. The trephine used is 5.1 mm. Simply align the probe through existing medial portal and line up the adjustable end of the guide to the medial malleolus. The guide arms

Fig. 16.8 Arthroscopic view of lateral shoulder and gutter

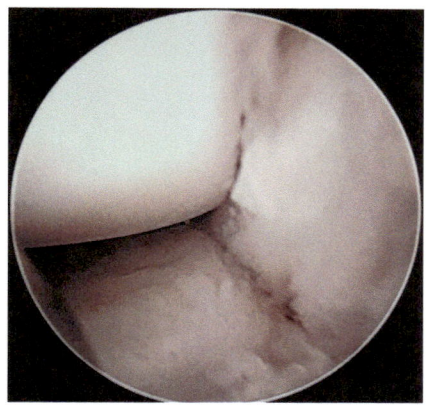

Fig. 16.9 Arthroscopic lateral to medial view

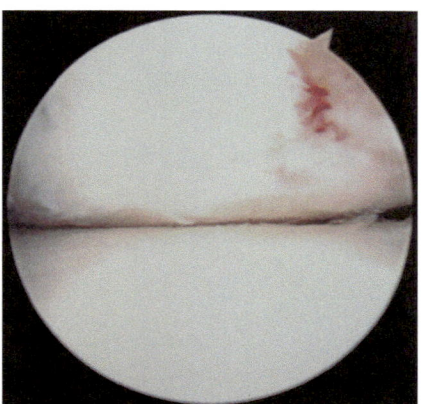

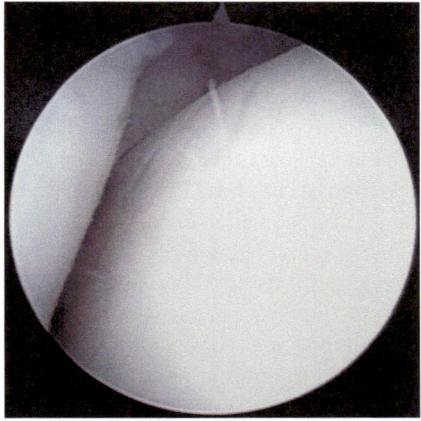

Fig. 16.10 Medial gutter from medial portal

Fig. 16.11 View through anteromedial portal prior to creation of trephine hole through medial malleolus

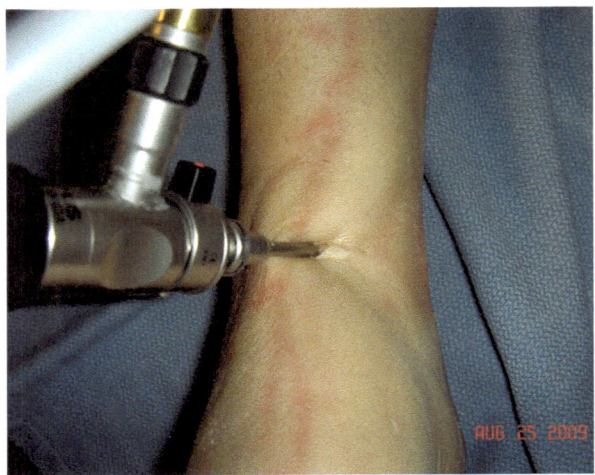

Fig. 16.12 Micro Vector™ drill guide arms intersecting

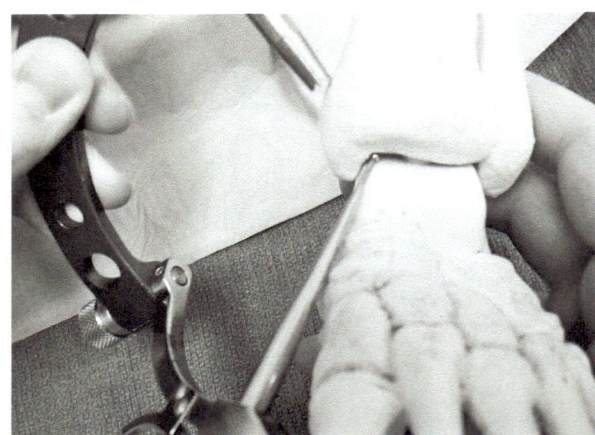

intersect (Fig. 16.12). Once the position is established, lock the hinge, and insert the 0.62 k-wire through the guide into the defect. Leaving the k-wire in place, remove the guide and bluntly dissect around the k-wire down to the medial malleolus. Next, a 5.1 mm trephine is placed over the k-wire and a core of bone is removed to access the ankle joint (Fig. 16.13). The defect should now be accessible for subchondral drilling using a 0.62 k-wire. This technique is designed to avoid potential "overheating" of bone which can occur during trans-malleolar and talar drilling (Fig. 16.14). Once completed, simply reinsert bony plug back into medial malleolus and repair periosteum using 3–0 vicryl. Next, release the joint distractor and suture the portal sites. The postoperative course should consist of a non-weight- bearing cast immobilization for 6–8 weeks if any windowing was performed. If the lesion was accessible via traditional portals, it is important to establish range-of-motion as soon as possible to prevent any adhesions from occurring and immediate weight-bearing is encouraged.[23,26,27] More detail on treatment of talar defects is found in Chap. 8 in the Sports Medicine section of this text.

Fig. 16.13 Trephine to remove bone plug

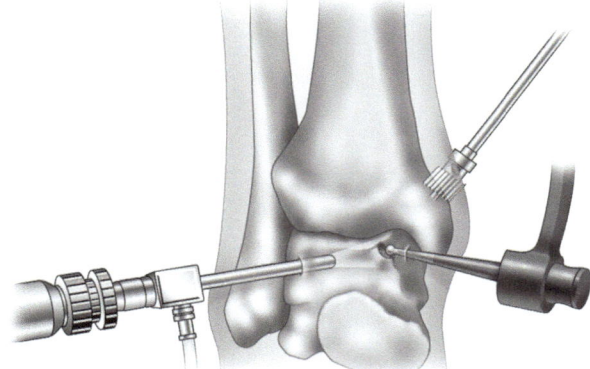

Fig. 16.14 Drilling lesion through medial malleolar hole

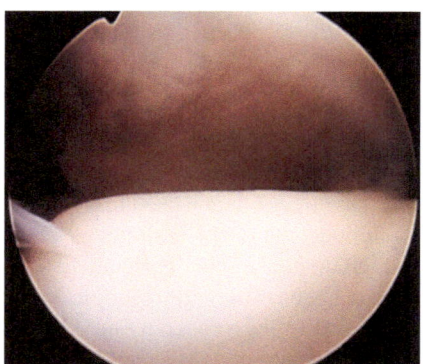

16.2   Discussion

Every surgical technique has complications and arthroscopy is no exception. The literature is scarce on this topic but several authors claim incidences as high as 17%, while others recording rates as low as approximately 1.8%.[23,27,28] Those authors with less complications attribute this to experience and good anatomic dissection. In our personal experience, early range of motion can also help reduce complication rates. The complications reported include nerve injury, infection, direct injury to the articular cartilage, hemarthrosis, vascular injury, thermal injury, accelerated degenerative joint disease, and instrument malfunction.[23,26,27,29,30] If an osteotomy is performed a nonunion becomes another postoperative concern. However, it has been the authors' experience that patients, if chosen correctly, do very well post operatively. Additionally, in 2008 Ferkel et al. performed a long-term follow-up study on arthroscopic treatment of chronic OCD of the talus and had very good results from 2 to 12 years later.[16] Depending on the severity of the pathology it will directly affect the patient's results. When dealing with lesions that are not routinely seen or are more difficult to access through traditional portals, a Micro Vector™ drill guide can be considered to access posterior medial lesions.

Fig. 16.15 Burring of degenerated cartilage

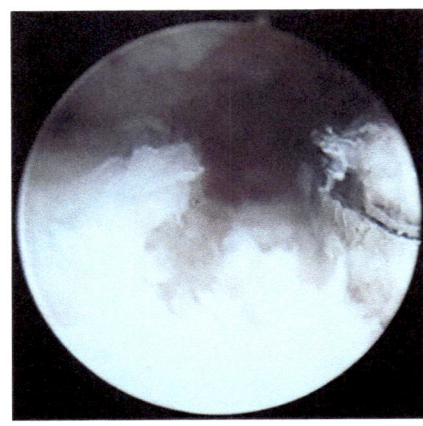

16.3 Arthroscopic Ankle Arthrodesis

The first description of the ankle joint arthrodesis by Albert is dated back to 1879. Since then, an ankle fusion technique has been evolving from external to internal fixation including numerous implanted devices and cancellous screws. The latter increased the number of successful fusions and diminished the rate of complications such as infections and pseudoarthroses.[31] More recently, advancement in arthroscopic technique has enabled surgeons to directly visualize the articular surface of joints which facilitated the debridement as well as subchondral bone resection techniques. The pioneer of the arthroscopic ankle arthrodesis was Schneider who was the first to describe the procedure in his video journal report in 1983.[32] Since then, the arthroscopic technique introduced many benefits over traditional open procedures.

16.3.1 Arthroscopic Ankle Arthrodesis Technique

Standard arthroscopic approaches as presented above are used. In addition, a posterolateral portal. An additional portal is created posterior-laterally. This is inserted through a guidance system whereby we put the obturator in through the anterior-lateral portal all the way through the posterior. When the point of the obturator is felt, we then make an incision right over the point. We then insert the cannula and obturator together through the posterior-lateral portal. This gives good visualization. This portal can be "free-handed" by making an incision just lateral to the Achilles tendon (thereby avoiding the sural nerve) and at the level 1 cm above the fibular tip. The posterior-medial portal is seldom used. The patient can be put in the prone position. Both posterolateral and posteromedial portals can be used in this position. This is discussed in Chap. 17.

Using the anterior-medial portal and a surgical abrader, the cartilage is denuded down to bleeding bone as shown in Fig. 16.15. It should be noted that we can only get to the middle of the talus through this portal. We then go ahead all the way across the medial side and the anterior-medial aspect. That is with the working channel medial

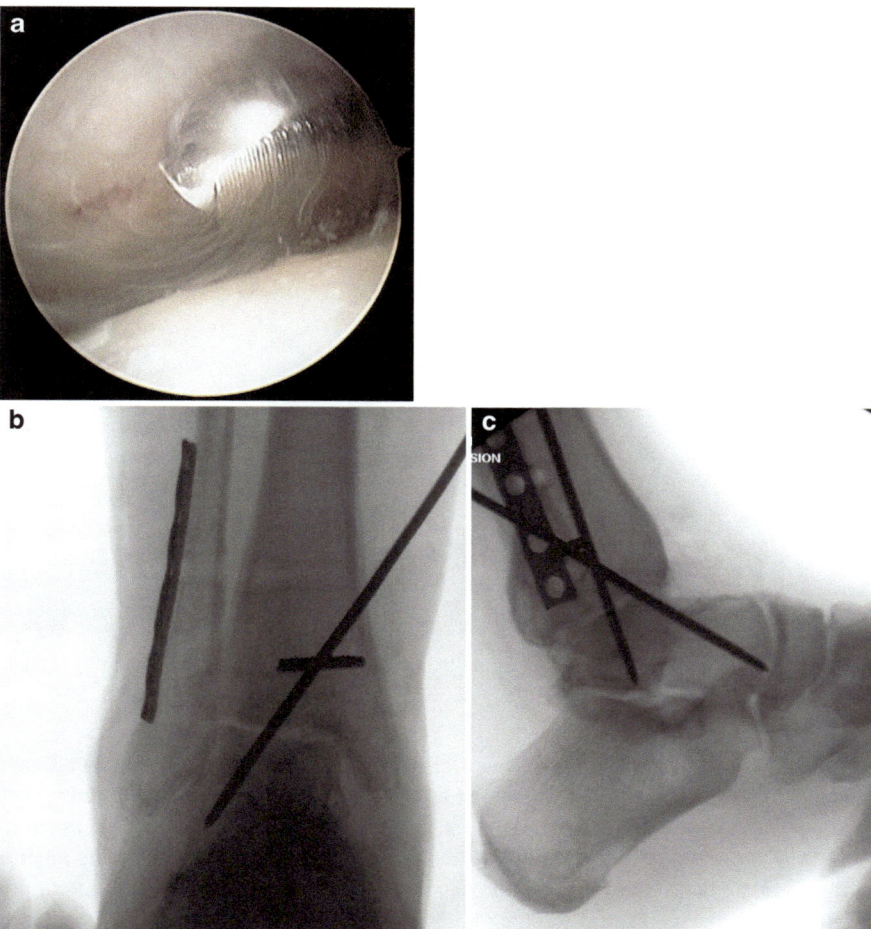

Fig. 16.16 Intra-operative guidewires for screw placement for arthroscopic ankle arthrodesis (Photos (**a**) – courtesy of Michael Lee, DPM; (**b, c**) – courtesy of Jack Schuberth, DPM)

and the scope laterally. We then switch the abrader laterally in the scope medially, and abrade the lateral-anterior aspect of the joint. Through the posterior incision described above, we then insert a working channel only. While visualizing from anteriorly, we are able to abrade the entire posterior cartilage down to bleeding bone. It should be noted that we can get up to 6.5 mm of distraction with the described technique of non-invasive distraction. This should be adequate to get the scope to at least seek when you reach the peak on the talus with the abrader. The patient may need to be positioned prone to remove all the posterior ankle cartilage if distraction and the posterolateral portal does not allow access. After the articular cartilage is removed, the subchondral surfaces are noted to be bleeding (suction is used to evacuate this), we then insert guide wires as shown, one medial and one lateral to the tibia, intersecting in the middle as show (Fig. 16.16). We then insert cannulated screws through percutaneous

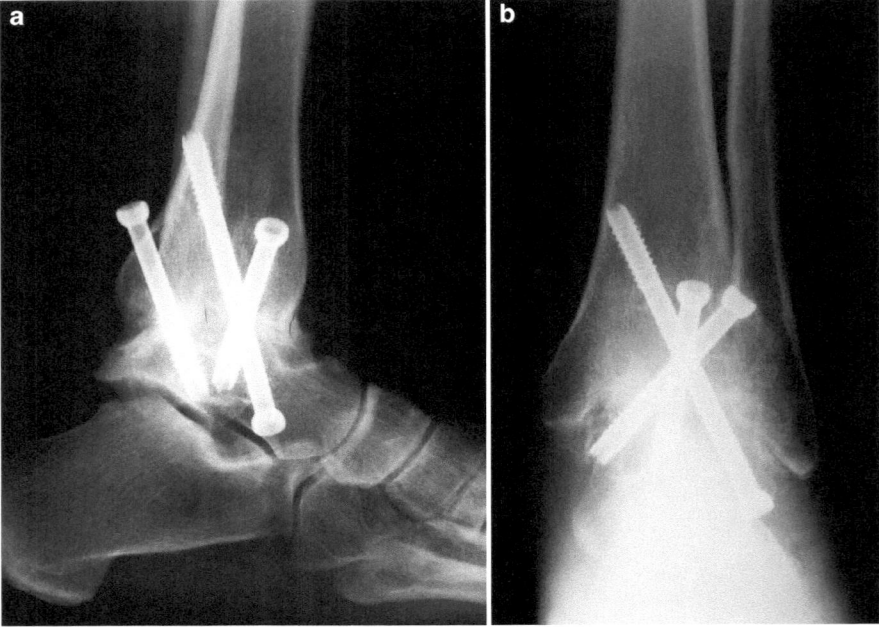

Fig. 16.17 (**a, b**) Screw placement after arthroscopic ankle arthrodesis (Photo Courtesy of Michael Lee, DPM)

incisions on the medial and lateral aspect of the tibia. After noting the placement is correct arthroscopically, we remove the arthroscope, compress the ankle, remove the distraction, compress the ankle (if an external fixator is used), and then we insert the screws in progressive fashion (Fig. 16.17). If one cannot achieve appropriate position with adequate dorsiflexion, it may be necessary to take more off anteriorly than posteriorly from the talo-tibial joint. Soft tissue posterior lengthening may need to be performed. This can be performed endoscopically of the Gastrocnemius in the supine position. Joint resection can be done either with an abrader or with an oval burr. After irrigation is performed at the end of the procedure, the incisions are then closed using one simple interrupted suture of 4–0 Prolene™. The wound is covered with Adaptic™ or Xeroform™, and 4×4 gauze sponges and a posterior splint is applied. Post-operatively, the patient is kept non-weight-bearing for 6 weeks followed by weight-bearing casting for the next month, after which time, if radiographic union has occurred, the patient may begin ambulating with an ankle brace.

16.3.2   Discussion

Ogilvie-Harris and colleagues were one of the first investigators who performed in depth analysis of the arthroscopic ankle fusion. The study "Arthroscopically Assisted

Arthrodesis for Osteoarthritic Ankle" published in 1993 reinforced the previous findings of Myerson and Quill in "Ankle Arthrodesis – a Comparison of an Arthroscopic and an Open Method of Treatment" published in 1991 and proved that procedure was, indeed, beneficial.[32,33] In addition, Ogilvie-Harris with coauthors established the average time of radiographic union and assessed functional results 2 years after the procedure. The authors carefully selected 19 patients with ankle arthritis who did not show evidence of frontal plane ankle deformities, rheumatoid arthritis, vascular or neural abnormalities in order to eliminate possible failures due to patients' comorbidities. Although the procedure protocol in many ways was similar to the modern techniques, no distraction device was used and the ankle alignment was achieved at 90° with respect to the tibial bisection without any frontal plane angulations. The results of the study showed striking decrease in postoperative pain and duration of hospitalization. Ten of 19 patients showed signs of radiographic union by the second postoperative month, 5 by the end of the third, 1 by the fifth and last by the sixth. Two patients developed a nonunion one of which was resolved with an open ankle arthrodesis. Among these patients, 2 had fair results, 4 had good results, and 12 had excellent results.[32]

In 1995, Corso and Zimmer introduced the study "Technique and Clinical Evaluation of Arthroscopic Ankle Arthrodesis" conducted between 1991 and 1993. They performed 16 ankle arthroscopic arthrodeses and achieved 100% fusion rate with average time of fusion of 9.5 weeks. The authors expanded inclusion criteria and performed an arthroscopic arthrodesis on the patient with a history of rheumatoid arthritis. Although the fusion had no complications, the patient continued to have diffuse pain in the foot. Thus, taking into consideration this limited experience, the authors remained uncertain whether patients with a history of rheumatoid arthritis were amenable to the arthroscopic procedure. They, however, acknowledged that the arthroscopic procedure may decrease risk of post operative wound complications in this patient group as well as patients with vascular compromise and history of prior surgeries.[31]

Around the same time, Turan et al. came out with the publication "Arthroscopic Ankle Arthrodesis in Rheumatoid Arthritis" which brought more clarity to the question posed by Corso and Zimmer. The arthroscopic technique utilized by the authors had been successfully used in seven patients with rheumatoid arthritis. The surgeons were able to achieve 100% fusion rate with average time until fusion of 10 weeks. There were no complications reported.[34]

In 1996, James Glick et al. published a prominent study "Ankle Arthrodesis Using an Arthroscopic Method: Long-Term Follow-Up of 34 Cases" that had been conducted between 1983 and 1989. This was the longest and, at that time, the largest study that involved 34 patients which were followed up for an average of 8 years. The authors reported 97% of the fusion rate with the average time until fusion of 9 weeks. Although the procedure was performed by four different surgeons, the attempt to standardize the procedure was accomplished by adhering to a similar surgical technique. One of the authors used Steimann pins for initial eight cases. Otherwise all the fusions were achieved with the crossed cancellous screws. There were two poor results; one was a nonunion and the other a malunion. The nonunion occurred due to the use of anterocentral portal which lead to formation of Dorsalis Pedis pseudoanurism. The malunion was due to intra-operative misalignment of the ankle joint. In addition to their findings, this article highlights authors' experiences with different fixation methods. Thus, Steinmann pins were found to be inadequate method of fixation and were replaced by noncannulated screws which in turn were abandoned in favor of cannulated screws when they became available.[35]

Kats et al. in 2003 published an improved arthroscopic technique that, according to the authors, had never been described in the past. In the article "Improvement in Technique for Arthroscopic Ankle Fusion: Results in 15 patients" the authors shared their promising results with bilateral distraction technique and deeper and parallel screw placement. In the group where the new technique was utilized, the average time until union was 12.5 weeks.[36]

Another noteworthy study was published by Gougoulias and colleagues in 2007. This study describes the first significant experience of the arthroscopic ankle arthrodesis in cases with prominent frontal plane deformities. Gougoulias et al. retrospectively evaluated 78 cases of arthroscopic fusions which included 30 ankles with varus or valgus deformities higher than 15°. The inclusion criteria in the study were ranging from posttraumatic osteoarthritis to rheumatoid arthritis, osteonecrosis of talus, osteochondral defect of the talar dome, and history of septic arthritis. In the group with significant frontal plane deformity the procedure was successful in 29 out of 30 (97%) patients. Postoperative tibiotalar alignment in the frontal plane in this group was ranging from 4 varus to 4 valgus. The postoperative complications in this group of patients (one nonunion, two painful subtalar joints, four painful hardware, one minor wound problem, and one pulmonary embolism) were comparable to the complications in the group of patients who underwent in situ arthrodesis.[37]

Over the years, an arthroscopic ankle arthrodesis has proved to be a safe and effective procedure. As the knowledge about the procedure advanced, surgeons significantly expanded a list of ankle joint pathology suitable for an arthroscopic fusion. There were successful experiences with an arthroscopic ankle arthrodesis on patients with autoimmune joint arthritis, avascular necrosis of talus, and, recently, with significant frontal plane joint deformities. Currently, main contraindications to an ankle arthroscopic fusion include neuropathic joints, active infectious process, and poor bone stock. Although a marked ankle deformity of higher than 10–15° of valgus or varus still remains one of the contraindications to many surgeons, evidence showed that such joints could be effectively treated with an arthroscopic procedure.[37]

The arthroscopic ankle arthrodesis procedure technique has also evolved. Nowadays, noninvasive joint distraction equipment is mainly preferred over previously used invasive devices. Also, the latest studies consistently report the use of standard anteromedial and anterolateral portals, while in the past some authors utilized anterocentral and additional posterior portals to facilitate ankle joint debridement. Accessory portals similar to those made for anterolateral and anteromedial impingent can aid in debridement of the ankle gutters (Fig. 16.18). The main difference, however, was noted in the positioning of an ankle joint prior to a fusion. While in the past the joint was positioned in neutral without frontal plane angulations, now

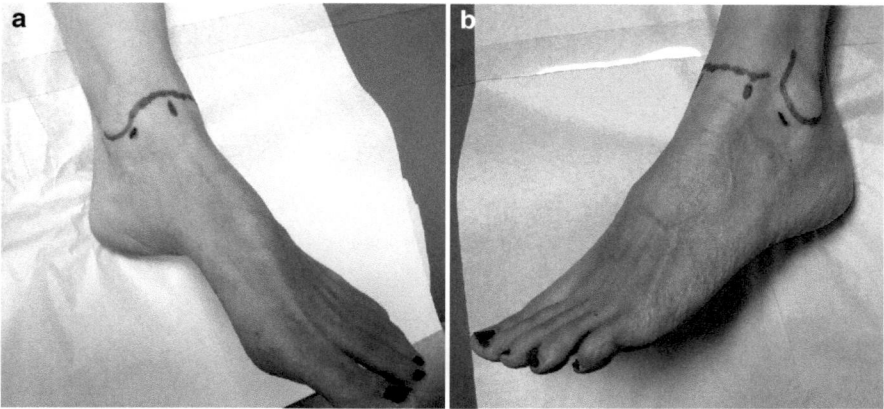

Fig. 16.18 (**a**) Accessory medial (*blue*) and (**b**) lateral portals (*blue*) in "safe zones" to gain access to "gutters"

it is fused in neutral in the sagittal plane with 0–5° rearfoot valgus and 5–10° of external rotation. The fixation is achieved with cannulated screws which could be placed either crossed or parallel and equally provide adequate fixation.

In conclusion, an arthroscopic ankle arthrodesis has demonstrated numerous advantages over an open technique including decrease in postoperative pain, reduced time to fusion, shorter hospital stay, and earlier patient mobilization. Although the procedure is a viable alternative to an open ankle arthrodesis, the successful outcome depends on surgeons' experience with the procedure, proper patient selection, and patients' compliance.

16.4   Arthroscopic Subtalar Arthrodesis

The arthroscopic subtalar arthrodesis emerged after encouraging outcomes of arthroscopic ankle fusions. The first arthroscopic subtalar arthrodesis took place in 1992. The procedure was reported as a preliminary review by Tasto later in 1994 at the annual meeting of the Arthroscopy Association of North America.[38]

16.4.1   Subtalar Arthroscopy Procedure

There are two main portals of entry of the subtalar joint. Both are lateral and right along the sinus tarsi. These exist approximately 1.5 cm distal to the fibula in the plane of where an Ollier's incision would be made (Fig. 16.19). Initially, we distend the subtalar joint using approximately 15 cc of saline (with great care not to "explode

Fig. 16.19 Incisions for subtalar arthroscopy

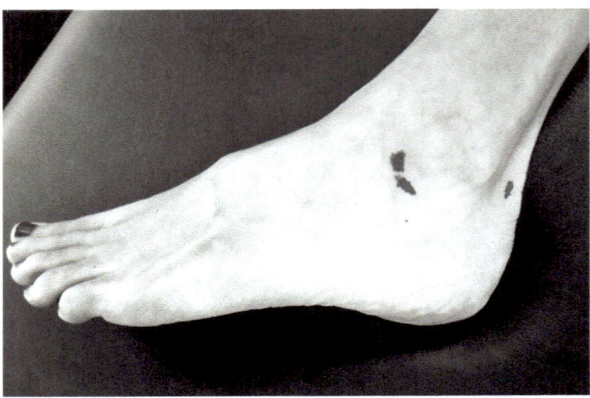

Fig. 16.20 Demonstration of distraction on a cadaver

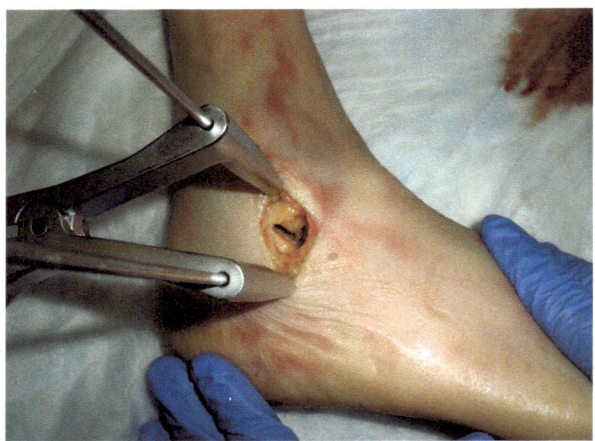

the synovium"). The needle is placed within the joint. Distraction can aid in arthrofibrotic joints as shown in Fig. 16.20. An incision is made and dissection is done bluntly down to the capsule with great care to examine for the sural nerve at the dorsal aspect of this incision. Dissection is then performed down to capsule, which is then incised with a trocar and cannula set up. Next, the trocar is removed and an obturator and cannula are placed into the joint as shown.(Fig. 16.21). This cannula is slipped into the posterior facet without doing damage to the posterior surface. This can be done with distraction or without distraction (Fig. 16.22). This distraction can be invasive (T-handle distracter) or it can be noninvasive, but this does not work well for the saddle configuration of the subtalar joint (Fig. 16.23). After putting in the cannula, the scope is inserted and the posterior facet can be observed. A second portal of entry is made just distal (Fig. 16.24). This is where the working channel is. Subsequently, the cannula and trocar are inserted to enter the sinus tarsi. The scope is then exchanged for the obturator and this is then slipped

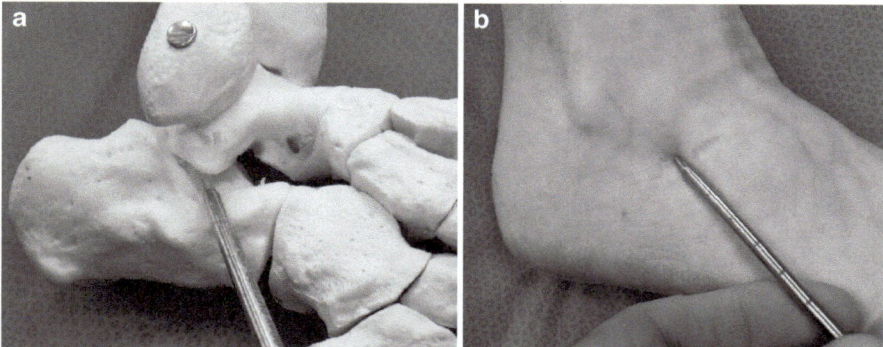

Fig. 16.21 (**a, b**) Insertion of obturator/cannula into subtalar joint

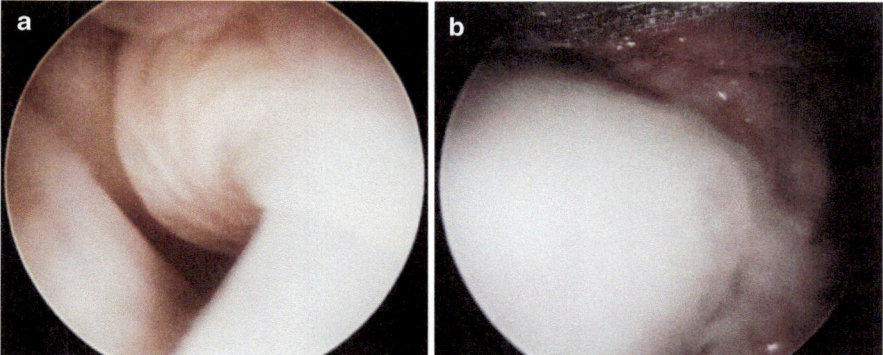

Fig. 16.22 Arthroscopic view of subtalar joint near intra-osseous ligament (**a**) and posterior subtalar joint (**b**)

into the joint. Now you have a scope looking at the posterior facet with the full radius resector to remove any synovitis that is there. If an osteochondritis dissecans exists, one can retrograde drill using a Micro Vector™ drill guide (Fig. 16.25). The other options are debridement of the posterior facet surfaces for arthrodesis (Fig. 16.26). When an arthrodesis is performed, the abrader is inserted and the entire cartilage and subchondral complex is abraded down to subchondral bone, both superiorly off the talar surfaces and superiorly off the calcaneal surface of the posterior facet. When subtalar arthrodesis is performed, arthroscopic burrs are used to denude all the articular cartilage from the posterior facet. Subchondral bleeding of the opposing surfaces is verified arthroscopically. Percutaneous wires are then inserted through the calcaneus from inferior-lateral to medial-superior into the talar body and another from the talar neck inferiorly into the calcaneus, ending in the calcaneus just before the cortical margin of the posterior-lateral surface of the calcaneus. This gives trans-sectional compression strength to the two cancellous screws used. It is not necessary when doing subtalar arthrodesis to fuse the middle or

Fig. 16.23 Region of the placement of the posterior portal of subtalar joint

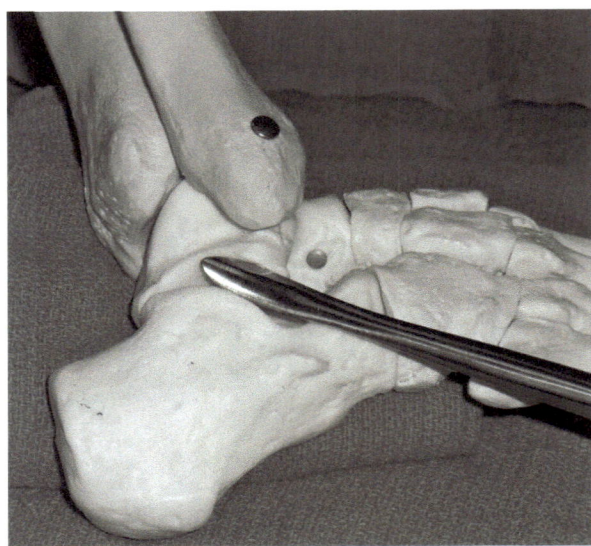

Fig. 16.24 Creation of second anterior ("working") STJ portal

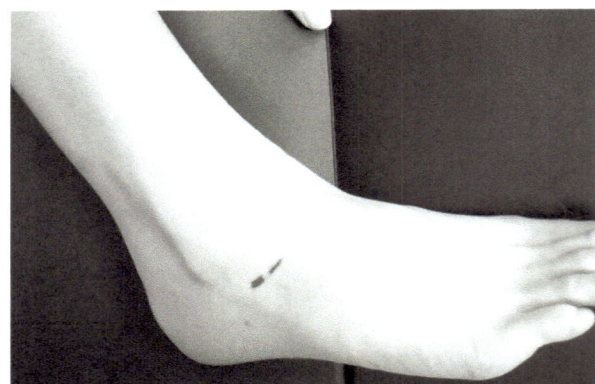

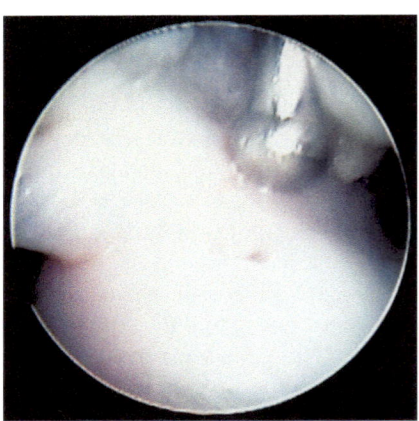

Fig. 16.25 Micro Vector™ drill guide for STJ OCD lesion

Fig. 16.26 Arthroscopic STJ debridement for arthrodesis

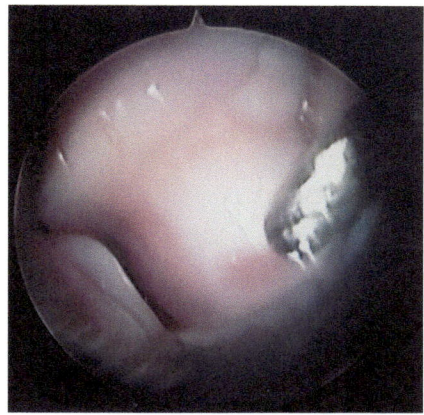

Fig. 16.27 Arthroscopic view of STJ anterior and middle facets

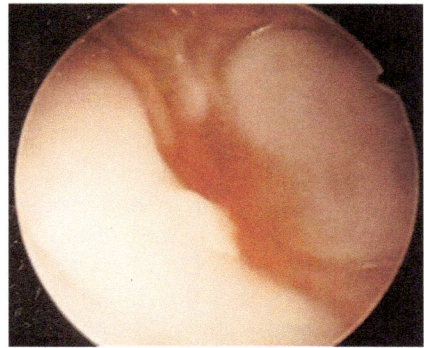

anterior facets. Nevertheless, using a scope, the middle and anterior facet can be visualized through the same approach using the sinus tarsi as the initial insertion of the scope. Once the obturator is inserted into the cannula, this can be slipped in to see the middle facet or the anterior facet (Fig. 16.27). It is difficult to put a working channel into the middle or anterior facet at the same time you are seeing it should there be pathology. Screw placement is performed with image control; however pin placements for cannulated screws are visualized arthroscopically. Typically one or two cannulated 6.5–7.3 mm screws are used (Fig. 16.28). Patients are kept non-weight-bearing for 4–6 weeks in a below-knee cast or boot; they weight-bear an additional 4–6 weeks in a below-knee boot and then begin physical therapy.

16.5 Discussion

Tasto reported nine cases of the arthroscopic subtalar arthrodesis that were followed on average for 17 months. The mean time to fusion was 10 weeks without complications.[38] Around the same time, Lundeen reported one case of arthroscopic subtalar

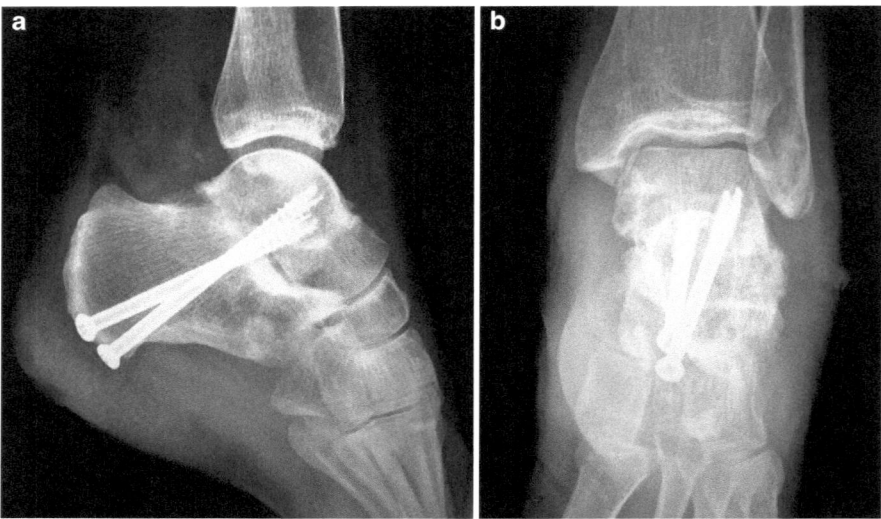

Fig. 16.28 (**a, b**) Post-operative screw placement for STJ fusion

arthrodesis in the article "Arthroscopic Fusion of the Ankle and Subtalar Joint."[39] Since then not many studies have been done. One of the few was the article by Scranton "Comparison of Open Isolated Subtalar Arthrodesis with Autogenous Bone Graft Versus Outpatient Arthroscopic Subtalar Arthrodesis Using Injectable Bone Morphogenic Protein-enhanced Graft" published in 1999. Scranton compared open subtalar arthrodesis to the arthroscopic procedure. His study had been conducted between 1990 and 1997 with the main goal being to compare the fusion rate, length of hospital stay, tourniquet time, and morbidity in patients who undergone standard versus minimally invasive procedure. Also, the author described his arthroscopic technique which included supine position of a patient, anterior sinus tarsi, middle and posterior portals and, prior to fusion, use of osteo-inductive gel. Scranton reported that length of hospital stay for the arthroscopic procedure was 1 night compared to 2–4 days for the open procedure. The tourniquet time was slightly longer (58 min versus 63 min) in the arthroscopic group. All arthroscopic subtalar arthrodesis patients showed evidence of union by 6 months after the procedure and at 1 year were pain-free with ambulation or subtalar stress. This work confirms that arthroscopic subtalar arthrodesis is an effective procedure; however, it does not state precise benefits over the traditional open technique.[40]

In 2000, van Dijk and colleagues in their case report "A 2-portal Endoscopic Approach for Diagnosis and Treatment of Posterior Ankle Pathology" described a new, posterior approach for subtalar joint arthroscopy.[41] In 2007, Carro et al. utilized the posterior approach for arthroscopically assisted subtalar arthrodesis with a patient in the prone position. There were two posterior portals used. One was lateral to the Achilles tendon and slightly superior or at the level of the lateral malleolus and the other was at the medial margin of the tendon approximately at the level of the lateral portal. The debridement of the joint was performed posterior to the interosseous ligament and only the posterior facet was fused with two percutaneous headless screws. The author reported four successful arthroscopic procedures performed between 2004 and 2005 utilizing the technique. The radiographic union was achieved at 8 postoperative weeks without complications. Carro et al. found that the posterior approach provided superior and safer access to the posteromedial aspect of the joint over the traditional technique. According to the authors, the lateral technique permitted visualization of the medial area of the joint only when the ligaments were lax. Also, the posterior approach allowed for better positioning of the joint prior to the fusion and facilitated correction of mild angular deformity.[42]

During the same year, Amendola et al. published "Technique and Early Experience with Posterior Arthroscopic Subtalar Arthrodesis" where they described their experience with 11 procedures using posterior approach and evaluated early results. Ten of 11 joints showed evidence of fusion by 10 weeks. One patient developed a nonunion. No other complications were reported. The article confirmed findings of Carro and colleagues about safety and dependability of the posterior arthroscopic arthrodesis technique.[43]

Another large and significant study was published by Glanzmann et al. in 2007. There were 41 arthroscopic subtalar arthrodeses performed. Patients were followed up on average for 55 months. The authors reported 100% fusion rate by 11 weeks with several complications which included peroneal tendonitis in one patient and persistent ankle pain in three patients.[44] These findings correlated with Scranton's experience in 1999 as well as Tasto's results in 2003 who reported 100% fusion rate in 25 patients following the procedure.

In 2009, Beimers et al. described a new three-portal approach for the arthroscopic subtalar fusion. The accessory portal was located at the sinus tarsi area and was used to distract the joint especially in the patient group who had limited joint space due to talocalcaneal coalition. It was also used for the debridement of the cartilage from the anterior facet of the joint. Three patients with a history of talocalcaneal coalition were operated on between March and July of 2006. The time of the procedure ranged from 52 to 65 min and the patients were discharged the following day. Patients demonstrated osseous union at 6 weeks after the surgery and had no complaints at the follow-up visits 24–28 months later. There were no complications reported. This article one more time emphasizes the safety of the approach and benefits of the accessory portal that allows for the sufficient joint distraction. In addition, this study showed the shortest time of osseous union (6 weeks) in all three patients.[45]

Today, the arthroscopic subtalar arthrodesis is an acceptable alternative to an open subtalar fusion. The minimally invasive nature of the procedure allows preservation of blood supply to the talus and calcaneus and contributes to high (91–100%) union rates. Decreased postoperative pain, preserved or minimally altered proprioception, a reduced hospital stay as well as shorter postoperative recovery are also benefits of arthroscopic procedure. Although effective, the arthroscopic subtalar fusion technique entails a learning curve (as with the other arthroscopic techniques described here), and proper candidate selection for a successful outcome.

References

1. Lundeen G. Historical perspectives of ankle arthroscopy. J Foot Ankle Surg. 1987;26:3–7.
2. Guhl JF. History and development of foot and ankle arthroscopy. 2nd ed. Thorofare: Slack Inc; 1993. p.1–6.
3. Takagi K. Arthroscopy of small joints. New York: Igaku-Shoin; 1982. p.3.
4. Lundeen RO. Manual of ankle and foot arthroscopy. New York: Churchill Livingstone; 1992.
5. Drez D, Guhl J, Gollehon DL. Ankle arthroscopy: technique and indications. Foot Ankle. 1981;2:138–42.
6. Parisien SJ, Shereff MJ. The role of arthroscopy in the diagnosis and treatment of disorders of the ankle. Foot Ankle. 1981;2:144–9.
7. Stienstra JJ. Intra-articular soft tissue masses of the ankle. Clin Podiatr Med Surg. 1994;11:371–83.
8. Stone JW, Guhl JF. Meniscoid lesions of the ankle. Clin Sports Med. 1991;10:661–76.
9. Bassett Fh, Gates HS, Billys JB, et al. Talar impingement by the anteroinferior tibiofibular ligament. J Bone Joint Surg Am. 1990;72:55–9.
10. Martin DF, Curl WW, Baker CL. Arthroscopic treatment of chronic synovitis of the ankle. Arthroscopy. 1989;5:110–4.
11. Lundeen RO. Ankle arthroscopy in the adolescent patient. J Foot Ankle Surg. 1990;29:510–5.
12. Lundeen RO. Arthroscopic anatomy of the anterior aspect of the ankle. J Am Podiatr Med Assoc. 1985;75:367–71.
13. Ray RG, Gusman DN, Christensen JC. Anatomical variation of the tibial plafond; the anteromedial tibial notch. J Foot Ankle Surg. 1994;33:419–26.
14. Berndt Al, Harty M. Transchondral fractures (osteochondritis dessicans) of the talus. J Bone Joint Surg Am. 1959;41:988.
15. Hamilton W. Differential diagnosis. In: Guhl J, editor. Ankle arthroscopy: pathology and surgical techniques. 2nd ed. Thorofare: Slack Inc; 1993.
16. Ferkel RD, Sgaglione NA, Del Pizzo W, et al. Arthroscopic treatment of osteochondral lesions of the talus: technique and results. Orthop Trans. 1990;14:172–3.
17. Meyer JM, Hoffmeyer P, Xavier X. High resolution computed tomography in the chronically painful ankle sprain. Foot Ankle. 1988;8:291–6.
18. Liu Sh, Nuccion Sl, Finerman G. Diagnosis of anterolateral ankle impingement. Am J Sports Med. 1997;25:389–93.
19. Deginder WL. Osteochondritis dessicans of the talus. Radiology. 1955;65:590.
20. Dipaola JD, Nelson DW, Colville MR. Characterizing osteochondral lesions by magnetic resonance imaging. Arthroscopy. 1991;7:101–4.
21. Palladino S. Distraction systems for ankle arthroscopy. Clin Podiatr Med Surg. 1994;11:499–511.
22. Cameron S. Technical note: noninvasive distraction for ankle arthroscopy. Arthroscopy. 1997;13:366–69.
23. Lamy CJ, Stienstra JJ. Complications in ankle arthroscopy. Clin Podiatr Med Surg. 1994;11:523–39.
24. Chen YC. Arthroscopy of the ankle joint. Arthroscopy. 1976;1–6.
25. Grady J, Hughes D. Arthroscopic management of talar dome lesions using a transmalleolar approach. J Am Podiatr Med Assoc. 2006;96(3):260–3.
26. Barber FA, Click J, Britt BT. Complications of ankle arthroscopy. Foot Ankle. 1990;10:263–6.
27. Lamy C, Stienstra JJ. Complications of ankle arthroscopy. Clin Podiatr Med Surg. 1994;11:523–39.
28. Martin DF, Baker C, Curl WW, et al. Operative ankle arthroscopy, long term follow-up. Am J Sports Med. 1989;17:16-23.
29. Armstrong RW, Bolding F, Joseph R. Septic arthritis following arthroscopy: clinical syndromes and analysis of risk factors. Arthroscopy. 1992;8:213–23.
30. Rodeo SA, Forster RA, Weiland AJ. Current concept review: neurologic complications due to arthroscopy. J Bone Joint Surg Am. 1993;75:917–26.

31. Corso S, Zimmer T. Technique and clinical evaluation of arhtroscopic ankle arthrodesis. Arthrosc J Arthroscopic Relat Surg. 1995;11(5):585–90.
32. Ogilvie-Harris DJ, Liberman I, Fitsialos D. Arthroscopically assisted arhtrodesis for osteoarthrotic ankles. J Bone Joint Surg Am. 1993;75:1167–74.
33. Myerson MS, Quill G. Ankle arthrodesis – a comparison of an arthroscopic and an open method of treatment. Clin Orthop Relat Res. 1991;268:84.
34. Turan I, Wredmark T, Fellander-Tsai L. Arthroscopic ankle arthrodesis in rheumatoid arthritis. Clin Orthop Relat Res. 1995;320:110–4.
35. Glick J, Morgan C, Myerson M, et al. Ankle arthrodesis using an arthroscopic method: long-term follow-up of 34 cases. Arthrosc J Arthroscopic Relat Surg. 1996;12(4):428–34.
36. Kats J, van Kampen A, de Waal-Malafijt M. Improvement in technique for arthroscopic ankle fusion: results in 15 patients. Knee Surg Sports Traumatol Arthrosc. 2003;11:46–9.
37. Gougoulias NE, Agathangelidis FG, Parsons SW. Arthroscopic ankle arthrodesis. Foot Ankle Int. 2007;28(6):695-706.
38. Tasto JP. Subtalar Arthroscopy. Operative Arthroscopy. 3rd ed. New York: Lippincott Williams and Wilkins; 2002:944–52.
39. Lundeen RO. Arthroscopic fusion of the ankle and subtalar joint. Clin Podiatr Med Surg. 1994;11(3):395-406.
40. Scranton PE. omparison of isolated subtalar arthrodesis with autogenous bone graft versus outpatient arthroscopic subtalar arthrodesis using injectable bone morphogenic protein-enhanced graft. Foot Ankle Int. 1999;20(3):162–5.
41. Van Dijk CN, Scholten PE, Krips R. A 2-portal endoscopic approach for diagnosis and treatment of posterior ankle pathology. Arthroscopy. 2000;16:871–6.
42. Carro LP, Golano P, Vega J. Arthroscopic subtalar arthrodesis: the posterior approach in the prone position. Arthrosc J Arthroscopic Relat Surg. 2007;23(4):445. e1–4.
43. Amendola A, Lee KB, Saltzman CL, Suh JS. Technique and early experience with posterior arthroscopic subtalar arthrodesis. Foot Ankle Int. 2007;28:298-302.
44. Glanzmann MC, Sanhueza-Hernandez R. Arthroscopic subtalar arthrodesis for symptomatic osteoarthritis of the hindfoot: a prospective study of 41 cases. Foot Ankle Int. 2007;28(1):2-7.
45. Beimers L, Leeuw P, van Dijk N. A 3-portal approach for arthroscopic subtalar arthrodesis. Knee Surg Sports Traumatol Arthrosc. 2009;17:830–4.

Chapter 17
Posterior Ankle Arthroscopy and Endoscopy

Peter A.J. de Leeuw, Maayke N. van Sterkenburg, Christiaan J.A. van Bergen, and C. Niek van Dijk

17.1 Introduction

Ankle arthroscopy has been developed and improved over the last three decades. Nowadays, this minimal invasive technique to treat a variety of ankle pathology is routinely used in a relatively safe and reliable manner. In 1931, Burman attempted the first ankle arthroscopy and concluded this joint not to be suitable for arthroscopy with respect to its narrow inter-articular access.[1] The technical improvements, such as smaller diameter arthroscopes and joint distraction methods, made it possible to report on a series of 28 ankle arthroscopies by Watanabe in 1972.[2]

Van Dijk et al. were the first to describe endoscopic access to the tendons by tendoscopy. These included tendoscopy of the posterior tibial tendon,[3] the peroneal tendons,[4,5] and Achilles tendon,[6] which was followed by endoscopic treatment for retrocalcaneal bursitis, called endoscopic calcaneoplasty.[7,8] In 2000, he introduced a two-portal endoscopic hindfoot approach.[9] Recently, the results of 55 consecutive patients with posterior ankle impingement were reported on with a good-to-excellent outcome in 74% of the patients.[10] This minimal invasive technique provides excellent access to the posterior aspect of the ankle and subtalar joint. Furthermore, extra-articular structures of the hindfoot such as the os trigonum, flexor hallucis longus, and the deep portion of the deltoid ligament can be assessed.[9] Based on these portals, recently, a minimally invasive groove-deepening technique for recurrent peroneal tendon dislocation was introduced.[11]

P.A.J. de Leeuw, M.Sc. (✉)
Department of Orthopaedic Surgery, Academic Medical Center,
Meibergdreef 9, Amsterdam 1105 AZ, The Netherlands
e-mail: p.a.deleeuw@amc.uva.nl

M.N. van Sterkenburg, M.D., M.Sc. • C.J.A. van Bergen, M.D., M.Sc. •
C.N. van Dijk, M.D., Ph.D.
Department of Orthopaedic Surgery, Academic Medical Center,
Amsterdam, The Netherlands

A. Saxena (ed.), *Sports Medicine and Arthroscopic Surgery of the Foot and Ankle*,
DOI 10.1007/978-1-4471-4106-8_17, © Springer-Verlag London 2013

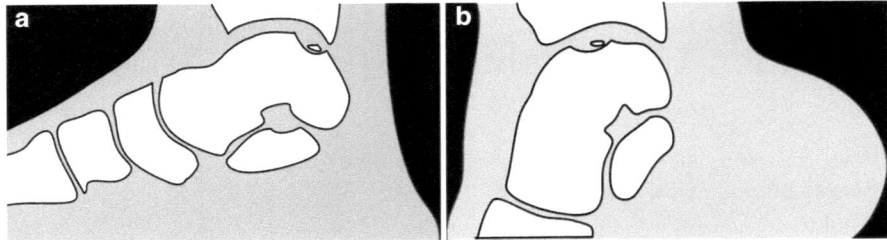

Fig. 17.1 Depending on the talar location of the osteochondral defect, the pathology can be addressed via anterior or posterior ankle arthroscopy. To determine whether the osteochondral defect can be approached via anterior ankle arthroscopy, the foot is forced in maximum plantarflexion. (**a**) Posteriorly located talar osteochondral defect with the foot in neutral position. (**b**) By forcing the foot in maximum plantar flexion, the osteochondral defect moves anteriorly. In this case, the osteochondral defect cannot be reached via anterior ankle arthroscopy but can be reached via posterior ankle arthroscopy

17.2 Contraindications/Indications of the Procedures

For each of the described endoscopic/arthroscopic procedures in this manuscript, there are no absolute contraindications. Caution must be taken into consideration with patients suffering from vascular diseases, such as diabetes. The different indications can be categorized according to the location of the pathology.

17.3 Articular Pathology

17.3.1 Posterior Compartment Ankle Joint

The main indications include both soft tissue and/or bony pathology. Soft tissue pathology mainly includes chronic synovitis, chondromatosis, and excessive scar tissue. Bony pathology includes loose bodies, ossicles, posttraumatic calcifications, avulsion fragments, and posterior tibial rim osteophytes. An osteochondral defect in the ankle joint, which cannot be approached by means of anterior ankle arthroscopy with the ankle in maximum plantar flexion, can be assessed through posterior ankle arthroscopy (Fig. 17.1). For lesions up to 15 mm, debridement and drilling is the treatment of choice.[12]

17.3.2 Posterior Compartment Subtalar Joint

The main indications are removal of osteophytes, treatment of degenerative changes in the subtalar joint, including talar cystic lesions, loose body removal, and a subtalar arthrodesis in case of osteoarthritis.[13-16] Intraosseous talar ganglions can also be treated arthroscopically.[17]

17.4 Periarticular Pathology

17.4.1 Posterior Ankle Impingement

Posterior ankle impingement syndrome is by definition a pain syndrome. The pain is present in the hindfoot during forced plantar flexion. The patients can be divided into an *overuse* and a *trauma* group based on the mechanism to produce this syndrome.

The *overuse* group is mainly composed of ballet dancers, downhill runners, and soccer players.[18-20] In professional ballet, the specific dancing steps force the ankle in hyper-plantar-flexion. The anatomic structures in between the calcaneus and the posterior part of the distal tibia thereby become compressed. Through exercise, the dancer will attempt to increase the range of motion and joint mobility, ultimately decreasing the distance between the calcaneus and the talus. The anatomical structures at the back of the ankle joint hereby can become compressed. During downhill running, the ankle is repetitively forced into plantar flexion, resulting in repetitive stress on the anatomical structures in this posterior area.[21] Kicking the ball with the foot in plantar flexion results in high forces on the anatomical structures in the hindfoot. These repetitive high forces can eventually cause posterior ankle impingement.

A hyper-plantar-flexion *trauma* and supination *trauma* can cause damage to the anatomical structures in the hindfoot and can finally lead to a chronic posterior ankle impingement syndrome.

A differentiation must be made between the two groups, since overuse trauma seems to have a better prognosis[22] and patients are more satisfied after arthroscopic treatment.[22] Congenital anatomic anomalies such as a prominent posterior talar process, an os trigonum, or a talus bipartitus[23] can facilitate the occurrence of the syndrome. An os trigonum is estimated to be present in 1.7–7% and occurs bilateral in 1.4% people.[24-26] These congenital anomalies in combination with a traumatic or overuse injury facilitate the occurrence of symptoms.[20,27-29] During plantar flexion, the soft tissue structures like synovium, posterior ankle capsule, or one of the posterior ligamentous structures can get pinched and compressed, eventually resulting in swelling, partial rupture, or fibrosis.

The diagnosis is clinical. The forced passive hyper-plantar-flexion test is positive when the patient experiences recognizable pain during the test (Fig. 17.2). A negative test rules out the posterior ankle impingement syndrome. A positive test is followed by a diagnostic infiltration with Xylocaine® (AstraZenica, Zoetermeer, The Netherlands) in the posterior ankle compartment. Disappearance of pain following infiltration confirms the diagnosis.

17.4.2 Deep Portion of the Deltoid Ligament/Cedell Fracture

Hyper-dorsiflexion or eversion trauma can result in avulsed fragments, posttraumatic calcifications, or ossicles in the deep portion of the deltoid ligament. The patient

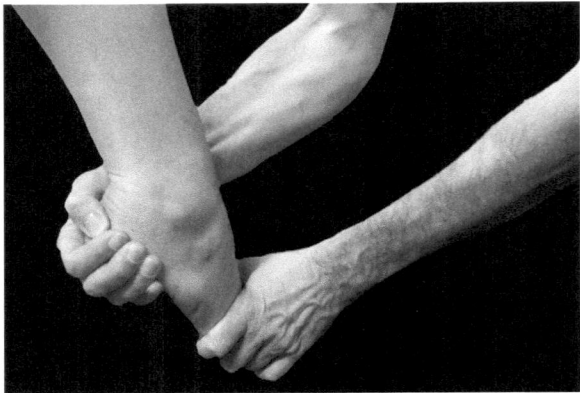

Fig. 17.2 The forced hyper-plantar-flexion test is performed with the patient sitting with the knee flexed in 90°. The test should be performed with repetitive quick passive hyper-plantar-flexion movements. The test can be repeated in slight external rotation or slight internal rotation of the foot relative to the tibia. The investigator can apply this rotational movement on the point of maximal plantar flexion, thereby "grinding" the (enlarged) posterior talar process/os trigonum in between tibia and calcaneus

typically presents with posteromedial ankle pain, which is aggravated by running and walking on uneven grounds. Ligament avulsion of the deep portion of the deltoid ligament from the posteromedial talar process was first described by Cedell.[30] A computed tomography (CT) scan is most often necessary to confirm the diagnosis.

17.4.3   Flexor Hallucis Longus

Posterior ankle impingement syndrome is often accompanied by tendinopathy of the flexor hallucis longus (FHL). The patient experiences posteromedial ankle pain. On physical examination, the tendon can be palpated behind the medial malleolus, just lateral to the flexor digitorum longus. By asking the patient to repetitively flex the big toe, the FHL tendon can easily be identified in between the medial and lateral talar processes while the ankle is in 10–20° plantar flexion. In patients with tendinopathy or paratendinopathy, crepitus and recognizable tenderness can be provoked by the examiner's finger placed over the tendon just behind the medial malleolus. In some patients, a painful nodule in the tendon can be palpated.

17.4.4   Achilles Tendon and Retrocalcaneal Bursa

A symptomatic inflammation of the retrocalcaneal bursa is caused by repetitive impingement of the bursa between the anterior aspect of the Achilles tendon and a bony postero-superior calcaneal prominence. A prominent postero-superior calcaneal rim in combination with retrocalcaneal bursitis was first described by Haglund in 1928.[31] Physical examination reveals swelling on both sides of the Achilles tendon at the level of the postero-superior calcaneal prominence. Pain is aggravated by palpating this area just medial and lateral to the Achilles tendon.

Retrocalcaneal bursitis can be accompanied by midportion and/or insertional tendinopathy. In case of insertional tendinopathy, there is pain at the bone–tendon junction, which gets worse after exercise. The area of maximal tenderness is often located in the central part of the insertion. Patients with tendinopathy of the main body of the Achilles tendon report pain and stiffness. A thick nodule is present 2–6 cm proximal to the insertion, which is tender on palpation.

17.4.5 Neurovascular Bundle

Entrapment of the posterior tibial nerve within the tarsal tunnel is commonly known as a tarsal tunnel syndrome.[32] Clinical examination should be sufficient to differentiate these disorders from an isolated posterior tibial tendon disorder.

17.4.6 Peroneal Tendons

Peroneal tendon disorders are an uncommon, under-recognized source of postero-lateral hindfoot pain and dysfunction. Pathology of the peroneal tendons is often overlooked because it is sometimes difficult to distinguish them from lateral ankle ligament disorders.[33]

Instability and dislocation are pathologies associated with the peroneal tendons and are often provoked by sports-related injuries. In 1803, Monteggia was the first describing peroneal instability in a ballet dancer.[34] There are two factors which can cause the tendons to dislocate. First, the superior peroneal tendon retinaculum can be too lax or disrupted.[35-37] The retinaculum normally tightly covers the peroneal tendons at the posterior distal fibula, maintaining the tendons at their anatomical site. In case of trauma, this function can be impaired. The second mechanism is a (congenital) flat/non-concave configuration of the posterior distal part of the fibula,[38,39] with or without an inadequate amount of cartilaginous rim.[36] In the normal situation, this part of the fibula is concave with a cartilaginous rim at the most distal part, nurturing the peroneal tendons behind the lateral malleolus. Superior peroneal retinacular dysfunction and an inadequate fibular groove often coexist in recurrent peroneal tendon dislocation.

Patients typically complain of a recurrent painful and snapping sensation at the lateral aspect of the ankle with a perception of ankle instability, especially when walking on uneven ground. The pain and dislocation can be provoked by combined dorsiflexion and eversion of the foot during physical examination.

17.5   Preoperative Planning

After history taking and physical examination, the diagnosis can be confirmed or rejected based upon different available imaging techniques. If history taking and the physical examination do not reveal abnormalities, additional diagnostics can be used to search for a clue or to rule out pathology, i.e., medico-legal reasons. Close consultation between the surgeon and the radiologist is necessary to decide upon optimal radiographic diagnostics.[40]

Always start with routine weight-bearing radiographs in an anteroposterior (AP) and lateral direction. In patients with an osteochondral defect, the standard weight-bearing radiographs may show an area of detached bone, surrounded by radiolucency. Initially the defect might be too small to be visualized. A heel rise mortise view may reveal a posteriorly located osteochondral defect.[41] For further diagnostic evaluation, CT and magnetic resonance imaging (MRI) have demonstrated similar accuracy.[41] A multi-slice helical CT scan is preferred to determine the extent of the defect and also to decide upon anterior or posterior arthroscopic approach for debridement and bone marrow stimulation.[41]

In patients with a posterior ankle impingement, the AP ankle view typically does not show abnormalities. Osteophytes, calcifications, loose bodies, chondromatosis as well as hypertrophy of the postero-superior calcaneal border can often be detected by the lateral ankle radiograph. In case of doubt for the differentiation between hypertrophy of the posterior talar process or an os trigonum, we recommend a lateral radiograph view with the foot in 25° external rotation in relation to the standard ankle view (Fig. 17.3). Especially in posttraumatic cases, a spiral CT scan can be important to ascertain the extent of the injury and the exact location of calcifications or fragments. In general, soft tissue pathology consequently can be visualized best using a MRI scan. Ultrasonography seems to be a good and relatively cheap alternative, with a positive predictive value of 100% for peroneal tendon dislocation.[42,43]

17.6   Operative Techniques

17.6.1   Posterior Ankle Arthroscopy

The procedure is carried out in an outpatient setting under general anesthesia or spinal anesthesia. The patient is placed in a prone position. The involved leg is marked by the patient with an arrow to avoid wrong side surgery, with a tourniquet inflated around the thigh, pressured 300 mmHg. A small support is placed under the lower leg, making it possible to move the ankle freely (Fig. 17.4). We use a soft tissue distraction device when indicated.[44]

For irrigation, normal saline is used, but Ringers solution is also possible. A 4.0-mm arthroscope with an inclination angle of 30° is routinely used for posterior ankle arthroscopy. Apart from the standard excisional and motorized instruments for treatment of osteophytes and ossicles, a 4-mm chisel and periosteal elevator can be useful.

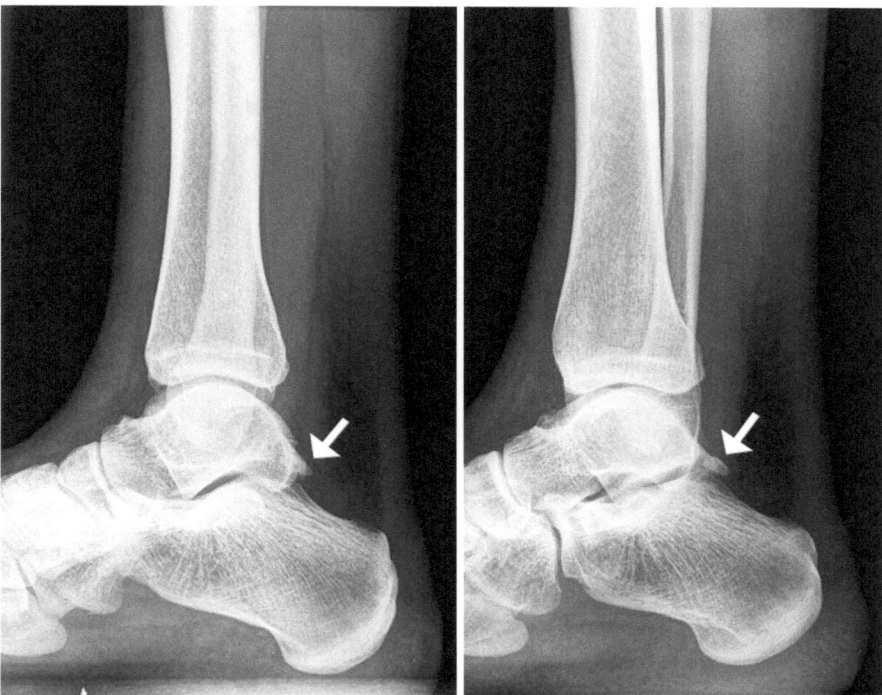

Fig. 17.3 A 27-year-old male patient presenting with posterior left ankle pain during plantarflexed movement of the foot. Hyper-plantar-flexion test is positive. (*Left*) The standard lateral radiograph shows a possible prominent posterior talar process (*arrow*). (*Right*) Lateral X-ray with the foot in 25° exorotation. An os trigonum can be recognized (*arrow*)

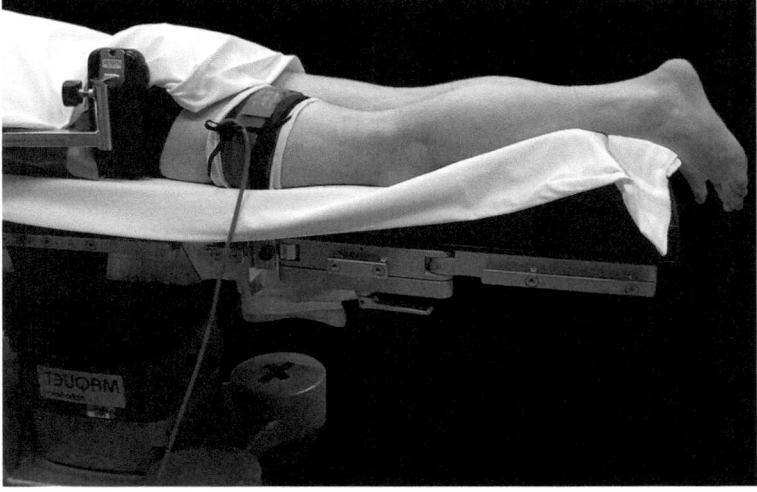

Fig. 17.4 For posterior ankle arthroscopy, the patient is placed in a prone position. A tourniquet is applied around the upper leg and a small support is placed under the lower leg, making it possible to move the ankle freely

Fig. 17.5 For marking the
anatomical landmarks that are
needed for portal placement,
the ankle is kept in a neutral
position. A hook can be useful
to determine the plane in which
the portal must be positioned.
A straight line is drawn from
the tip of the lateral malleolus
to the Achilles tendon, parallel
to the foot sole. The
posterolateral portal (*arrow*) is
made just above the line from
the tip of the lateral malleolus
to the interception with the
Achilles tendon

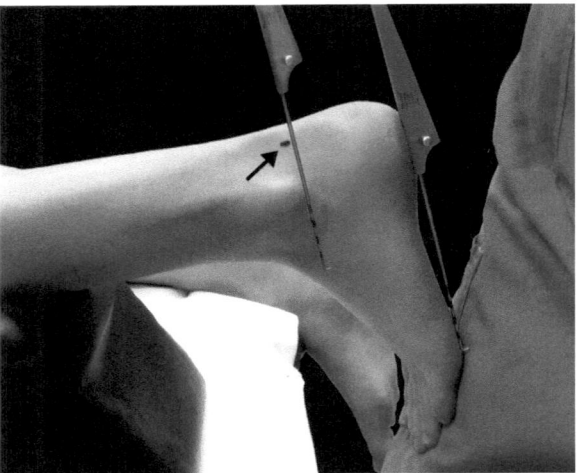

The anatomical landmarks on the posterior ankle are the lateral malleolus, medial and lateral border of the Achilles tendon, and the foot sole. The ankle is kept in a neutral position. A straight line is drawn from the tip of the lateral malleolus to the Achilles tendon, parallel to the foot sole (Fig. 17.5).

The posterolateral portal is made directly in front of the Achilles tendon just proximal to this line. After making a vertical stab incision, the subcutaneous layer is split by a mosquito clamp. The mosquito clamp is directed anteriorly, pointing toward the interdigital webspace, in between the first and second toes (Fig. 17.6a). When the tip of the clamp touches the bone, it is exchanged for a 4.5-mm arthroscopic shaft with the blunt trocar pointing in the same direction (Fig. 17.6b). By palpating the bone in the sagittal plane, the level of the ankle joint and subtalar joint can often be distinguished since the prominent posterior talar process or os trigonum can be felt as a posterior prominence in between the two joints. The trocar is situated extra-articularly at the level of the ankle joint. The trocar is exchanged for the 4-mm arthroscope with the direction of view 30° to the lateral side.

The posteromedial portal is made at the same level, just above the line from the tip of the lateral malleolus, but just in front of the medial aspect of the Achilles tendon (Fig. 17.7). After making a vertical stab incision, a mosquito clamp is introduced and directed toward the arthroscope shaft in a 90° angle (Fig. 17.6c). When the mosquito clamp touches the shaft of the arthroscope, the shaft is used as a guide to "travel" anteriorly in the direction of the ankle joint, all the way down while contacting the arthroscope shaft until it reaches the bone (Fig. 17.6d). The arthroscope is now pulled slightly backward and slides over the mosquito clamp until the tip of the mosquito clamp comes into view (Fig. 17.6e). The clamp is used to spread the extra-articular soft tissue in front of the tip of the lens. In situations where scar tissue or adhesions are present, the mosquito clamp is exchanged for a 5-mm full radius shaver. The tip of the shaver is directed in a lateral and slightly plantar direction toward the lateral aspect of the subtalar joint.

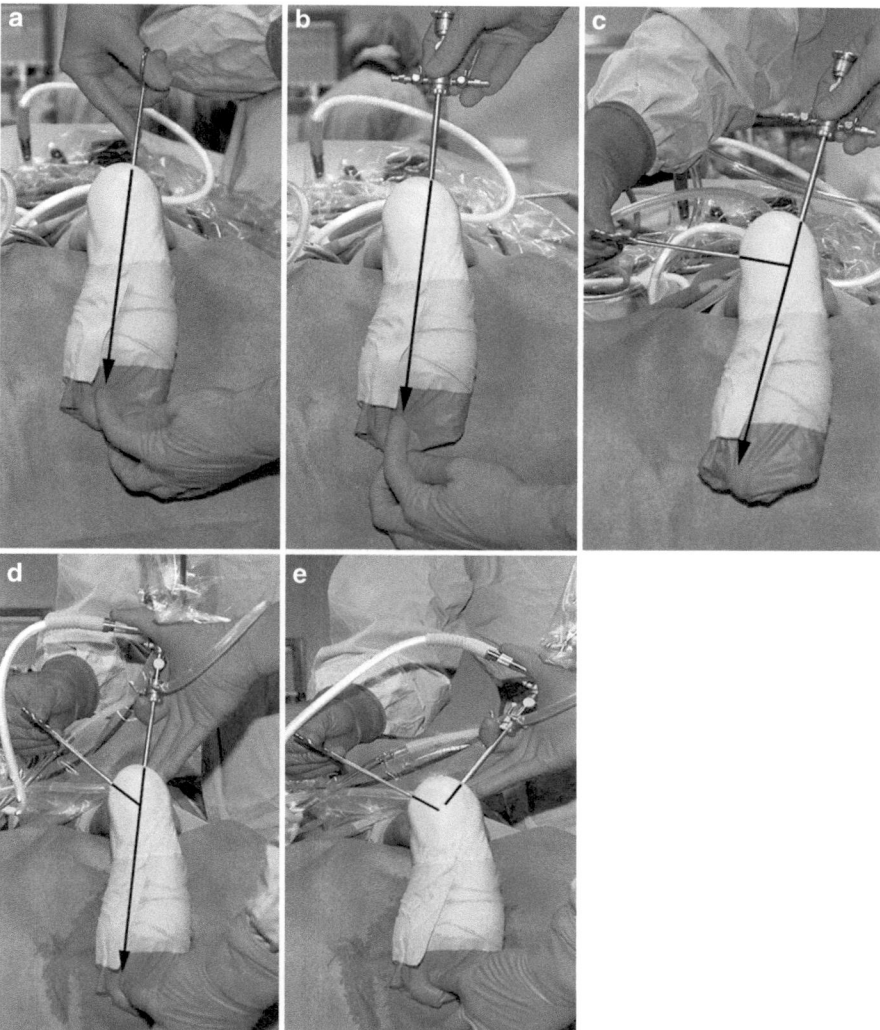

Fig. 17.6 Macroscopic image of a right ankle indicating the stepwise portal placement for hindfoot endoscopy. (**a**) After making a vertical stab incision, the subcutaneous tissue is bluntly divided by a mosquito clamp in the direction of the first interdigital webspace. (**b**) The mosquito clamp is exchanged for the blunt trocar, still the direction is toward the interdigital webspace. (**c**) After the medial portal has been created, a mosquito clamp is introduced, directed toward the arthroscopic shaft in a 90° angle. (**d**) The arthroscopic shaft is used as a guide to travel anteriorly with the mosquito clamp toward the bone. (**e**) The arthroscope is slightly pulled back until the clamp comes into view

The joint capsule and fatty tissue can be removed. After removal of the very thin joint capsule of the subtalar joint, the posterior compartment of the subtalar joint can be inspected. At the level of the ankle joint, the posterior tibiofibular ligament is recognized and the posterior talofibular ligament is recognized. The cranial part

Fig. 17.7 The anatomical
landmarks for posterior ankle
arthroscopy are marked on a left
ankle. The posterolateral portal
(*PL*) is made just above a
horizontal line drawn from the
tip of the lateral malleolus (*L*)
to the Achilles tendon (*AT*),
parallel to the foot sole with the
foot in the neutral position. The
posteromedial portal (*PM*) is
created at the same level, just
medial to the Achilles tendon.
M medial malleolus,
C calcaneus)

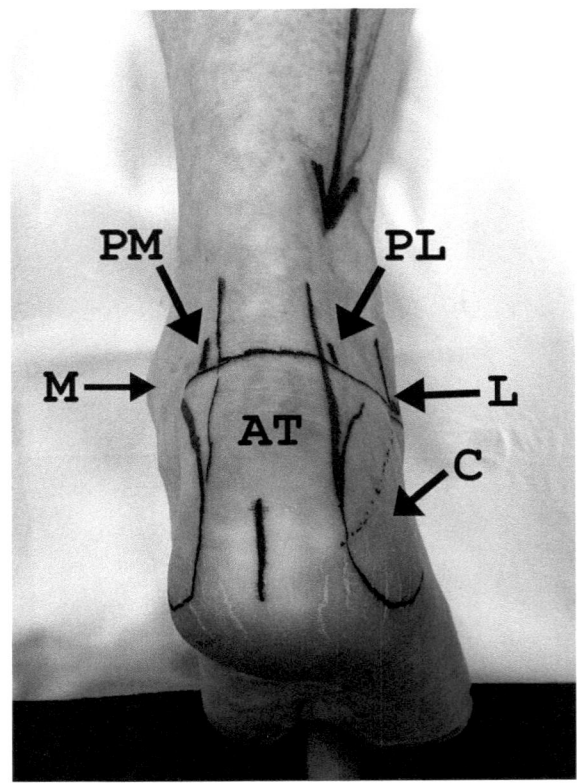

of the posterior talar process is now freed from scar tissue, and the FHL tendon is identified. Before addressing the pathology, the FHL tendon should always be inspected. The FHL tendon is an important safety landmark, since the neurovascular bundle runs just medial from this tendon. In case of a FHL tendinopathy, the flexor retinaculum and the tendon's sheet can be opened to release the tendon (Fig. 17.8). After removal of the thin joint capsule of the ankle joint, the intermalleolar and transverse ligament can be lifted in order to enter and inspect the ankle joint.

On the medial side, the tip of the medial malleolus and the deep portion of the deltoid ligament can be visualized. By opening the joint capsule from inside out at the level of the medial malleolus, the tendon sheath of the posterior tibial tendon can be opened when desired, and the arthroscope can be introduced into the tendon sheath. The posterior tibial tendon can be inspected. The same procedure can be done for the flexor digitorum longus tendon.

By applying manual distraction to the os calcis, the posterior compartment of the ankle opens up and the shaver can be introduced into the posterior ankle compartment. We prefer to apply a soft tissue distractor at this point.[44] A synovectomy and/or capsulectomy can be performed when indicated. The talar dome can be inspected over almost its entire surface as well as the complete tibial plafond.

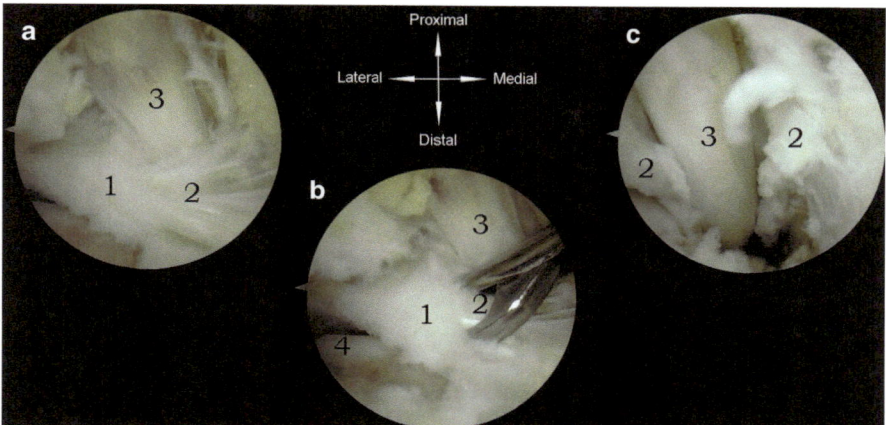

Fig. 17.8 A 23-year-old female patient presenting with posteromedial left ankle pain during plié. Clinically, the pain could be provoked by active/passive flexion of the great toe and palpation just behind the medial malleolus. (**a**) Endoscopic image displaying the flexor hallucis longus tendinopathy (3). The flexor hallucis longus tendon is located just medial to the posterolateral talar process (1) and is fixated by the flexor retinaculum (2) in between the posteromedial and posterolateral talar process. (**b**) The flexor retinaculum is released using a punch. (4 = level of the subtalar joint). (**c**) Postoperative endoscopic image showing a complete release of the flexor hallucis longus

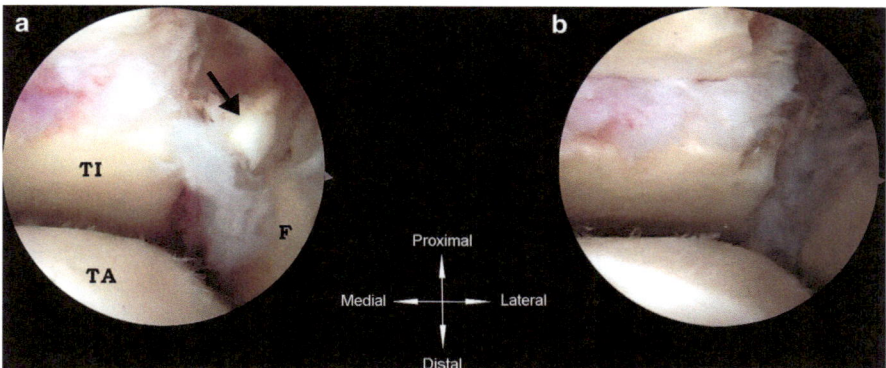

Fig. 17.9 A 43-year-old male patient with persisting deep right ankle pain. (**a**) Arthroscopic image showing fibrotic syndesmotic ligaments and a loose body. The syndesmotic ligaments are visualized with the arthroscope through the posteromedial portal. (*TI* tibia, *TA* talus, *F* fibula). (**b**) Postoperative arthroscopic image showing the debrided syndesmotic ligaments

An osteochondral defect or subchondral cystic lesion can be identified, debrided, and drilled. The posterior syndesmotic ligaments are inspected and debrided if fibrotic or ruptured (Fig. 17.9). The syndesmotic stability can easily be tested with a hook. Also loose bodies in the syndesmotic ligament complex can be released and subsequently removed.

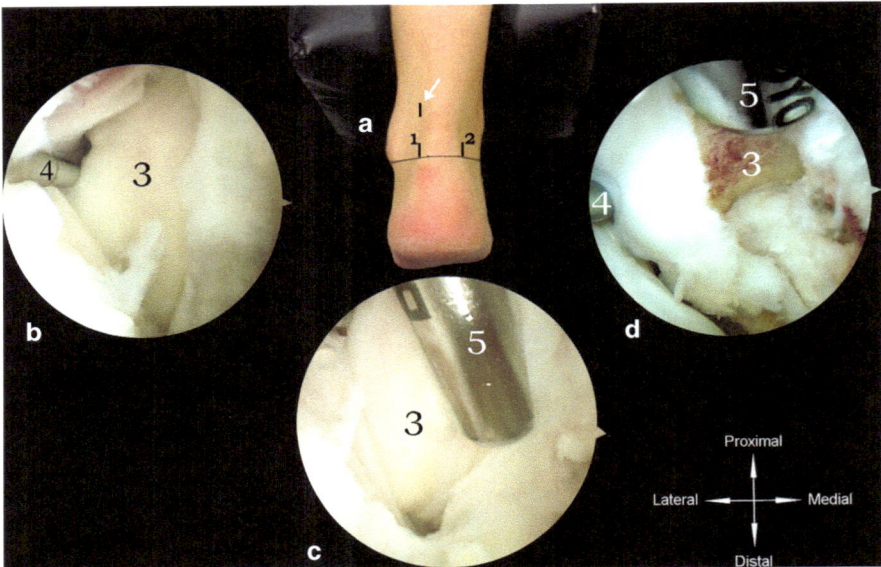

Fig. 17.10 (**a**) Macroscopic image of a left ankle indicating the portal placement for endoscopic groove-deepening in case of peroneal tendon dislocation. Regular hindfoot portals are indicated: posterolateral (1) and posteromedial portal (2). An accessory portal is positioned 4 cm proximal to the posterolateral portal (*arrow*). (**b**) Endoscopic image of a left ankle. By using a hook (4), introduced through the posterolateral portal, the peroneal tendons are dislocated, freeing the non-concave fibular groove (3). (**c**) A bonecutter shaver (5) is introduced through the accessory portal to deepen the fibular groove. (**d**) The fibular groove is deepened up to 6–7 mm in width and 5 mm in depth. These figures can be judged upon the 5.5-mm outer diameter of the shaver

Removal of a symptomatic os trigonum, a nonunion of a fracture of the posterior talar process or a symptomatic large posterior talar prominence involves partial detachment of the posterior talofibular ligament and release of the flexor retinaculum, which both attach to the posterior talar prominence. Release of the FHL tendon involves detachment of the flexor retinaculum from the posterior talar process. The tendon sheath can now be entered with the scope, following the tendon under the medial malleolus and a further release can be performed.

Bleeding is controlled by electrocautery at the end of the procedure. To prevent sinus formation, the skin incisions are sutured with 3.0 Ethilon. The incisions and surrounding skin are injected with 10 ml of a 0.5% bupivacaine/morfine solution. A sterile compressive dressing is applied (Klinigrip, Medeco BV, Oud Beijerland, The Netherlands). Prophylactic antibiotics are not routinely given.

17.6.2   *Endoscopic Groove-Deepening for Recurrent Peroneal Tendon Dislocation*

The patient is positioned similar as in posterior ankle arthroscopy. Standard posteromedial and lateral portals are made as described above (Fig. 17.10a). A 30° 4.0-mm arthroscope is introduced through the posterolateral portal while introducing a punch through the posteromedial portal. With the arthroscope at the level of the lateral part of the subtalar joint, looking 30° to the lateral side, the peroneal tendon sheath can be identified. The peroneal tendon sheath can now be opened using the punch. The tendon sheath can subsequently be bluntly released with a probe, after which it is exchanged through the posteromedial portal for the punch and the peroneal tendons can be inspected.

The arthroscope is now removed from the posterolateral portal and is introduced through the posteromedial portal. A probe is introduced through the posterolateral portal. This probe is subsequently used to dislocate the peroneal tendons laterally and anteriorly over the lateral edge of the lateral malleolus, thus leaving the fibular groove empty (Fig. 17.10b). We sometimes introduce a second probe through the same posterolateral portal to dislocate the peroneal tendons, at a higher level, thus exploring a larger portion of the groove. Now, 4 cm proximal to the posterolateral ankle portal, a vertical stab incision is made (Fig. 17.10a). The subcutaneous tissue is split, with a mosquito clamp, until it is positioned into the fibular groove. Then a 5.5-mm full radius bonecutter shaver is introduced, pointing inferiorly down to the level of the most distal part of the fibular bony groove (Fig. 17.10c). Subsequently, under direct arthroscopic view, the fibular groove can be deepened (Fig. 17.10d). Since the outer diameter of this shaver is 5.5 mm, the width and depth of the groove can be judged, aiming for 6–7 mm and a depth of 5 mm. After deepening and widening the groove, the potential sharp edges are smoothened. The probes and shaver are retracted and the peroneal tendons are positioned back into their newly created fibular groove. By manipulating the foot, the stability of the peroneal tendons can be checked under direct arthroscopic examination.

To prevent sinus formation, at the end of the procedure, the skin incisions are sutured with 3.0 Ethilon. The incisions and surrounding skin are injected with 10 ml of a 0.5% bupivacaine/morfine solution. A sterile compressive dressing is applied. Prophylactic antibiotics are not routinely given.

17.7   Postoperative Management and Rehabilitation

17.7.1   Posterior Ankle Arthroscopy/Endoscopic Groove-Deepening Technique

The patient can be discharged the same day of surgery and weight-bearing is allowed as tolerated. After an endoscopic groove deepening, partial weight bearing is advised for 5 days. The patient is instructed to elevate the foot when not walking to prevent edema. The dressing is removed 3 days postoperatively, and the patient is permitted to shower. Performing active range-of-motion exercises at least three times a day for 10 min each is encouraged. Following endoscopic groove deepening, a soft brace is applied for 4–6 weeks with the permission to fully bear weight. With satisfaction of the surgeon and patient, no further outpatient department contact is necessary. Patients with limited range of motion are directed to a physiotherapist.

17.8   Technical Alternatives and Pitfalls

17.8.1   *Posterior Ankle Arthroscopy/Endoscopic Groove-Deepening Technique*

In the hindfoot, the crural fascia can be quite thick. This local thickening is called the ligament of Rouvière.[45] This ligament needs to be at least partially excised or sectioned, using arthroscopic punch or scissors, to reach the level of the subtalar joint. The position of the arthroscope is important; the view should always be to the lateral side. Initially the arthroscope must be pointed in the direction between the first and second toes to be in a safe area. The FHL tendon is an important landmark. The working area is laterally with respect to the FHL tendon. The FHL tendon can safely be identified by shaving on top of the posterior talar process while the opening of the shaver is pointing toward the bone. While staying in contact with the bone, the tip of the shaver should be moved slowly and slightly twisted to the medial side, so that the opening of the shaver is to the lateral side and thus the blunt back of the shaver blade is turned toward the FHL tendon. The contour of the posterior talar process is followed until the shaver suddenly drops in between the posterior talar process and the FHL tendon. Shaving should be stopped at this moment, and the FHL tendon must be identified. The opening of the shaver should always be directed away from the tendon at this point. The FHL tendon should only be passed medially with a mosquito clamp if a release of the neurovascular bundle is required (posttraumatic tarsal tunnel syndrome). If a hypertrophic posterior talar process is removed by using a chisel, care must be taken not to place the chisel too far anteriorly. Only the infero-posterior part of the process should be removed with the chisel. The remnant of the process can be taken away with a bonecutter shaver. If initially the chisel is placed too much anteriorly, it is hard to avoid taking away too much bone at the level of the subtalar joint.

Loose bony particles can easily be created with the microfracture awl in case of puncturing the subchondral plate in osteochondral defects. They can become detached upon withdrawal of the awl. If the particles are not removed properly, they may act as loose bodies and should therefore be removed.[46]

Deepening the fibular groove can potentially damage the ligamentous structures. Medial from the groove, the posterior syndesmotic ligaments and the posterior talofibular ligament are located. The contour of the groove must be followed from proximal to distal. The calcaneofibular ligament inserts more anteriorly in the most distal part of the lateral malleolus. The fibular groove must be deepened anteriorly and distally, while the shaver is directed medial from the calcaneofibular ligament insertion.

The depth of the fibular groove needs to be sufficient in order to prevent redislocation of the peroneal tendons and should approximately be 5 mm. At the end of the procedure, the ankle is manipulated to check whether sufficient bone is excised. Removing too much fibular bone could induce weakening, which could eventually result in a fracture of the remaining lateral rim. It is important to smoothen the created lateral edge of the groove in order to prevent it from causing peroneal tendon (length) ruptures.

The advantage of a two-portal procedure[9] and also of the three-portal endoscopic groove-deepening technique[11] with the patient in the prone position is the working space that can be created in between the Achilles tendon and the back of the ankle and subtalar joint. The position is ergonomic for the surgeon. Soft tissue distraction can easily be applied.[40]

17.9   Discussion/Consideration

Arthroscopy has become common practice in today's modern medicine. It is an important operative technique in treating a wide variety of ankle pathology and provides a minimally invasive approach as a good alternative to the existing open surgical approaches. The surgeon must be familiar with the anatomy and must try to use routine portals in ankle arthroscopy. Ideally, these routine portals can be used to treat the vast majority of pathology, without the need for additional portals.

The authors feel that the posteromedial and posterolateral portal, as described in 2000, possess the criteria, as discussed above.[9] Also portals must provide a safe access, as is anatomically demonstrated to be the case for these posterior endoscopic portals.[47,48]

Recently, a retrospective study was published in which 16 posterior ankle arthroscopies were evaluated.[49] The patients all had a good functional and clinical outcome at a mean follow-up of 32 months. One patient had a temporary numbness in the region of the scar. Similar results were published in a prospective study by the senior author.[10] In total, 55 posterior ankle arthroscopies were assessed. All patients had a posterior ankle impingement syndrome. Good to excellent functional and clinical outcomes were reported on in 74% of the cases. One complication occurred, being a temporary sensational loss of the posteromedial heel. The two-portal endoscopic hindfoot approach compares favorably to open surgery with regard to less morbidity and a quicker recovery.[10]

The technique has now expanded to other areas in the hindfoot. The endoscopic groove-deepening technique for recurrent peroneal tendon dislocation, as described in this manuscript, is one of these new possibilities.[11]

References

1. Burman MS. Arthroscopy of direct visualisation of joints. An experimental cadaver study. J Bone Joint Surg. 1931;13:669–95.
2. Watanabe M. Selfoc-arthroscope (Watanabe no 24 arthroscope) monograph. Tokyo: Teishin Hospital; 1972.

3. van Dijk CN, Kort N, Scholten PE. Tendoscopy of the posterior tibial tendon. Arthroscopy. 1997;13(6):692–8.
4. Scholten PE, van Dijk CN. Tendoscopy of the peroneal tendons. Foot Ankle Clin. 2006;11(2):415–20, vii.
5. van Dijk CN, Kort N. Tendoscopy of the peroneal tendons. Arthroscopy. 1998;14(5):471–8.
6. Steenstra F, van Dijk CN. Achilles tendoscopy. Foot Ankle Clin. 2006;11(2):429–38, viii.
7. Scholten PE, van Dijk CN. Endoscopic calcaneoplasty. Foot Ankle Clin. 2006;11(2):439–6, viii.
8. van Dijk CN, van Dyk GE, Scholten PE, Kort NP. Endoscopic calcaneoplasty. Am J Sports Med. 2001;29(2):185–9.
9. van Dijk CN, Scholten PE, Krips R. A 2-portal endoscopic approach for diagnosis and treatment of posterior ankle pathology. Arthroscopy. 2000;16(8):871–6.
10. Scholten PE, Sierevelt IN, van Dijk CN. Hindfoot endoscopy for posterior ankle impingement. J Bone Joint Surg Am. 2008;90(12):2665–72.
11. de Leeuw PAJ, Golano P, van Dijk CN. A 3-portal endoscopic groove deepening technique for recurrent peroneal tendon dislocation. Tech Foot Ankle Surg. 2008;7(4):250–6.
12. Zengerink M, Szerb I, Hangody L, Dopirak RM, Ferkel RD, van Dijk CN. Current concepts: treatment of osteochondral ankle defects. Foot Ankle Clin. 2006;11(2):331–59, vi.
13. Amendola A, Lee KB, Saltzman CL, Suh JS. Technique and early experience with posterior arthroscopic subtalar arthrodesis. Foot Ankle Int. 2007;28(3):298–302.
14. Carro LP, Golano P, Vega J. Arthroscopic subtalar arthrodesis: the posterior approach in the prone position. Arthroscopy. 2007;23(4):445.e1–e4.
15. Glanzmann MC, Sanhueza-Hernandez R. Arthroscopic subtalar arthrodesis for symptomatic osteoarthritis of the hindfoot: a prospective study of 41 cases. Foot Ankle Int. 2007;28(1):2–7.
16. Tasto JP. Arthroscopic subtalar arthrodesis. Tech Foot Ankle Surg. 2003;2(2):122–8.
17. Scholten PE, Altena MC, Krips R, van Dijk CN. Treatment of a large intraosseous talar ganglion by means of hindfoot endoscopy. Arthroscopy. 2003;19(1):96–100.
18. Hamilton WG, Geppert MJ, Thompson FM. Pain in the posterior aspect of the ankle in dancers. Differential diagnosis and operative treatment. J Bone Joint Surg Am. 1996;78(10):1491–500.
19. Hedrick MR, McBryde AM. Posterior ankle impingement. Foot Ankle Int. 1994;15(1):2-8.
20. van Dijk CN, Lim LS, Poortman A, Strubbe EH, Marti RK. Degenerative joint disease in female ballet dancers. Am J Sports Med. 1995;23(3):295–300.
21. Maquirriain J. Posterior ankle impingement syndrome. J Am Acad Orthop Surg. 2005;13(6):365–71.
22. Stibbe AB, van Dijk CN, Marti RK. The os trigonum syndrome. Acta Orthop Scand. 1994;Suppl 262:59–60.
23. Weinstein SL, Bonfiglio M. Unusual accessory (bipartite) talus simulating fracture. A case report. J Bone Joint Surg Am. 1975;57(8):1161–3.
24. Bizarro AH. On sesamoid and supernumerary bones of the limbs. J Anat. 1921;55(pt 4):256–68.
25. Lapidus PW. A note on the fracture of os trigonum. Report of a case. Bull Hosp Joint Dis. 1972;33(2):150–4.
26. Sarrafian SK. Anatomy of the foot and ankle: descriptive, topographic, functional. Philadelphia: Lippincott; 1983.
27. Brodsky AE, Khalil MA. Talar compression syndrome. Am J Sports Med. 1986;14(6):472–6.
28. Hamilton WG. Stenosing tenosynovitis of the flexor hallucis longus tendon and posterior impingement upon the os trigonum in ballet dancers. Foot Ankle. 1982;3(2):74-80.
29. Howse AJ. Posterior block of the ankle joint in dancers. Foot Ankle. 1982;3(2):81–4.
30. Cedell CA. Rupture of the posterior talotibial ligament with the avulsion of a bone fragment from the talus. Acta Orthop Scand. 1974;45(3):454–61.
31. Haglund P. Beitrag zur Klinik der Achillessehne. Zeitschr Orthop Chir. 1928;49:49–58.
32. Coughlin MJ, Mann RA. Surgery of the foot & ankle. Tarsal tunnel syndrome. Surgery of the foot and ankle. St. Louis: Mosby; 1993.
33. Molloy R, Tisdel C. Failed treatment of peroneal tendon injuries. Foot Ankle Clin. 2003;8(1):115–29, ix.

34. Monteggi GB. Instituzini Chirurgiche. Italy: Milan; 1803:336–41.
35. Brage ME, Hansen ST Jr. Traumatic subluxation/dislocation of the peroneal tendons. Foot Ankle. 1992;13(7):423–31.
36. Eckert WR, Davis EA Jr. Acute rupture of the peroneal retinaculum. J Bone Joint Surg Am. 1976;58(5):670–2.
37. Zoellner G, Clancy W Jr. Recurrent dislocation of the peroneal tendon. J Bone Joint Surg Am. 1979;61(2):292–4.
38. Edwards ME. The relations of the peroneal tendons to the fibula, calcaneus and cuboideum. Am J Anat. 1928;42:213–53.
39. Poll RG, Duijfjes F. The treatment of recurrent dislocation of the peroneal tendons. J Bone Joint Surg Br. 1984;66(1):98–100.
40. van Dijk CN, de Leeuw PA. Imaging from an orthopaedic point of view. What the orthopaedic surgeon expects from the radiologist? Eur J Radiol. 2007;62(1):2–5.
41. Verhagen RA, Maas M, Dijkgraaf MG, Tol JL, Krips R, van Dijk CN. Prospective study on diagnostic strategies in osteochondral lesions of the talus. Is MRI superior to helical CT? J Bone Joint Surg Br. 2005;87(1):41–6.
42. Rockett MS, Waitches G, Sudakoff G, Brage M. Use of ultrasonography versus magnetic resonance imaging for tendon abnormalities around the ankle. Foot Ankle Int. 1998;19(9):604–12.
43. Waitches GM, Rockett M, Brage M, Sudakoff G. Ultrasonographic-surgical correlation of ankle tendon tears. J Ultrasound Med. 1998;17(4):249–56.
44. van Dijk CN, Verhagen RA, Tol HJ. Technical note: resterilizable noninvasive ankle distraction device. Arthroscopy. 2001;17(3):E12.
45. Rouviere H, Canela Lazaro M. Le ligament peroneo-pstragalo-calcaneen. Annales d'anatomie Pathologique. 1932;7(IX):745–50.
46. van Bergen CJ, de Leeuw PA, van Dijk CN. Potential pitfall in the microfracturing technique during the arthroscopic treatment of an osteochondral lesion. Knee Surg Sports Traumatol Arthrosc. 2009;17(2):184–7.
47. Lijoi F, Lughi M, Baccarani G. Posterior arthroscopic approach to the ankle: an anatomic study. Arthroscopy. 2003;19(1):62–7.
48. Sitler DF, Amendola A, Bailey CS, Thain LM, Spouge A. Posterior ankle arthroscopy: an anatomic study. J Bone Joint Surg Am. 2002;84-A(5):763–9.
49. Willits K, Sonneveld H, Amendola A, Giffin JR, Griffin S, Fowler PJ. Outcome of posterior ankle arthroscopy for hindfoot impingement. *Arthroscopy*. 2008;24(2):196–202.

Chapter 18
Postoperative Physical Therapy for Foot and Ankle Surgery

Amol Saxena and Allison N. Granot

Evidence-based studies for foot and ankle rehabilitation mainly focus on preventative and nonsurgical rehabilitation of Achilles and ankle injuries. Postoperative protocols have not been studied for many of the surgical procedures in this text. Only ankle stabilization surgery has been studied comparing 6 weeks of below-knee casting versus earlier range of motion (ROM) with shorter periods of casting. Karlsson et al. studied a randomized group of patients undergoing surgery for chronic (greater than 6 months) ankle instability and found an earlier return to sports and work when patient began controlled ankle ROM at 3 weeks post-surgery and formalized strengthening at 5 weeks, as compared to those who started physical therapy after 6 weeks of below-knee casting.[1] We consider this study a good basis for all types of foot and ankle procedures and therefore use it as justification for our various protocols, i.e., initiation of active ROM at 3 weeks post-surgery and some form of strengthening by 5–6 weeks post-operative, (and often earlier).

When reviewing other studies, postoperative care is often mentioned by authors; however, they state "generically" that physical therapy "is initiated" or "is performed" but do not say exactly what is performed and which modalities or exercises are used. Therefore, the aim of this chapter is to give examples of exercises that we currently utilize for most of the postoperative protocols in our clinics. It is our practice to have patients initiate "home" exercise regimen daily with icing, elevating, and early active ROM exercises even prior to initial evaluation by the therapist, generally at 3 weeks post-operation.

A. Saxena, D.P.M. (✉)
Department of Sports Medicine, PAFMG-Palo Alto Division,
Clark Bldg., 3rd Flr, 795 El Camino Real,
Palo Alto, CA 94301, USA
e-mail: heysax@aol.com

A.N. Granot, P.T., M.P.T., O.C.S., C.S.C.S.
Dept of Physical Therapy, Palo Alto Medical Foundation,
Palo Alto, CA, USA

A. Saxena (ed.), *Sports Medicine and Arthroscopic Surgery of the Foot and Ankle*,
DOI 10.1007/978-1-4471-4106-8_18, © Springer-Verlag London 2013

Fig. 18.1 Stationary bike
with cast boot

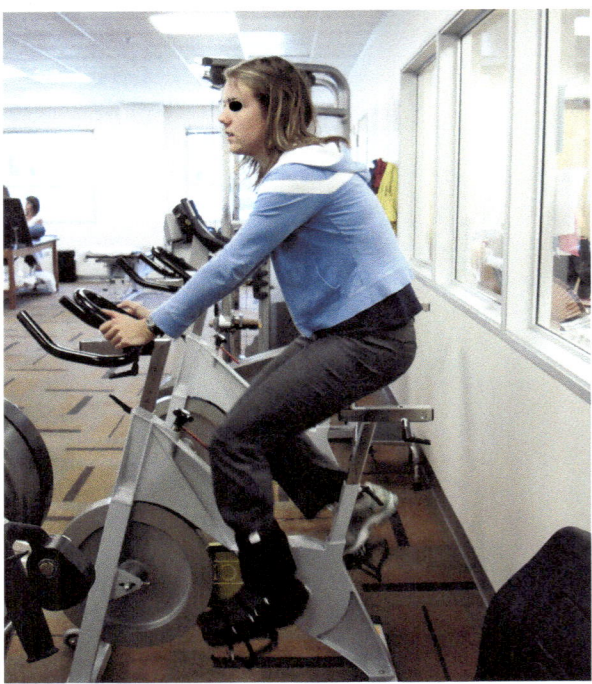

Typical immediate postoperative home instructions include the following:

- Ice for 15 min with an ice pack behind or above the knee (because the surgical dressings insulate and do not allow for vasoconstriction) 4×/day.[2]
- Icing directly with nonchemical ice packs (ice cubes in water) or ice bucket immersion can occur as determined by wound healing and the need for postoperative dressings. Caution with diabetic and neuropathic patients is needed.
- Elevate operative limb, but not above heart (avoids elevation ischemia),[3] and no direct pressure on surgical site such as resting on the heel region after retrocalcaneal surgery.
- When tolerated due to pain and surgically stable, stationary bicycling with the cast or boot on, using the heel region on the pedal, is permitted 15–30 min/day (this can range from less than one to up to 6 weeks post-surgery) (Fig. 18.1).
- When stable and suitable healing has taken place, ankle and foot range-of-motion exercises are initiated using a towel (this can range from less than one to up to 6 weeks post-surgery) (Fig. 18.2).

Formalized physical therapy visits are initiated generally from 2 to 12 weeks post-surgery with an evaluation by a physical therapist.[4-12] In the United States, patients are typically seen 2–3 times/week. A detailed assessment is performed by the physical therapist including history of the injury and surgical procedure, which regions should be protected and not be mobilized (such as with arthrodesis procedures), location of hardware or implants, and generalized situation of the patient.

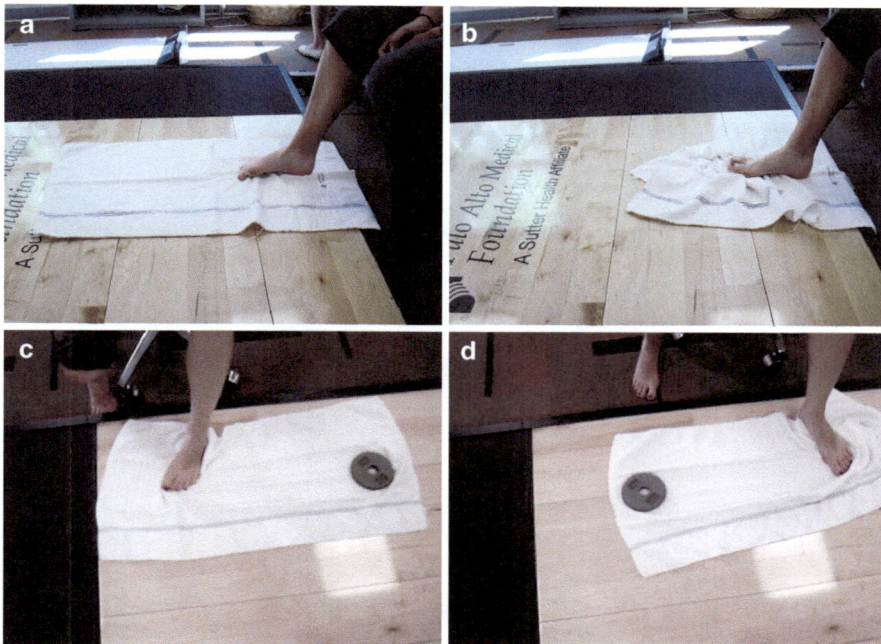

Fig. 18.2 Towel curls for toe (**a**) flexion and (**b**) extension; (**c, d**) Towel "swishes" for ankle inversion/eversion

Table 18.1 Assessment by physical therapist

1. History of injury, date, and type of surgery
2. Length of protection with boot, i.e., when can patient get out of the boot "OOB"
3. Length of protection due to healing such as tendon, fusion site, or bone graft
4. Location of hardware and implants
5. Restriction of motion to be maintained such as with arthrodesis procedures
6. Patients home, work, and activities including sports
7. Degree of pain, swelling, warmth, color of surgical site, presence of external sutures.
8. Disability (needs assistive aids), aggravating and easing factors
9. Patient's current amount of activity, icing, and exercising
10. Patient's goals/sports/occupation
11. Current functional status: ROM, strength, gait, balance, and proprioception
12. Surgeon's expected return to activity "RTA" for procedure
13. Consider objective foot scoring device (i.e., American Orthopedic Foot and Ankle Society, Foot and Ankle Assessment Module, Maryland Foot Score)

Note should be taken as to timing of protection with boots and braces. An appreciation for the stage of the healing must be understood before the therapist determines the effective treatment plan. Different procedures will require strategically timed protection/pain control, while others will call for early motion (Table 18.1).

Fig. 18.3 Game Ready™ ice device and elevation

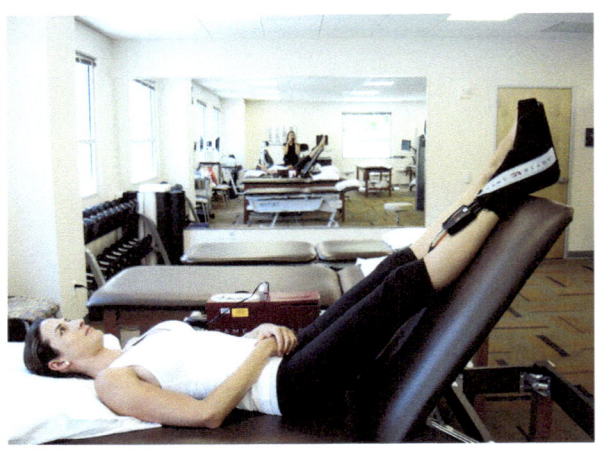

Fig. 18.4 Kinesio™ tape for ankle swelling

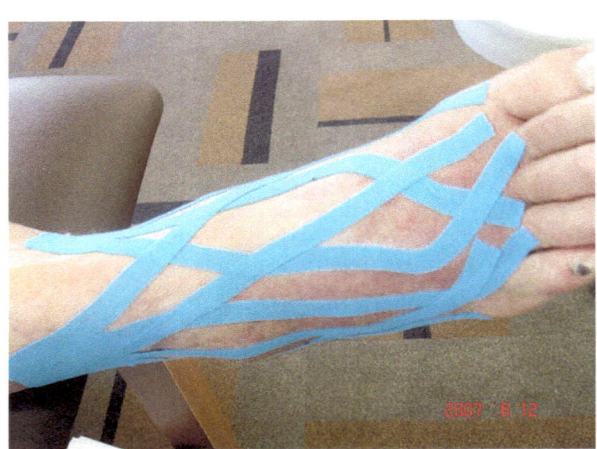

Modalities used postoperatively (such as ultrasound, phono- and iontophoresis, and interferential current) have not been critically studied, and therefore not often used post-surgically in our clinics. Though use of electrical stimulation and ultrasound is common and may be helpful, (for swelling and adhesions, respectively) firmly established protocols have not been performed. Postoperative edema reduction can be enhanced by ice compression devices such as the GameReady™ and Aircast Cryo Cuff™ in a controlled setting (Fig. 18.3).[2] Taping techniques such as Kinesio™ tape for edema control and ankle protection can be helpful (Fig. 18.4). Lymph massage has been proven as helpful and is utilized as needed. This is particularly helpful in patients having multiple surgeries, incisions, and venous stasis.[10]

Ergonomic equipment such as stationary bikes and elliptical trainers is utilized at appropriate times. Strengthening programs have primarily been studied post-ankle sprain and for nonsurgical treatment of Achilles tendonopathy often, with good success. The eccentric programs for Achilles tendonopathy have not been studied

Fig. 18.5 Runner on
Alter-G™ treadmill

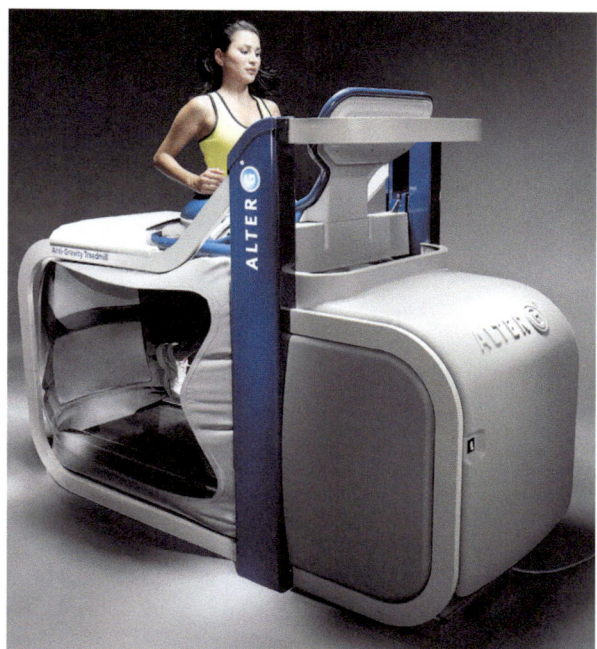

Table 18.2 Concentric heel raise progression (on successive days if pain-free):	
3 sets of 10 repetitions single-legged, pain-free
4 sets of 10 repetitions single-legged, pain-free
5 sets of 10 repetitions single-legged, pain-free
3 sets of 15 repetitions single-legged, pain-free
4 sets of 15 repetitions single-legged, pain-free
5 sets of 15 repetitions single-legged, pain-free
3 sets of 20 repetitions single-legged, pain-free
4 sets of 20 repetitions single-legged, pain-free
5 sets of 20 repetitions single-legged, pain-free
3 sets of 25 repetitions single-legged, pain-free
4 sets of 25 repetitions single-legged, pain-free
5 sets of 25 repetitions single-legged, pain-free

post-surgery. We therefore initiate rehabilitation with concentric strengthening programs post-surgery.[7,8,13,14] Eccentric exercises can be utilized in the later phases of rehabilitation after gait is normalized.[15-18] We also recommend hip stabilization exercises as recent studies point to hip weakness as a factor in ankle injuries.[18-20]

A recent device we have found helpful for lower extremity strengthening and rehabilitation is the "Alter-G™ Treadmill" (Alter-G, Milpitas, CA USA) (Fig. 18.5). This specialized treadmill allows adjustment and reduction of bodyweight such that if a patient is unable to perform lower extremity tasks such as heel raises or walking, the machine can be calibrated to allow them to do so. In our clinic, we typically reduce the body weight 30–50% and initiate single-legged concentric heel raises and restore normal gait (Table 18.2).[8]

Fig. 18.6 (**a, b**)
Plantarflexion exercises with
towel

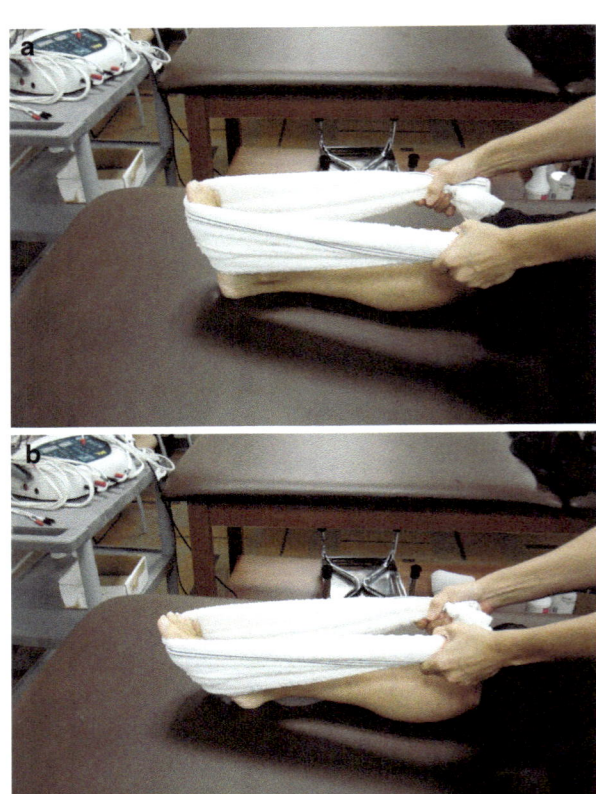

Rehabilitation Programs Used for Ankle Procedures

This program is followed after ankle procedures, i.e., Achilles, posterior tibial tendon reconstruction procedures, peroneal tendon repair, ankle stabilization or fracture repair, and osteochondral defect repair (with bone graft) or chondral lesion (micro-fracture).

Active ROM is allowed at 3 weeks (generally after cast removal) working on plantarflexion and inversion/eversion with a towel (Fig. 18.6). A below-knee cast boot that is maintained for immobilization is removed for exercise. Patients may be non-weight-bearing from 2 to 6 weeks depending on the procedure. Formal physical therapy is initiated between 8 and 10 weeks ("slower healing" procedures start later), though cross-training on a stationary bike is allowed with the boot/cast (with the heel on the pedal) as soon as 1 week post-surgery.[6,7] Swimming is allowed (without flip-turns) between 4 and 6 weeks post-surgery. Physical therapy includes progressive strengthening with visits on a bi-weekly basis with a physical therapist. It should be noted that stretching, thought to be appropriate post-injury, may have a limited role post-surgery. It must be done under proper supervision.[14,21]

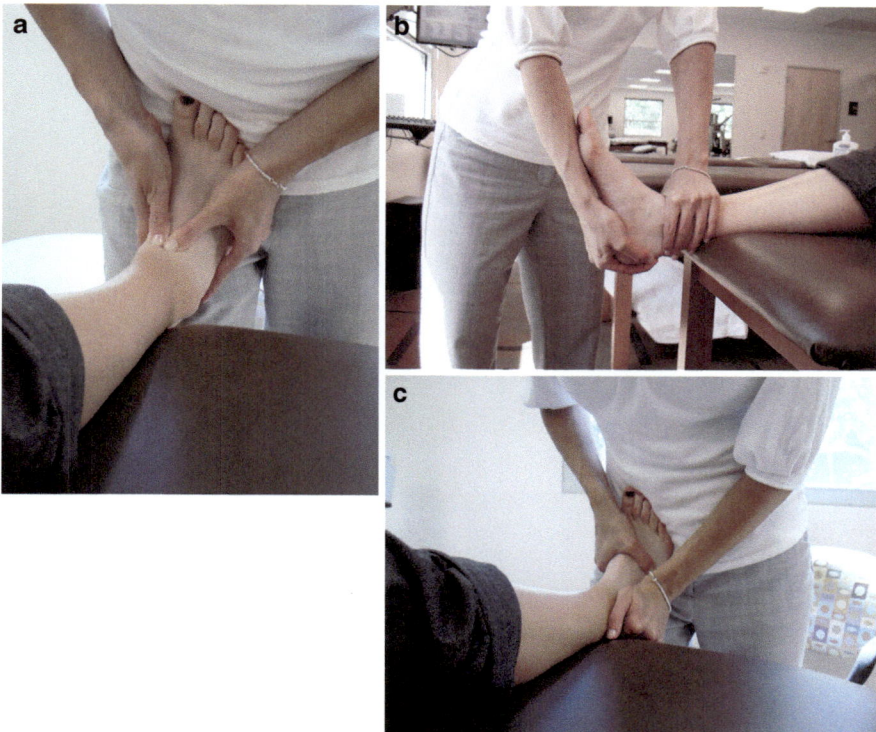

Fig. 18.7 (**a–c**) Distraction with anterior and posterior "glides" (mobilization) of the subtalar joint

Phase 1

Weeks 8–10 Post-surgery

- Initial evaluation;
- Protected mobilization, i.e., dorsiflexion to tolerance with Achilles procedures, no eversion beyond neutral with posterior tibial/medial stabilization, no inversion beyond neutral with peroneal/lateral stabilization procedures. Also, note, no mobilization of fused joints; (Figs. 18.7 and 18.8).
- Non-weight-bearing ankle strengthening with surgical tubing (inversion, eversion, dorsiflexion and plantarflexion) (Fig. 18.9).
- Cross-friction massage to incision (once fully healed) and posterior ankle (Fig. 18.10).
- Seated and standing calf stretch (Fig. 18.11).
- Introduce single-limb proprioception (Fig. 18.12).
- Bilateral concentric heel raises (can start in a pool, Alter-G™ or on leg press machine if patient is unable to do it on flat ground) (Fig. 18.13).
- Home instruction on strengthening with a towel.
- Cryotherapy for 15 min at session end.

Fig. 18.8 Mobilization (PA glide) of the subtalar joint

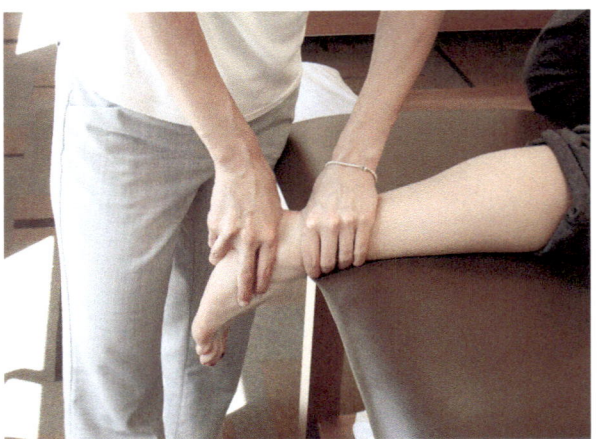

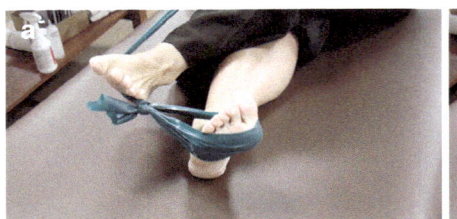 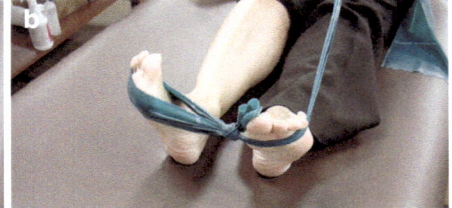

Fig. 18.9 (**a**) Ankle/STJ inversion (*right foot*) and (**b**) Ankle/STJ eversion (*right foot*) with elastic tubing

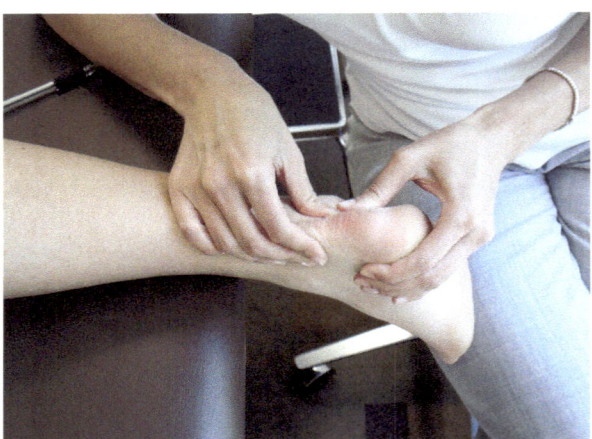

Fig. 18.10 Cross-friction massage of ankle tendons

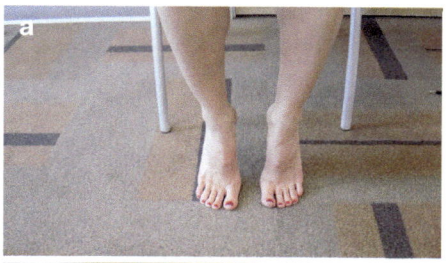

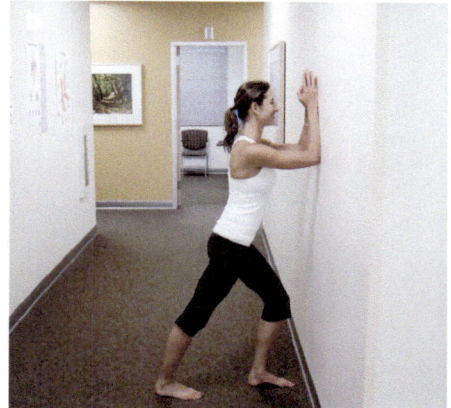 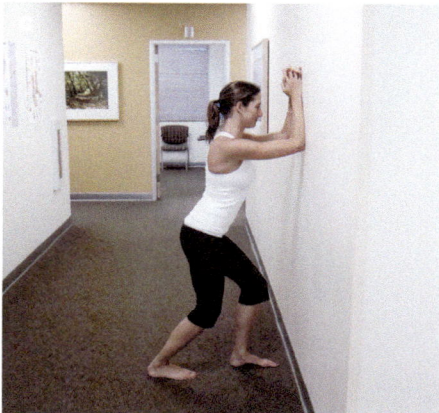

Fig. 18.11 Seated (**a**) and standing with knee straight (**b**) and knee bent (**c**) calf stretch

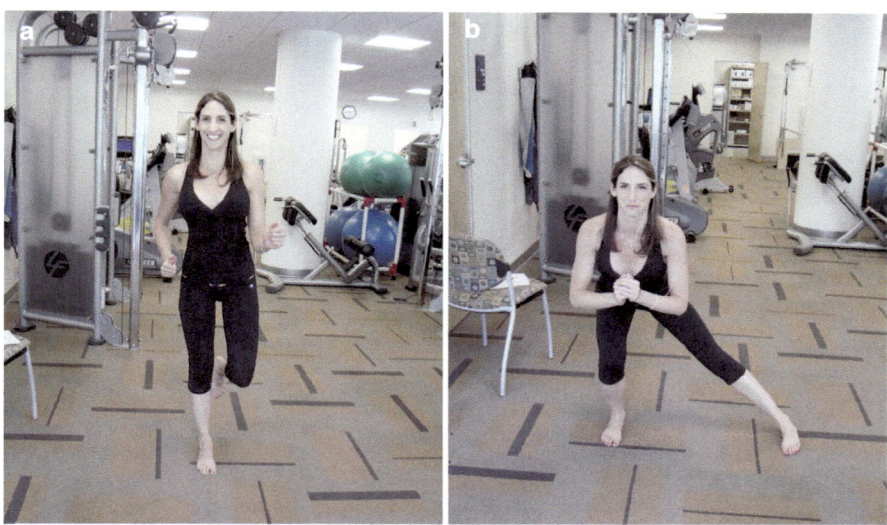

Fig. 18.12 (**a–c**) Single leg, side squat/lateral lunge, back to single leg ankle stability exercise on flat surface, for gluteal strengthening

Fig. 18.12 (continued)

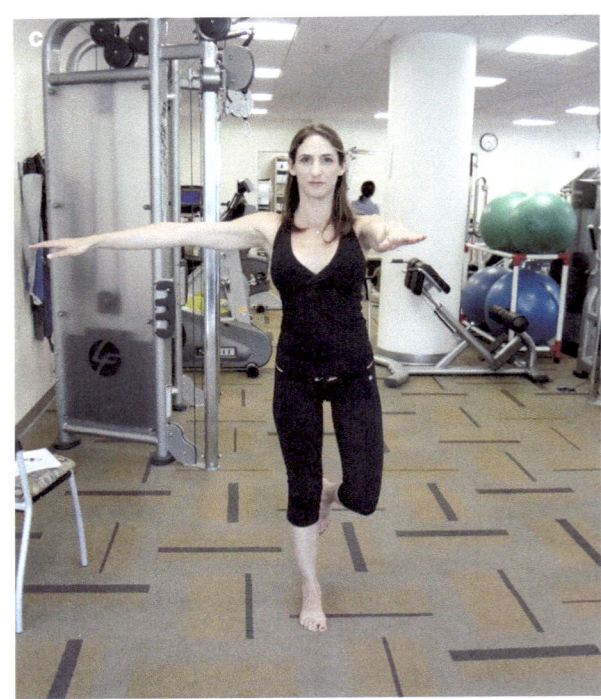

Fig. 18.13 Bilateral
concentric heel raise

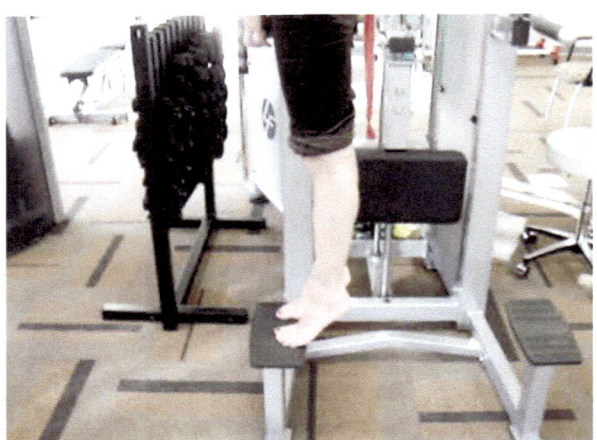

Weeks 10–12+ Post-surgery

Same as above, plus:

- Soft-tissue massage to calf muscle and posterior ankle tendons (Figs. 18.14 and 18.15)
- Mobilization of subtalar joint (unless fused) (Fig. 18.8)

Fig. 18.14 (a, b)
Mobilization of ankle

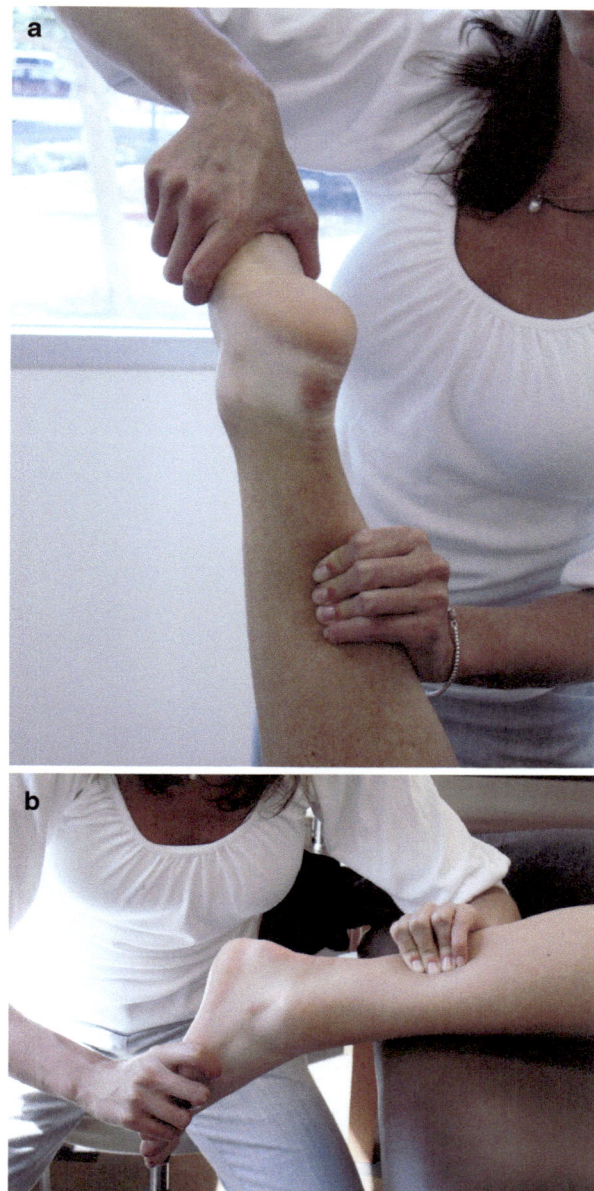

- Gluteal strengthening; (Figs. 18.16 and 18.17)
- Unilateral concentric strengthening at 60% bodyweight (BW) in Alter-G™; (Fig. 18.18)
- Stationary bike without boot
- Modalities such as ultrasound and electrical stimulation if needed
- Walking on Alter-G™ @ 40% (BW) for 10 min (minimum). (Can substitute pool workouts)

Fig. 18.15 (**a**, **b**) Mobilization of calf

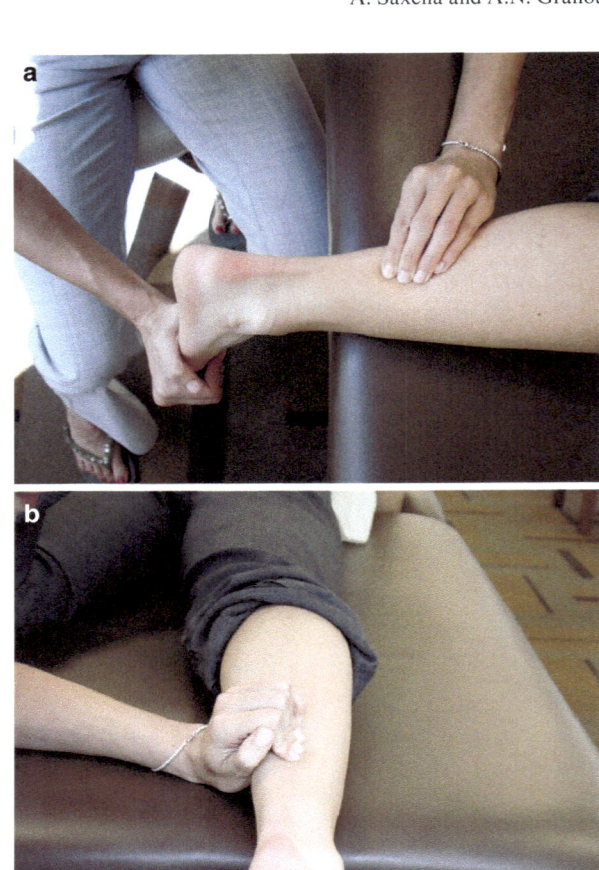

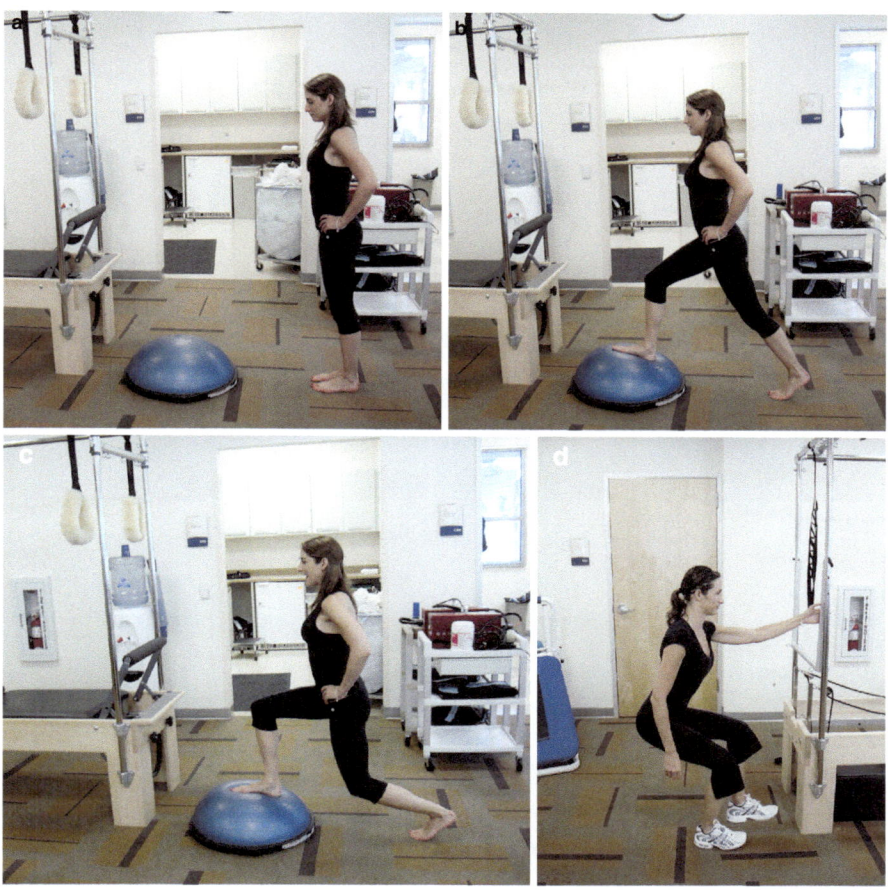

Fig. 18.16 (**a–c**) "1/4" Squats with (**d**) showing 2-legged version for assistance if needed

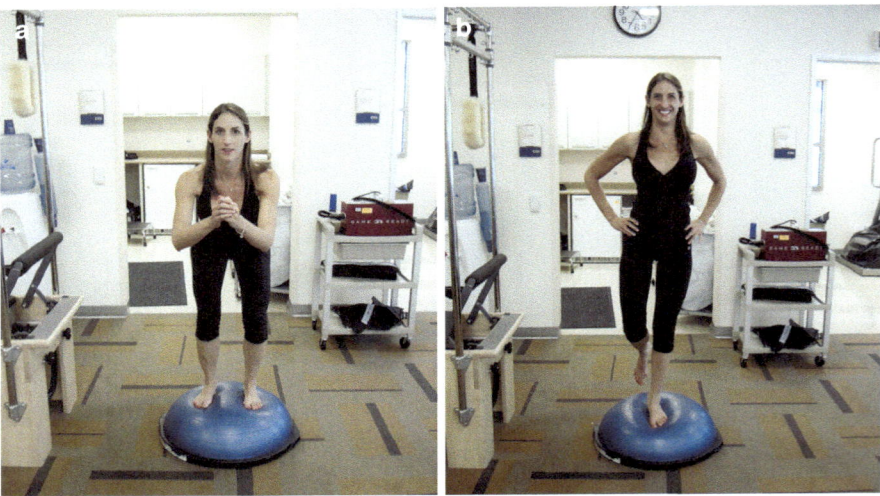

Fig. 18.17 (**a**, **b**) Double and single legged BOSU™ ball exercise

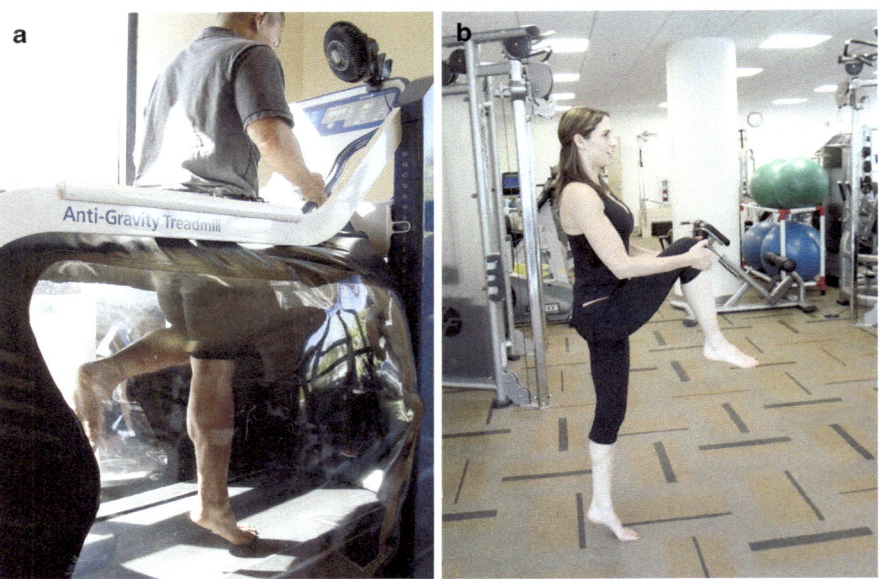

Fig. 18.18 (**a**) Unilateral leg strengthening on flat surface (shown utilizing Alter-G™ to reduce body weight or can do in shallow swimming pool if needed) (**b**) More advanced single-legged strengthening and balance

Fig. 18.19 Hip abduction
with elastic band

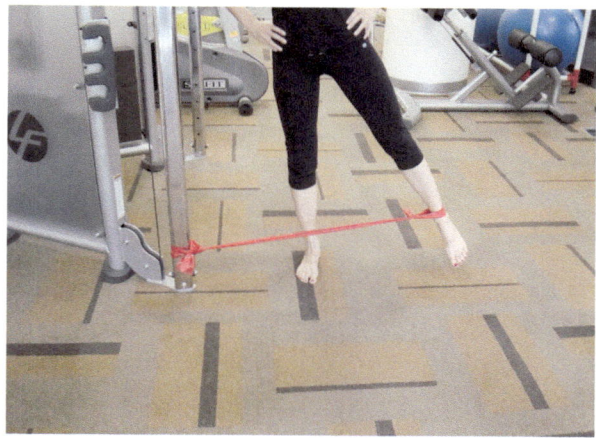

Phase 2

Approximately Week 12 or Later Post-surgery

Same as above plus:

- Standing hip Theraband™ 4 way; (Fig. 18.19)
- Gym ball exercises progressed from above (Fig. 18.20)
- Side steps with tubing (Fig. 18.21)
- Pilates Reformer ™ (leg press, calf raise, hamstring arcs and circles) (Fig. 18.22)
- Ankle proprioceptive neuromuscular facilitation PNF (Fig. 18.23) mobilization of great toe (Fig. 18.24)
- Progression to walking/running at 70% BW in Alter-G™ for 10 min
- Increase home program strengthening

Phase 3

Approximately Week 14 or Later Post-surgery

Same as above with:

- Progression of single-limb strengthening from 70% to 90% BW in Alter-G™ or in pool (starting w 3× 10 reps, progress to 5× 25).
- Walking/running up to 2 mi at 70% BW.
- Depending on patient's individual progress: dynamic balance and BOSU™ squats (Figs. 18.25 and 18.26); step-downs; calf eccentrics if pain-free, first with the knee straight and can progress to knee bent (Fig. 18.27); lunges; single leg heel raises and leg press and ankle PNF as shown above.

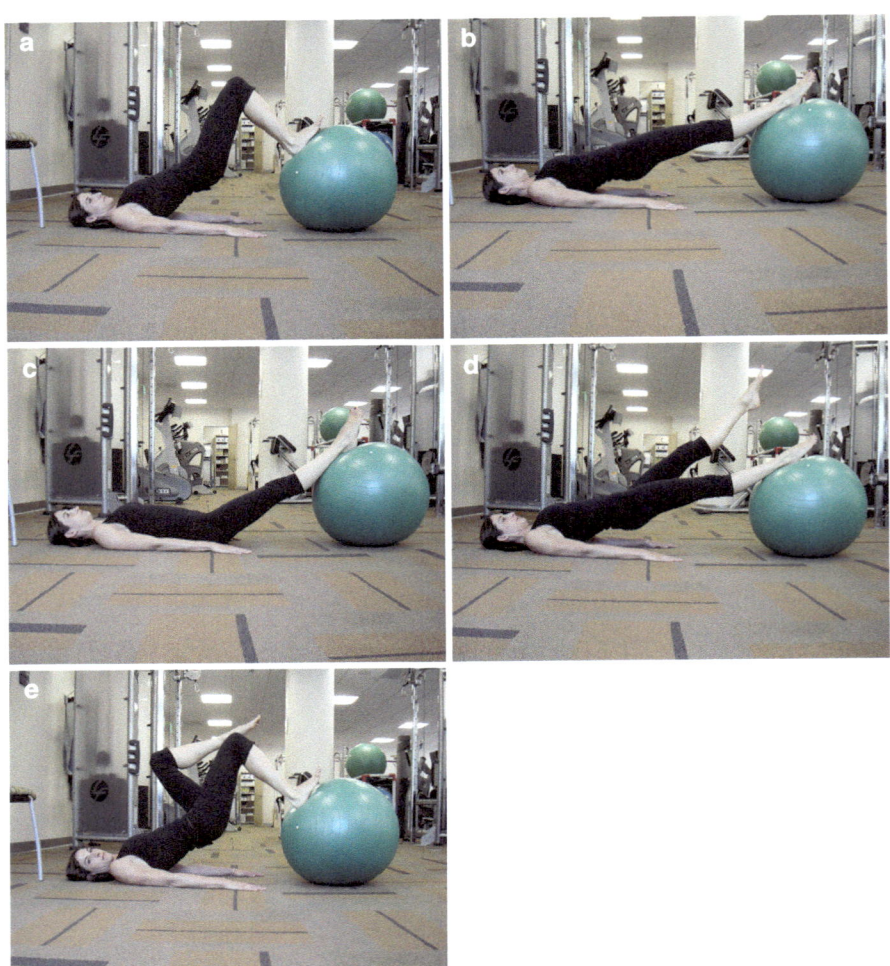

Fig. 18.20 (**a–e**) "Gym ball" hamstring strengthening

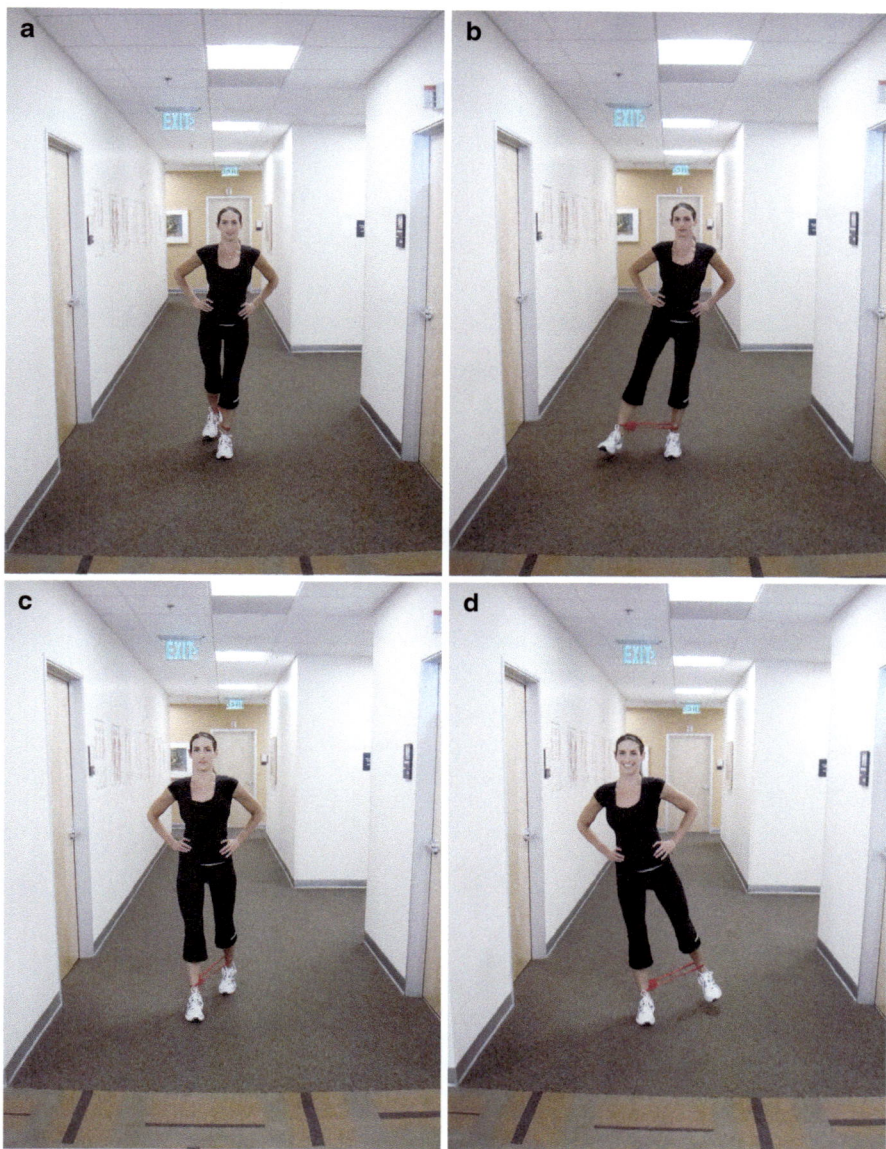

Fig. 18.21 (**a–d**) Figure-of-eight walk with elastic band

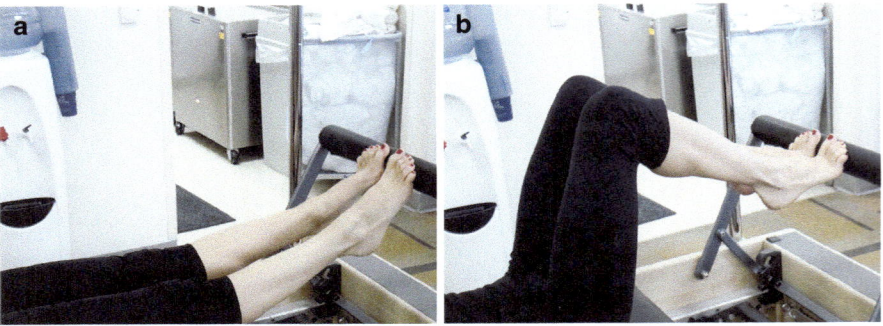

Fig. 18.22 (**a**, **b**) Pilates Reformer™ exercises

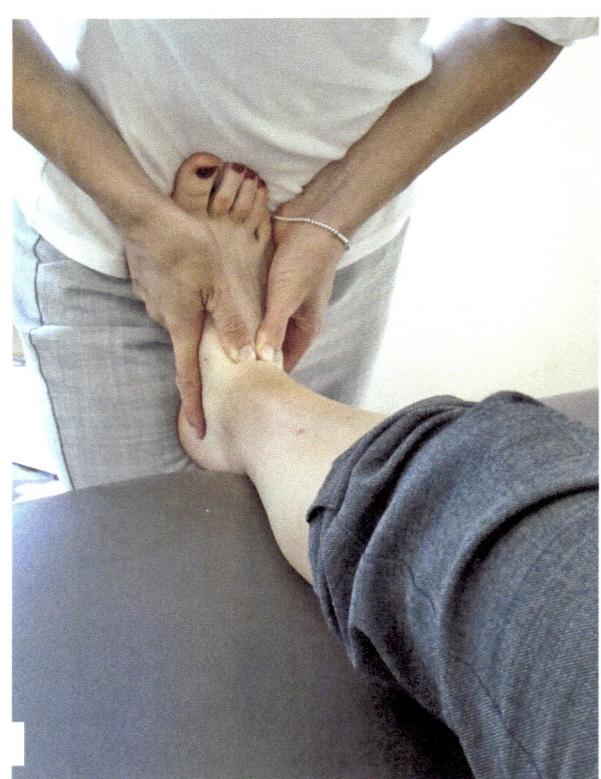

Fig. 18.23 Talar AP
mobilization

Fig. 18.24 Mobilization of first MPTJ

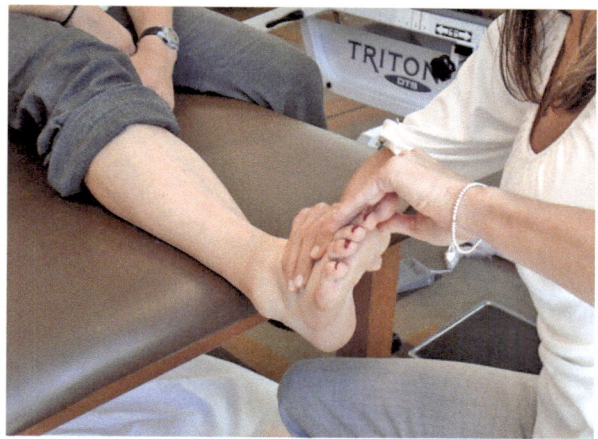

Fig. 18.25 Ankle stability on pillow. Rotating an object increases the "demand." Ball sports athletes can throw a ball against a wall or rebounding apparatus and try to catch it, which further improves balance

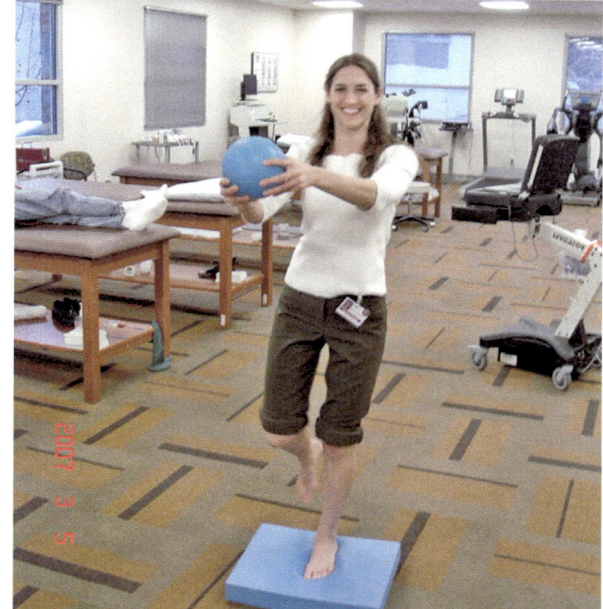

Fig. 18.26 (**a**, **b**) Ankle
stability on balance board

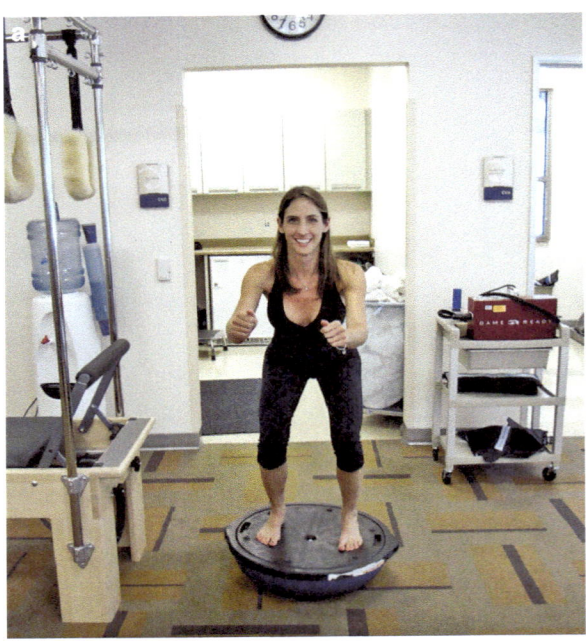

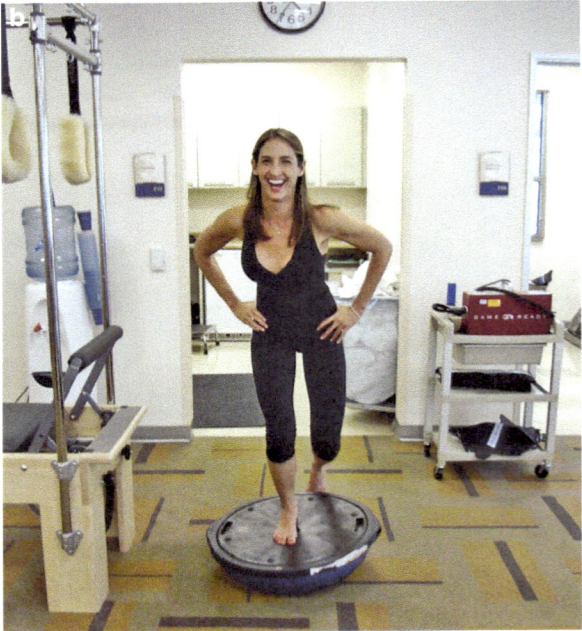

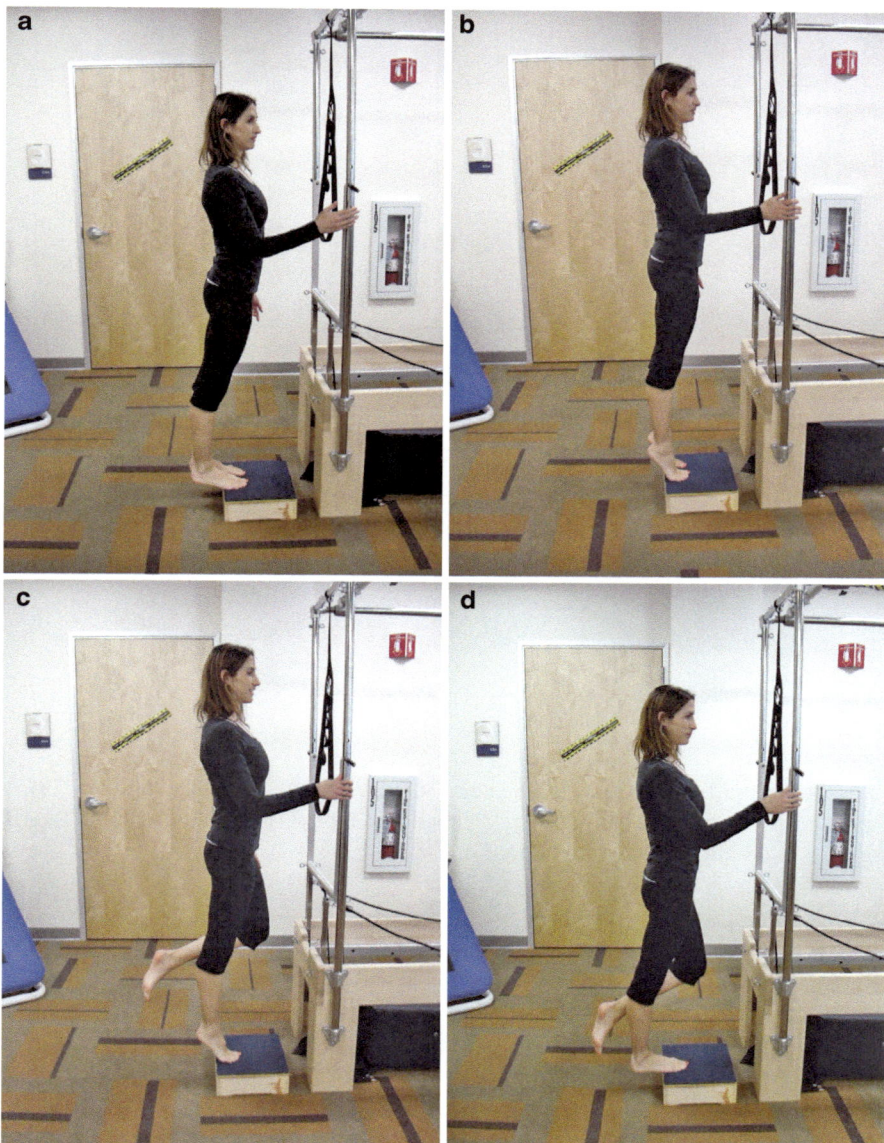

Fig. 18.27 Eccentric strengthening with knee straight. Heel raise with two legs, and lowering with one leg below the platform (achieve negative heel). (**a** through **d**) Side and (**e** through **g**) front views. Start with three sets of 10 repetitions

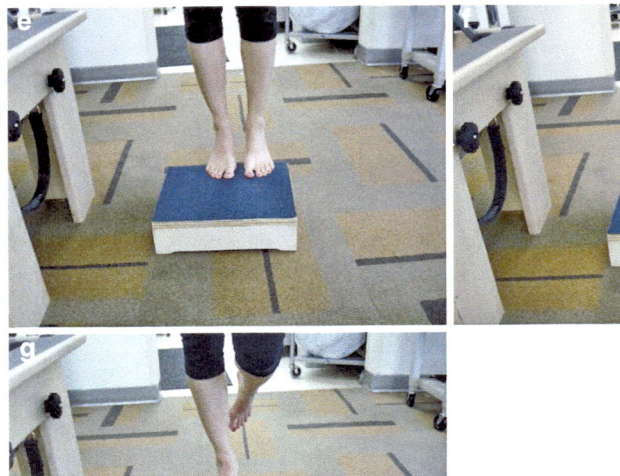

Fig. 18.27 (continued)

Taping may be helpful either laterally (Fig. 18.28), medially (Fig. 18.29), or posteriorly (Fig. 18.30) as necessary with elastic tape (Darco Body Armour Tape™, Darco International, West Virginia, USA).

Week 15 or Later Post-surgery

Same as above with progression to walking/running 75–85% BW in G-trainer or in pool for 30 min. Increase strengthening concentrically full bodyweight with surgical limb including active hip stabilization (Fig. 18.31).

Week 16 or Later

Same as above plus begin walk/jog program progress 75–85% BW in G-trainer for 10–20 min or in pool 30–40 min. Patients are typically discharged at this time with their home program of strengthening, proprioception, stretching, and cryotherapy to be maintained until they are able to return to their full activity level. Please see the respective chapters in this text for more specifics as to typical return to activity (RTA) time frames as many reconstructive procedures require up to a year to return to full activity. Athletes often have an accelerated RTA, as have been found in some

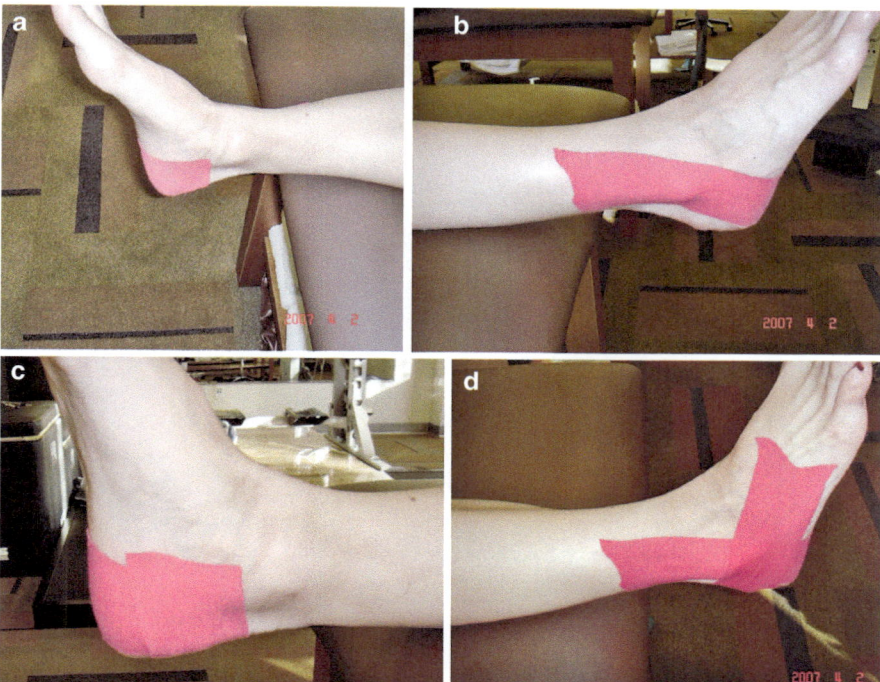

Fig. 18.28 (**a, b**) Taping from medial to lateral with Kinesio™ tape for lateral ankle stability. (**c, d**) Applying a second layer of tape perpendicular to the 1st, again medial to lateral

studies.[5,6,8] A continuation of specific strengthening and proprioception for the entire lower quarter is continued for over a year postoperatively.

Rehabilitation of Midfoot Surgeries and Fusions (Lisfranc's Injuries, Navicular Injuries, and Lapidus Procedure)

Postoperative course is nearly identical to the surgeries discussed above. Patients may be non-weight-bearing from 4 to 6 weeks. Formalized appointments start generally around 8–10 weeks post-surgery (Phase 1), when alignment and/or bony consolidation is confirmed. Similar postoperative rehabilitation progression as above with the exception that no mobilization is performed on the midfoot, and barefoot proprioception is delayed especially on the BOSU™ ball. Seated heel raises (Fig. 18.32) and first metatarsal–phalangeal joint (MPJ) mobilization techniques described in the next section are utilized for the Lapidus procedure. The physical therapy progression is similar as above, though patients with Lisfranc's injuries, particularly those requiring significant reconstruction, may take more than 6 weeks of sessions. Therefore, patients may not enter Phase 2 until 16 or more weeks post-surgery. Phase 3 may take 26 or more weeks.

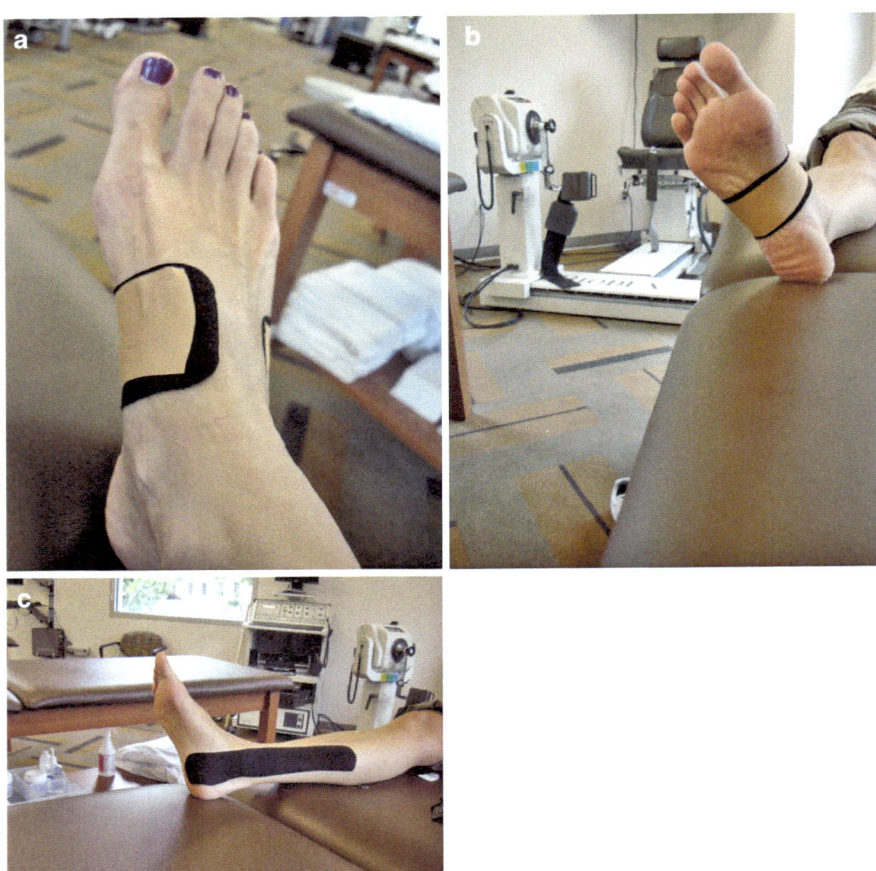

Fig. 18.29 Kinesio (TM) tape for medial arch support (**a**, **b**) and for posterior tibial support (c)

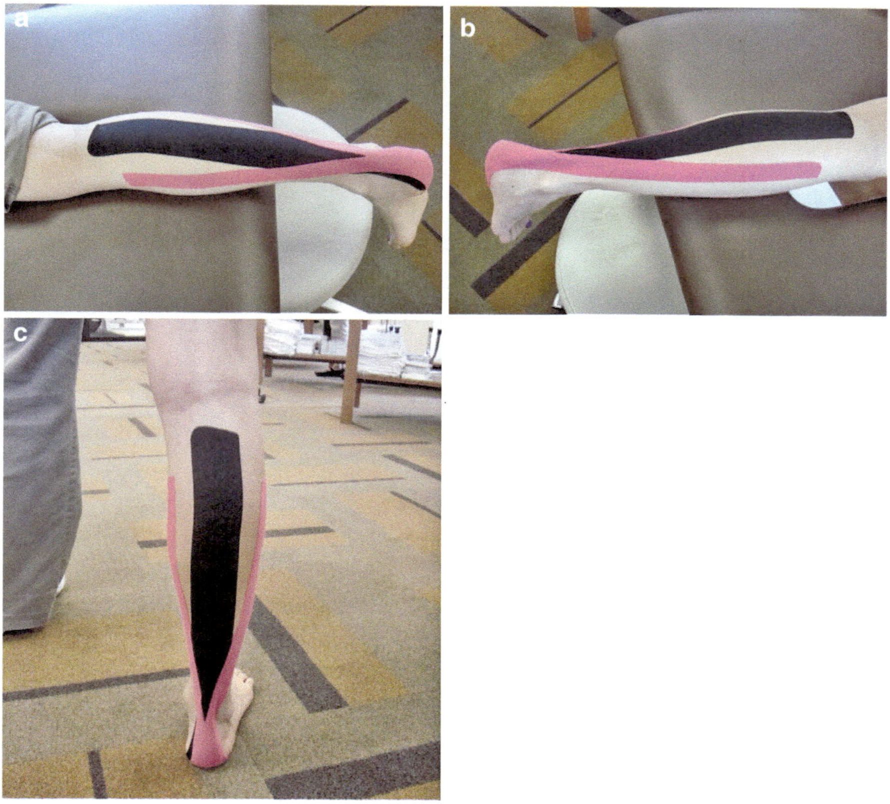

Fig. 18.30 (**a**–**c**) Kinesio™ tape for Achilles support

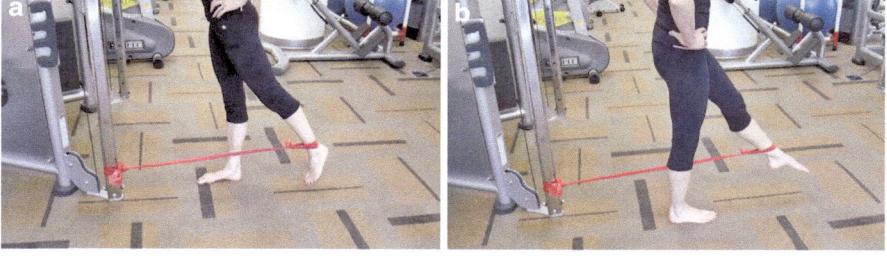

Fig. 18.31 Hip extension (**a**) and flexion (**b**) with elastic tubing for Core/dynamic strengthening

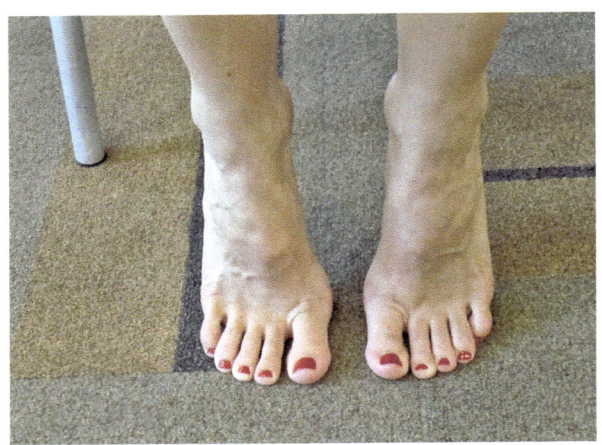

Fig. 18.32 Seated dorsiflexion for MPTJs

Rehabilitation of Forefoot Surgeries

The program for forefroot surgeries (i.e.,hammertoe, neuroma, bunionectomy/hallux rigidus surgery with or without osteotomy, lesser metatarsal osteotomy, and sesamoidectomy) is similar to the postoperative rehabilitation described above, though cast or boot immobilization may be shorter or not needed. Patients are able to use a stationary bike with a cast, cast boot, or even athletic shoe often within the first postoperative week with their heel on the pedal. Between 2 and 3 weeks post-surgery, patients begin towel exercises including curling, and seated dorsiflexion exercises. Patients with some forefoot procedures may be weight-bearing within 2–5 days, such as with hammertoe or primary neuroma surgeries; other forefoot surgeries may non-weight-bearing for 3 weeks. Formalized physical therapy sessions begin between 4 and 6 weeks post-op, (Phase 1), except for the Lapidus procedure discussed above in "Midfoot." Postoperative mobilization and physical therapy gains also focus on improving metatarsophalangeal motion. This may be assisted by applying mobilization (Figs. 18.33 and 18.34). The progression of the physical therapy sessions is similar as described above, though may be more rapid, and sometimes courses for 3–4 weeks duration for some more minor forefoot procedures starting at 6 or more weeks post-surgery. Phases 2 and 3 occur around 10 and 12 weeks or later post-surgery. Arch taping/support may be helpful for some procedures postoperatively (Fig. 18.35).

Return to Running Sports

Lower extremity rehabilitation postoperatively includes not only surgical site strengthening but core stabilization as well. We are including diagrams of exercises to be considered post foot and ankle surgery. Combination of some of these and

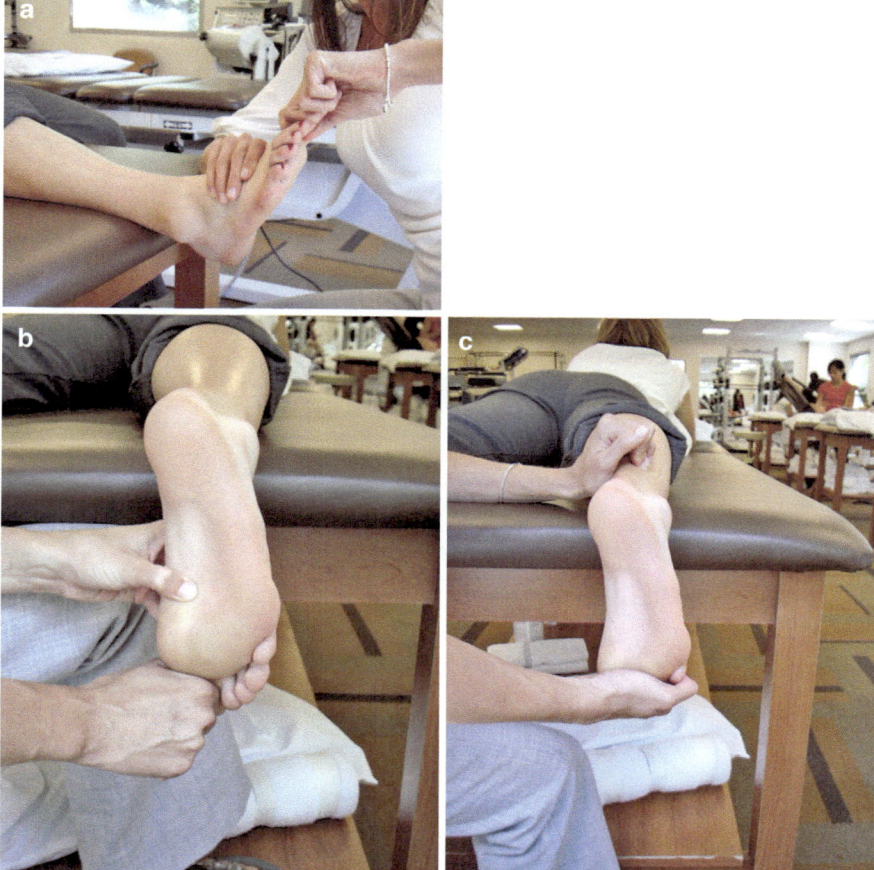

Fig. 18.33 Mobilization of the first MPTJ (**a, b**) and FHL/soleous (**c**)

individualization of the treatment plan should be determined by the surgeon and therapist as needed. The criteria for returning to sports have not been firmly established for all types of foot and ankle surgeries.[6,15] We utilize the following parameters based on research on rehabilitation of the Achilles tendon to clear patients to return to running sports[6-8]:

- Calf girth within 5 mm of nonoperative limb measured 10 cm distal to an adult's tibial tuberosity.
- Affected joint ROM within 5° of nonoperative limb.
- Ability to perform 5 × 25 concentric heel raises pain-free with operative limb.
- Include vertical leap testing and broad jump testing (3 hop test). The patient should be able to show you they can and are willing to bound on that leg prior to release.[18]
- 10 step-downs from an 8-in. step without discomfort.[18]

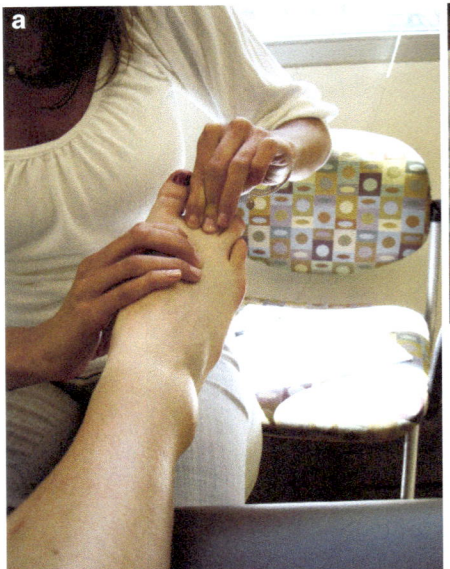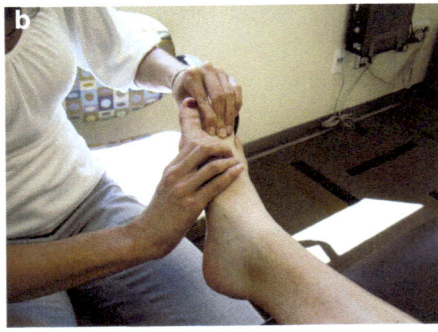

Fig. 18.34 (**a**, **b**) Mobilization of lesser MPTJ

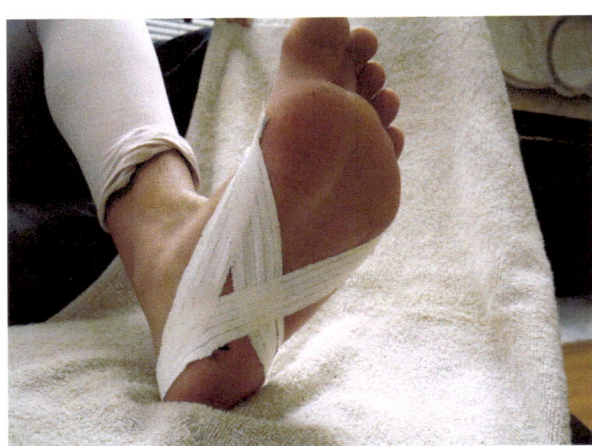

Fig. 18.35 Arch taping

Table 18.3 Sample return to "LAND" running

Day 1 (min)	Day 2	Day 3 (min)	Day 4	Day 5	Day 6	Day 7 (min)
15	Rest	15	Rest	20 min	Rest	20
20	Rest	25	Rest	25 min	Rest	30
20	Rest	30	Rest	40 min	Rest	40
20	Rest	40	Rest	50 min	Rest	50
20	Rest	50	30 min	Rest	60 min	20

Table 18.4 Sample return to running using the Alter-G™ treadmill

	Outside running		Alter-G time (min)	Alter-G body weight (%)		
Week 1			30–>40	70–>85		
Week 2			30–>60	75–>90		
Week 3	20 min qod 3 days		40–60	75–90		1 day off
Week 4	30–40 min qod 3 days		60–75	75–90		1 day off
Week 5	40–50 min qod 3–4 days		60–90	75–90		1 day off
Week 6	50–60 min 4 days	Strides on grass	60–90	75–90		1 day off
Week 7	60+ min 4 days	Strides on grass	60–90	75–90	Tempo/speed on alter-g	1 day off
Week 8	60+ min 4 days	Strides on grass	60–90	75–90	Tempo/speed on alter-g	1 day off
Week 9	Gradual → Full training					

qod = every-other day

A typical return to running program would be as follows: Have the patient alternate walking and jogging for 2 min each, completing four cycles (16 min of total activity). Have them take a rest day and then reassess 2 days later. If they felt challenged, have them repeat this every-other day for a week. If this was not challenging, then have the patient alternate 3-min jogging with 1-min walking, again for four cycles. Again have the patient reassess and repeat this every-other day for a week. If the patient experiences any increase in pain accompanied by swelling, they should refrain from running until the symptoms subside. Running can then be re-initiated.

As the running program progresses, the patient and therapist should monitor symptoms of compensatory symptoms such as lateral foot pain after first MPJ procedures or excessive contra-lateral limb soreness from favoring the surgical side or "vaulting." Once the patient can run every-other day, they can begin other sports drills. Increased ball handling skills can be performed. If running is the primary sport, the patient can begin with the running schedule outlined in Table 18.3. If the therapist has access to an Alter-G™ treadmill, they can utilize Table 18.4 as a guideline.

Summary

Postoperative physical therapy is often currently done in a non-structured approach across the world. In our clinic, we are currently establishing protocols based on surgical rationale, published RTA of common procedures, and previous evidence-based findings on other studies with ankle rehabilitation. A good dialogue between therapist, surgeon, and patient, including a fundamental understanding of the procedure and goals, is needed. We hope to verify our protocols in the future, and therefore, for now, use the above guidelines as suggestions and to provoke more study.

Acknowledgments   The authors would like to thank Matt Richardson, DPT and Marc Guillet, MSPT for their assistance with this chapter.

References

1. Alfredson H, Pietila T, Jonsson P, Lorentzon R. Heavy-load eccentric training for the treatment of chronic Achilles tendinosis. Am J Sports Med. 1998;26:360–366.
2. Cook JL, Purdam CR. Rehabilitation of Achilles and patellar tendinopathies. Best Pract Res Clin Rheumatol. 2007;21:295–316.
3. Saxena A, O'brien T. Post-operative physical therapy for podiatric surgery. J Am Podiatr Med Assoc. 1992;82(8):417–423.
4. Saxena A. Retrospective review of 91 surgeries for chronic achilles pathology. J Am Podiatr Med Assoc. 2003;93(4):283–291.
5. Saxena A. Results of achilles tendon surgery in elite and sub-elite track athletes. Foot Ankle Int. 2003;24(9):712–720.
6. Hansen ST. Acute compartment syndromes. "Elevation ischemia". In: Functional Reconstruction of the Foot and Ankle. Philadelphia: Lippincott; 2000:37, chap 2.
7. Knight K. Orthopedic surgery and cryotherapy. In: Cryotherapy in Sports Injury Management. Champaign: Human Kinetics; 1995:99–105.
8. Saxena A, Guillet M, Maffulli N. Rehabilitation of the operated Achilles Tendon: parameters for predicting return to activity. J Foot Ankle Surg. 2011;50(1):37–40.
9. Saxena A, Granot A. Use of a novel treadmill in the rehabilitation of the operated Achilles tendon: a pilot study. J Foot Ankle Surg. 2011;50(5): (epub).
10. Adler SS, Beckers D, Buck M. Proprioceptive Neuromuscular Facilitation in Practice: An Illustrated Guide. 3rd ed. Berlin: Springer; 1993.
11. Voss DE, Ionta KI, Myers BJ. Proprioceptive Neuromuscular Facilitation. 3rd ed. Philadelphia: Harper and Row; 1985.
12. Proprioceptive Neuromuscular Facilitation 1: the functional approach to proprioceptive neuromuscular facilitation. Institute of Physical Art. Course Notes Jan 1992.
13. Karlsson J, Lundin O, Lind K, Styf J. Early mobilization versus immobilization after ankle ligament stabilization. Scand J Med Sci Sports. 1999;9(5):299–303.
14. Donatelli R, Hall W, Prell B, Ferkel R. Lateral ligament repair. In: Maxey L, Magnusson J, eds. Rehabilitation for the Postsurgical Orthopedic Patient. 2nd ed. St. Louis: Mosby; 2007:401–432.
15. Donatelli R, Hall W, Prell B, Ferkel R. Open reduction and internal fixation of the ankle. In: Maxey L, Magnusson J, eds. Rehabilitation for the Postsurgical Orthopedic Patient. 2nd ed. St. Louis: Mosby; 2007:433–446.
16. Cozen D, Ferkel R, Maxey L. Ankle arthroscopy. In: Maxey L, Magnusson J, eds. Rehabilitation for the Postsurgical Orthopedic Patient. 2nd ed. St. Louis: Mosby; 2007:447–460.

17. Zachazewski J, Gruber J, Giza E, Mandelbaum B. Achilles tendon repair. In: Maxey L, Magnusson J, eds. Rehabilitation for the Postsurgical Orthopedic Patient. 2nd ed. St. Louis: Mosby; 2007.
18. Prelaz C. Transitioning the jumping athlete back to the court. In: Maxey L, Magnusson J, eds. Rehabilitation for the Postsurgical Orthopedic Patient. 2nd ed. St. Louis: Mosby; 2007:513–524.
19. Nicholas JA, Marino M. The relationship of injuries of the leg, foot, and ankle to proximal thigh strength in athletes. Foot Ankle. 1987;7:218–228.
20. Friel K, McLean N, Myers C, Caceres M. Ipsilateral hip abductor weakness after inversion ankle sprain. J Athl Train. 2006;41:74–78.
21. Small K, McNaughton L, Matthews M. A systematic review into the efficacy of static stretching as part of a warm-up for the prevention of exercise-related injury. Res Sports Med. 2008;16(3):213–231.

Index